Robert Douglas

General View of the Agriculture of the Counties of Roxburgh and

Selkirk

Robert Douglas

General View of the Agriculture of the Counties of Roxburgh and Selkirk

ISBN/EAN: 9783741184383

Manufactured in Europe, USA, Canada, Australia, Japa

Cover: Foto ©Lupo / pixelio.de

Manufactured and distributed by brebook publishing software
(www.brebook.com)

Robert Douglas

General View of the Agriculture of the Counties of Roxburgh and Selkirk

GENERAL VIEW

OF THE

AGRICULTURE

OF THE

COUNTIES

OF

ROXBURGH AND SELKIRK;

WITH

OBSERVATIONS ON THE MEANS OF THEIR IMPROVEMENT.

DRAWN UP FOR THE CONSIDERATION OF

THE BOARD OF AGRICULTURE,

AND INTERNAL IMPROVEMENT.

BY THE REV. ROBERT DOUGLAS, D.D.

MINISTER AT GALASHIELS.

————in Nature's bounty rich,
In herbs and fruits; whatever greens the spring
When Heaven descends in showers; or bends the boughs
When summer reddens, and when autumn beams;
Or in the wintry ... be whatever lies
Concealed, and fattens with the richest sap;
These are not wanting; nor the milky drove
Luxuriant, spread o'er all the lowing vale;
Nor bleating mountains ————
THOMSON.

LONDON:

PRINTED FOR RICHARD PHILLIPS, BRIDGE STREET,
BLACKFRIARS;

SOLD BY FAULDER & SON, BOND STREET; REYNOLDS, OXFORD
STREET; J. HARDING, ST. JAMES'S STREET; J. ASPERNE,
CORNHILL; BLACK, PARRY, & KINGSBURY, LEADENHALL
STREET; CONSTABLE & CO. EDINBURGH; BRASH & REID,
GLASGOW; BROWN, ABERDEEN; J. ARCHER, DUBLIN; &
ALL OTHER BOOKSELLERS;
BY D. M'MILLAN, BOW STREET, COVENT GARDEN.

1798.
[*Price Seven Shillings in Boards.*]

GENERAL VIEW

OF THE

AGRICULTURE

IN THE COUNTY OF

ROXBURGH.

YE generous Britons, venerate the plough!
And, o'er your hills and long withdrawing vales,
Let Autumn spread his treasures to the sun,
Luxuriant and unbounded. ———— ————
'Tis Beauty all and grateful song around,
Join'd to the low of kine, and num'rous bleat
Of flocks thick nibbling thro' the clovered vale.

THOMSON.

INTRODUCTION.

THIS work was undertaken at the united request of Sir John Sinclair, and of several gentlemen in both counties. Great pains have been taken to ascertain facts, and to state them with plainness and brevity. Provincial phrases have been studiously avoided or explained, and such words only used as, it is hoped, will be generally understood.

There may, however, be several omissions, mistakes, and errors. The information principally relied upon may have been in some instances partial, inaccurate, or not rightly apprehended. Averages and calculations may not always be formed on sound principles, and on sufficient grounds, or free from numerical mistakes. A few typographical errors may have escaped notice and correction; and perhaps peculiarities or improprieties of language may occur.—All of which are to be imputed, to my ignorance of some of the prescribed subjects, and my imperfect acquaintance with others, to my studies lying in a different line, and to much of my time and thoughts being neceſſarily occupied by the duties of my office, all the while that I was collecting materials and preparing this publication for the preſs.

I lie under great obligations to ſeveral intelligent friends ; ſome of whom came v luntarily forward with liberal communications, and others were put to no ſmall trouble in ſatisfying my inquiries. To them are to be aſcribed moſt of the uſeful obſervations, which the reader will find, on the prevalent modes of huſbandry and of the information relative to the botany and natural hiſtory of both counties. My acknowledgments are likewiſe due to Mr Ure and Mr Johnſton, whoſe Agricultural Surveys of Roxburgh and Selkirk ſhires I have frequent occaſion to quote, and whoſe previous labours have in different reſpects facilitated mine. I have alſo derived aſſiſtance, from the Statiſtical Accounts of ſeveral pariſhes, from the Agricultural Reports of different counties, and particularly from the reprinted one of Mid-Lothian, from Mr Culley's " General View of the " Agriculture of Northumberland," from his " Treatiſe on " Live Stock," and from the converſation and letters of ſeveral gentlemen unconnected with either county. I forbear to mention many reſpectable names, who have favoured me with their correſpondence, leſt I ſhould incur the imputation of oſtentatious vanity, offend the modeſty of ſome, and inadvertently omit others out of the liſt. I muſt requeſt ſeveral of them to forgive the liberty, which I was obliged to take, of abridging the ſubſtance and altering

the

the arrangement of their letters, and of making ſtatements,
not according to the information tranſmitted by any in-
invidual, but from the reſult of comparing the accounts
received concerning the ſame particulars from different
corners of the county.

Where oppoſite opinions or repreſentations were given
on any point by perſons of reſpectability, that, which ſeem-
ed moſt probable in itſelf, and was ſupported by the greateſt number of authorities, is inſerted in the text; and ſome
notice is generally taken of the other either there or in the
notes. The public may be aſſured, that nothing is advanced confidently, except upon the moſt undoubted information or perſonal knowledge. For, from a reſidence of thir-
ty-ſix years in the one county or the other, and from frequent intercourſe with well informed gentlemen and farmers in both, much ſurely may be ſeen and learned without great pretenſions to talents or application.

On ſome branches of the plan adopted by the Board,
which have frequently engaged my attention, I have ventured to throw out a few obſervations. For theſe, and for
all incidental ſtrictures on the practices of either county, I
alone am reſponſible. Whatever praiſe or blame they may
deſerve muſt fall upon me and not upon my employers. I
wiſh it, however, to be underſtood, that my commendations
and cenſures are to be applied, not to men, but to meaſures, and to ſuch meaſures only as belong ſtrictly to my
ſubject—to ſubſtantial improvements of every kind favourable to agriculture, by whomſoever they have been introduced,—

duced,—and to foolish prejudices and abfurd maxims which retard the melioration of the country, by whomfoever they are retained. For however prepofterous it may be, to venture upon innovations, which require the furrender of real good, for the vifionary profpect of catching fomething better; is it not equally prepofterous, to carry veneration for ancient ufages fo far, as to reject obftinately thofe alterations, which are found to be falutary and ufeful by unbiaffed experience?

To my charge, likewife, muft be laid any omiffions, defects, or errors in the maps or plates. The engravers were abundantly ready to make every alteration that was fuggefted. The maps were accurately reduced from the large and correct ones of Stobie and Ainflie. In that of Roxburghfhire, nothing is inferted, but the names of parifhes, towns, villages, fuch places as are mentioned in the work, and a few on the confines which jut out into other counties. With regard to Selkirkfhire, there being few parifh churches or villages, and not many farms deferving particular notice in an agricultural view, had the fame rule been rigidly followed, a large track of it would have appeared uninhabited; to prevent which, the feats of the refiding proprietors, the places from whence others take their titles, and fome of the moft extenfive farms, are named in the map. The principal mountains have the word *law*, or *fell*, or the letter *H*, added to them; and every place is carefully marked, where marl is dug, lime is burned for fale, or coals are wrought. In delineating the roads, and diftin-

guifhing,

guishing, by different colours, the arable, the green pasture, and the heath lands, I have received much assistance from persons of accurate local observation in very distant parts of the counties, but was still reduced to the necessity, in several cases, of being guided by my own geographical knowledge, in which I am far from desiring the reader to place entire confidence. The plate which contains the implements of husbandry, requiring some explanation, could not stand so conveniently in the place to which it naturally belongs, as at the end of the work. I regret that the ruts in the harrows are not at such equal distances as could be wished.

It may be proper to inform the reader, that the principal part of what relates to Roxburghshire was written in the months of June, July, and August 1796, and went to the press about the end of that year; and that what relates to Selkirkshire, and the concluding chapters, were written at different intervals during the course of 1797. This will enable him to understand the precise time to which I allude, when I speak of the present season, without specifying the year. And this has rendered it necessary to add a few pages, for the sake of inserting some interesting particulars, which either occurred since the greatest part of the work was printed, or did not reach me in time to claim earlier notice. In these *addenda*, mention may be made of places not to be found in the maps.

He

He is particularly requested to supply the following omissions, and to correct the following errors:

P. 3. l. 4. *Note. after* Smaillholm *insert* Stitchill.

P. 12. l. 1, 2. *The mark of reference should be at* Ednam, l. 2. *where there is clay marl, not at* Selkirk, l. 2. *where there is none.*

P. 12. L. 16. *after* Whitrigg *insert* in.

P. 29. l. 24. *for* knead *r.* kneaded.

P. 63. l. 2. *for* fix, seven, or at most eight, *r.* fix and an half or at most nine.

P. 85. l. 5. *after* faint *insert* cast.

P. 88. l. 2. *for* which are, *r.* which is. *Note,* l. 2. *for* fickle *r.* fcythe.

P. 91. l. 28. &c. *The sentence should run thus:* " order, " five are fufficient, viz. one before winter, one acrofs about " the beginning or middle of April, a third in May in the " fame direction with the firft, a fourth to form the drills, " or more properly the ridges, in June, or as foon afterwards " as circumftances permit, and a fifth to cover the dung " immediately before the feed is fown."

P. 92. l. 23. *for* 1500 or 1600 cwt. *r.* 15 or 16 cwt.

P. 130. l. 16. *I underftand feveral judicious farmers think drains should be covered with a lefs depth of foil than eight or ten inches, that they may be more eafily opened by the plough, to let away furface-water.*

P. 189. L. 5. *for* 36 *by* 1 yards, *r.* 36 yards by 1.

P. 199. l. 23. *for* Newton toll-bar *r.* Newtown toll-bar.

P. 207. l. 8. *after* wholefale *add* here.

P. 210. l. 3. *A mark of reference is improperly placed before the words,* " at 16 s." *it should be deleted.*

—— l. 14. *for* price *r.* produce; l. 27. *for* L. 114,900, *r.* L. 114,900 : 8 : 0.

Note,

Note, l. 4. *for* 413,823, *r.* 413,831, *and for* 9673 *r.* 9665.

P. 222. *In this Statistical table* Exp. *should be in the same column with and immediately over* L. 300, *and,*

For Galashiels $\frac{1}{7}$, *r.* Galashiels $\frac{1}{4}$.

P. 232. l. 26. *after* shells, *insert* upon them.

P. 244. l. 3. *for* four proprietors *r.* five proprietors.

P. 258. l. 9. *for* who *r.* which.

—— l. 26. *In calculating the interest of* L. 1179, *there is a palpable error. Instead of* L. 55, 4 s. *as in the text, it should be* L. 58, 19 s. *which increases the expenditure,* L. ult. *to* L. 521, 9 s. *and reduces the gain,* p. 255. l. 9. *to* L. 105, 11 s. *Owing to this error in the calculation of interest, the sum to be deducted,* p. 26. l. 15. *is* L. 52, 19 s. *Hence the expenditure,* l. 22. *should be* L. 507, 19 s. *and the profit,* p. 261. l. 12. *should be only* L. 62, 11 s.

P. 291. Note 3. l. 1. *for* Hairmofs *r.* Hatemofs.

P. 295. Note, l. 30. *for* without marl, *r.* without repeating marl.

P. 305. l. 14. *for* milk *r.* fuck.

P. 326. l. 19. *Two articles are here confounded, and the amount of one of them omitted. They must be separately stated as under, and the sum total,* l. 24. *will then be right.*

Wool, 36,000 fleeces, at 11 d.	L. 1650
Cheese, about — —	800

P. 334. l. 5. *after* who do not, *insert* reside in the parish or

I forbear to point out some errors, evidently typographical, such as p. 68. l. penult. *tha* for *that*; p. 131. l. 16. *inverten* for *inverted*; p. 268. *gredually* for *gradually*, &c.

These

Thefe every reader will be able to correct. Nor muſt all thoſe in the preceding liſt be laid wholly to the charge of the printer. I have no doubt that moſt of them were owing to my inadvertence; and I perfuade myſelf, that they would have been fewer and leſs material, had it not been for my inconvenient diſtance from the preſs.

GALASHIELS,
Jun. 15. 1798.

Tᴜᴇ diverſity of ᴡᴇɪɢʜᴛs and ᴍᴇᴀsᴜʀᴇs through the kingdom muſt render it very eligible, in a work of this nature, to reduce thoſe, which are moſt generally uſed in the counties, to ſome known ſtandard.

The Engliſh pound of 16 oz. Avoirdupois; their ſtone containing 14 of theſe lbs.; their hundred weight confiſting of 8 of theſe ſtones; and their ton of 20 cwt. are all pretty generally known through the whole iſland. In relation to theſe, the weights in Roxburgh and Selkirk ſhires, ſtand as under:

IN ROXBURGHSHIRE,

Hay, wool, lint, butter, cheeſe, tallow, and raw hides are ſold by

The Scotch Tron ſtone = 24 lbs. Engliſh, or Avoirdupois.

This ſtone contains 16 lbs. Scotch Tron, and the lb. = 24 oz. Engliſh, or Avoirdupois.

IN

IN SELKIRKSHIRE,

The ftone, by which the above articles are fold, contains only 23 lbs. 8 oz. Englifh, or Avoirdupois.

N.B. A pack of wool confifts of 12 of thefe ftones.

IN BOTH COUNTIES,

All kinds of grain, meal, flour, pot-barley, iron, cattle, butcher meat and fifh, are fold by

The Scotch, Troy, or Dutch ftone = 17¼ lbs. Englifh or Avoirdupois.

This ftone contains 16 lbs. Troy or Dutch, and the lb. is = 17¼ oz. Englifh, or Avoirdupois.

N.B. Grain and cattle are rarely fold by weight, but their value is commonly computed and fpoken of by this ftandard. Flour, when bolted and dreffed, is fold by the Englifh ftone of 14 lbs. The boll or load of meal, is 16 Scotch Troy ftones.

All other articles are fold by the Englifh or Avoirdupois weight; but the ftone of it, in fome places, and in all places with refpect to fome articles, confifts of 16 lbs. Avoirdupois, and not of 14 lbs. as in England.

The Linlithgow firlots are the ftandard meafures in Scotland for all grains. There are two of them; one for wheat, rye, peafe, beans, and white falt; the other for barley, oats, and malt. The former contains 2197,335 folid inches, and 21¼ pints, each pint being 103,404 folid inches. The latter contains 3205,524 folid inches, and 31 of the fame
pints.

pints. The Winchester bushel, being 2150,420 solid inches, is very little less than the Scotch firlot for wheat, &c. Relative to these standards, the measures of Roxburgh and Selkirk shires, are as follows :

IN ROXBURGHSHIRE,

Wheat, pease, beans and rye, are sold by the boll of five firlots, each firlot containing 2274,888 cubic inches, and 22 pints, being 3 Scotch mutchkins, or nearly $1\frac{1}{10}$ English quart, above the Scotch standard. The boll is $=$ 5 firlots $3\frac{1}{2}$ pints Scotch standard, and $=$ 5 bushels 3 pecks 2 pints, and a fraction English standard.

IN SELKIRKSHIRE,

The firlot is $\frac{1}{10}$ of a pint larger, which gives only a very trifling increase in the boll.

N. B. In both counties this boll is falling into disuse, and in the following work has reference only to the *fiars*, and average monthly returns of the prices of grain to Government. These grains are commonly sold by the boll of 6 firlots instead of 5. To this boll I uniformly refer, except as above ; and the reader will see that in Roxburghshire it is precisely equal to 4 of the county firlots for oats, barley and malt as under.

IN ROXBURGHSHIRE,

Oats, barley and malt, are sold by the boll of 5 firlots, each firlot containing 3412,332 cubic inches, and 33 pints, being 2 pints (near 3 English quarts) above the standard.

This boll is $=$ 5 firlots 10 pints Scotch standard measure, and is $=$ 7 bushels 3 pecks 11 pints and a fraction English, ditto.

IN

IN SELKIRKSHIRE,

This boll confifts of 10 *fulls*, each *full* containing 1615,685 cubic inches. Two of thefe fulls make a firlot of 3221,370 cubic inches, and five of thefe firlots make a boll = 5 firlots 1¼ pints Scotch ftandard, and = 7 bufhels 2 pecks and a fraction Englifh ditto.

N. B. Little or no malt is now fold. And meal is never fold by meafure. The Roxburghfhire firlot is ufed in many places of Selkirkfhire. Of this firlot 4 is the moft common, both of wheat and peafe, and 5 of oats and barley in both counties, though there are many exceptions.

This boll, viz. of 4 Roxburghfhire firlots for wheat and peafe, and of 5 of the fame firlots for oats and barley, is always to be underftood in the following work, where no exception is exprefsly mentioned.

Land is always meafured by the Englifh ftatute acre, and roads by the Englifh ftatute mile.

AGRI.

AGRICULTURAL SURVEY

OF

ROXBURGHSHIRE.

CHAP. I.

GEOGRAPHICAL STATE AND CIRCUMSTANCES.

SECT. I.—*Situation and Extent.*

ROXBURGHSHIRE, called alfo TEVIOTDALE, from the river Teviot running through its moft extenfive dale, is fituated in N. lat. from 55° 7' to 55° 42', and between 1° 39' and 2° 36' W. long. from London. Its fouthern point, known by the name of Liddefdale, ftretches out between Dumfriesfhire and Cumberland, being feparated from the former by the tops of mountains, and the Mare-burn, which falls into Liddal-water; and from the latter, firft by that water, and afterwards by Kerfhope, to its fource, from whence the boundary with Northumberland, except in a very few fpots, runs along the fummit of a lofty ridge, in various curves E. and N. E., towards the eaftern and higheft part of Cheviot, where it turns N. and N. W., croffing Bowmont-water, and proceeding with feveral irregularities towards the river Tweed, at its junction with Carham-burn:

Following

Following thefe curvatures, this county borders with England about 60 miles. It is divided from Berwickfhire for
a fhort way by Tweed; but about a mile above the mouth
of Carham-burn it croffes that river, and includes the parifhes of Ednam, Stitchill, Kelfo, Smaillholm, and Makerf-
toun. At the weftern extremity of this laft parifh, Tweed
again becomes the boundary, until it receives the water of
Leeder on the N. Here a fpace of about 5 miles fquare
juts out northward, between Berwickfhire and Selkirkfhire,
till it meets the fouthern angle of Mid-Lothian on the N. W.
From Selkirkfhire, on the W. it is feparated fucceffively
by Gala, Tweed, and Ettrick Waters, and afterwards by a
line running moftly S. S. W. in a moft crooked and whim-
fical manner towards the confines of Dumfriesfhire, comprehending a part of the parifhes of Galafhiels, Selkirk, Afhkirk, and Roberton. Its greateft length, from the junction
of the Mare-burn with Liddal to the junction of Carham-
burn with Tweed, is 41 miles: and its greateft breadth, by
a line croffing the above at right angles, is 29 miles. Its
medium length is about 30, and its medium breadth a little
more than 22 miles, making its contents nearly 672 fquare
miles, or 430,080 fquare acres; of which about three-fifths,
or 268,048 acres are in fheep-pafture, and the remaining
two-fifths, or 172,032 acres are occafionally under the
plough, except about 8000 acres occupied in woods, pleafure-grounds, and the fites of towns and villages. It contains
29 complete parifhes, befides part of the 4 already mentioned, and the old parifh of Stitchill, to which that of
Home in Berwickfhire is now annexed.   •

Sect. II.—*Division.*

THE only agricultural divifion, of which this county admits, is into pafture and arable lands. A line, drawn from
the point where the boundary with England croffes Bow-
mont-

mont-water, W. S. W. by Jedburgh and the N. of Dunian
and Rubers-law to Hawick, and turning N. from thence
along the turnpike-road to Selkirk, will nearly separate the
former of these on the S. from the latter on the N., with the
exception of the small tract N. of Tweed betwe : Leader
and Gala Waters, the largest half of which is allotted to
sheep. In the one, there are many fertile vales in tillage,
which greatly overbalance the pasture hills in the other.
Two of these hills, in the arable district, attract the notice of
travellers; Minto, with two flat tops, on the N. of Teviot,
858 feet, and Eildon, immediately S. of Tweed, near Melrose, whose three conical tops, though only 1330 feet, are
seen at a great distance. In the pasture district there are
many hills of considerable height. The Dunian, 1021 feet,
and Ruberslaw, 1419 feet, are, like Eildon, conspicuous
from their situation and shape, though much lower than
Wisp and Tidhope, each of which is 1830 feet; Millen-
wood-fell and Windhead, each of which is computed, from
an observation taken by the theodolite, to be 2000 feet [*]; and
Hownamlaw, Windburgh, Maidenpaps, and Greatmoor,
whose measurements are not known. On the confines of
Northumberland, Carter-fell is 1602 feet, and Chillhill must
be rather upwards of 2000 feet, as it stands near the highest
top of Cheviot, which is 2682 feet. These heights are all
taken from the level of the sea, by a barometer, and may
not be perfectly exact.

For the purposes of justice and police, the county is divided into four districts [†], in each of which the Justices of

Peace

[*] See Statistical Account of Castletown, vol. xvi. p. 63.

[†] Viz. The district of Jedburgh, comprehending the parishes of Jed-
burgh, Crailing, Oxnam, Southdean, Hobkirk, Bedrule, Minto, and Ancrum.
The district of Kelso,—Kelso, Sprouston, Linton, Yetholm, Morebattle,
Hownam, Eckford, Roxburgh, Makerstown, Smailholm, and Ednam. The
district of Melrose.—Melrose, St Boswells, Maxton, Lilliesleaf, Bowden,
Galashiels, and Selkirk: And the district of Hawick,—Hawick, Wilton,
Cavers, Kirktown, Castletown, Roberton, and Ashkirk.

Peace hold courts quarterly, or oftener if bufinefs requires. They take cognizance chiefly of caufes between mafters and ervants, trefpaffes againft the game-laws, public nuifances, and crofs roads; with all of which the interefts of agriculure have a nearer or more remote concern.

Sect. III.—*Climate.*

Some fields in this county being only about 90, and feveral hills about 2000 feet above the level of the fea; the greateft part of it declining towards the E. and a fmall part towards the W.; the climate muft, of courfe, be extremely various. In proportion to the elevation of the ground, the air is more moift and fharp; and through the whole ifland, the weftern coaft is more expofed to wind and rain than the eaftern. In the Tranfactions of the Royal Society of Edinburgh, vol. i. there is a comparative table of the quantity of rain which fell at Dalkeith, Branxholm, and Langholm, for the following years :

	Dalkeith.	Branxholm.	Langholm.	Wool or Wall.
1773,	25.473	32.652	38.850	34.022
1774,	27.925	29.250	34.405	30.688
1775,	29.550	38.573	39.300	39.177
1776,	20.650	26.295	34.161	27.579
1777,	22.025	29.533	36.950	
	125.623	156.303	183.665	

Langholm and Dalkeith are not in this county; but the former, being in the neighbourhood of Liddefdale, cannot differ much from it in climate; nor can the latter be much drier than Kelfo in the lower part of Roxburghfhire. It appears, that, in five fuccellive years, there was about one-fifth lefs rain at Dalkeith than at Branxholm, and about one-fixth lefs at Branxholm than at Langholm. Now as Branxholm (near Hawick) is nearly equidiftant from Langholm and Kelfo, there can be no material error in fuppofing,

that

that about one-sixth less rain falls at the latter place than at
Branxholm, especially as this still allows to Kelso a more
humid climate than Dalkeith. After the most diligent inquiry, I cannot learn that a diary of the weather has been
kept in any other part of the county, except at Wool, about
7 miles N. from Branxholm, in a higher exposure. From
it I was favoured with the additional column in the above
table, and also with the following abstract of the medium
state of the barometer, thermometer, and rain, for the year
1780, which is placed opposite to an abstract of these particulars at Branxholm that year :

	Branxholm.			Wool or Wall.		
	Bar.	Ther.	Rain.	Bar.	Ther.	Rain.
January,	29.160	35.625	Frost.	29.390	29.620	1.120
February,	29.020	31.290	1.250	28.250	34.370	1.110
March,	29.070	42.61	2.650	28.612	43.000	2.780
April,	28.903	46.70	2.500	28.710	46.850	4.085
May,	29.090	50.126	4.613	25.912	51.520	3.530
June,	29.217	55.007	2.100	29.097	52.507	1.860
July,	29.280	58.155	1.050	29.995	60.050	1.630
August,	29.430	59.000	.150	29.310	61.000	.500
September,	29.000	54.900	3.35	25.630	56.140	4.415
October,	29.217	44.200	4.70	25.71	45.050	4.060
November,	28.180	34.607	1.975	29.150	36.850	1.417
December,	29.550	35.700	.30	29.440	35.025	.540
			25.510			27.170

This table shows, that in the more elevated situation there
is both greater heat and more rain than in the lower one;
and it confirms the general opinion, that July and August
are the warmest and driest months in the year, although
sometimes prodigious thunder-showers fall in both. The
weather in September and October admits of every possible
variation. It is often serene and pleasant : But excessive
rains, winds, and frosts, even hail and snow, are by no
means uncommon, and have done incredible damage to the
crops in different years November is nearly of the same
complexion. December is in general more moderate and
uniform. Frost and snow are seldom severe, or of long duration

ration, before Chriſtmas. January and February are the months when ſnow is moſt common, and when froſt is moſt intenſe. With ſome ſhort interruptions, they have been known to remain until diſſipated by the influence of the ſun in March. During that month, froſty mornings are ſucceeded, ſometimes by clear ſunſhine, at other times by a hurricane of wind, rain, and ſleet, and not unfrequently by piercing northerly blaſts, accompanied with hail. Cold eaſterly winds prevail very much in April and May, often too in June, either bringing conſtant rains for a ſucceſſion of days, or exhaling moiſture ſo quickly from the earth, as to ſtunt the tender ſtalks both of corn and graſs. But every one of theſe general aſſertions has been at times reverſed. After an open and ſoft winter, great quantities of ſnow have fallen in March, April, and May. In other years, April has been wonderfully mild, May and June the warmeſt, July and Auguſt the wetteſt, and September and October the moſt ſettled months. This extreme uncertainty of the weather makes farmers deſirous of ſowing wheat, eſpecially on clay lands in fallow, early in September, or as ſoon thereafter as the ſtate of the ground will permit. After beans, peaſe, and clover, it is ſown whenever the crop can be removed, and the field can be ploughed, generally in October; and after potatoes, in the end of that month, or beginning of November. Of late, a good deal of ſpring-wheat is ſown after turnips eaten by ſheep. Beans, and *cold* or late peaſe, are ſown, in favourable ſeaſons, as early as February, but more commonly about the beginning of March; oats, during the whole of that month, and in the two firſt weeks of April; *hot* or early peaſe, towards the middle and end of that month; and barley, from the middle of it till Whitſunday. Harveſt, in the lower parts of the arable diſtrict, has been known to commence in July, but has very ſeldom become general, even there, till the middle of Auguſt, and

is

is moftly over about the beginning of October. In the higher grounds it is a fortnight or three weeks later. Much corn has been feen in the fields in November.

Sect. IV.—*Surface and Soil.*

The furface is finely diverfified, and exhibits many fcenes that are truly beautiful, few that are romantic or fublime. The hills have moftly floping fides, and are covered with a green fward to the very top. Very few of them are bleak, and none rugged or tremendous. The profpects from their fummits are extenfive, variegated, and delightful. The numerous vales, whether of narrow or wide extent, are all watered by limpid ftreams; many of them are naked, and many fringed with wood. Some afford excellent pafture; others are in high cultivation. They are, in general, inclofed by gentle declivities, though feverals are hemmed in by fteep banks, over-run with brufhwood, or adorned with lofty trees, which form a fcenery rather agreeable than magnificent. In a county, fo large, and on the whole fo elevated, the proportion of heath and mofs * is very inconfiderable, but cannot be calculated with any degree of exactnefs,

as

* *Mofs*, in Scotland, is equivalent to *morafs* or *bog* in England, when thefe contain the black or dark-coloured fubftance formed by ftagnant water from corrupted vegetables, which is fometimes in a fluid ftate, and fometimes dry and porous. In a fluid ftate, a variety of water plants fhoot forth from it; when dry and porous, it is covered with a tough fward of heath and coarfe graffes, capable of bearing the weight of fheep, and even of cattle. In this ftate, the furface is, in many places, made into *turf*, and the black fubftance beneath is dug with a fpade contrived for the purpofe, and dried into *peats*, both for fuel. Under it marl is often found, when the water, detained in it, is favourable to the production of thofe animals, out of whofe fhells and decayed bodies, that manure is now underftood to be compofed. A curious fact, illuftrative of this theory relative to the formation of marl, is inferted in the Agricultural Report of the neighbouring county of Selkirk.

as they are scattered every where, in portions of unequal size. In Liddesdale, where improvement has hitherto made flow progress, patches of moss are seen by the edges, and even in the middle of fertile vales. There are indications of this having been once the case in other parts of the county, on which industry has now wrought a happy change.

In the pasture district the soil is dry, wet, or heathy. To the eastward of Jed Water, the hills are mostly composed of red granite, and covered with a thick sward of rich and sweet grass; there is very little heath; the marshes are not numerous or extensive, and interfected by a multitude of drains. The dry soil, west of Jed Water including Liddesdale, is either on limestone or gravel; there are many *mosses*, a great deal of fenny land, a deficiency of drains; and a large tract of stubborn clay, lying on a cold impenetrable till *, stretches from the S. W. skirt of Rubers-law to the confines of Liddesdale. That detached corner †, whose value only begins to be known, is almost wholly pastoral,. and though unquestionably the wettest part of the county, has no small proportion of dry land, and many spungy fields producing coarse grass, which are susceptible of great improvement by draining; yet much of its best soil is thickly interspersed with spots or stripes of moss, which cannot easily be removed, or turned to any solid advantage. There is

not

* " The most general signification of till seems to be, a very hard clay, " impenetrable by the roots of plants, and but in a small degree by water. " Frequently, in this clay, are imbedded a great number of small stones, " like coarse gravel; these are often so firmly combined by the clay, or " other cementing matter, that they are not easily disunited. Such is the " till that prevails in Roxburghshire. It may be converted into soil; but " in order to render it fertile, no small pains, and a considerable length of " time, are necessary." Mr Ure, p. 9, 10.

† It is 18 miles by 14; but being a triangle, one half of the produce makes its contents about 30,000 acres.——Stat. Acc. of Castletown, vol. xvi. p. 61.

not much heath and moor in proportion to the extent of the
pasture lands.   But in these, and indeed through the district
at large, the dry and sound soil greatly predominates.

In the arable district, the soil is partly light, and partly
heavy.   The light consists of rich loam, or mixtures of loam
and sand, of loam and gravel, of sand or gravel and clay, in
every various proportion.   The loam, gravel, sand, and
clay, also, are of very different qualities, or degrees of excellence.   It is also to be distinguished, according as it is incumbent on till, clay, gravel, sand, freestone, limestone, and
different kinds of granite.   Where it is shallow, some of
the substratum, being ploughed up and by frequent culture
incorporated with the soil, may partly occasion the medley
which the surface exhibits :   And deep spots in low lands
are probably composed of decayed vegetables, and rich
particles of earth, carried down and deposited by the rivers.
The heavy soil is chiefly clay of different depths and degrees of stiffness, or mixtures where clay prevails, placed
on till, or other matter, retentive of water.   In a very few
spots this surface lies on a dry bottom ; and not unfrequently different and opposite soils are strangely blended in
the same field.   The light soil, however, is in general
found on low and level lands near the beds of rivers and
their branches ; and also on several eminences of considerable extent, especially in the parishes of Linton, Eckford,
Crailing, Ancrum, Maxton, and Melrose.   The heavy soil
rarely appears on the vallies, and chiefly occupies the higher grounds.   The largest track of it lies immediately S. of
Eildon Hills, including nearly the whole of Minto, Lilliesleaf, and Bowden parishes, and a great part of Melrose, St
Boswell's, Ancrum, Maxton, and Roxburgh.   Stretching
in a straight line about 10 miles, and being, at an average,
above 4 miles broad, it must comprehend about 10,000
acres ; of which at least one half is shallow, cold, and un-
kindly,

B

kindly, difficult to labour, and uncertain in its produce; on which account, upwards of 1000 acres have properly been planted with trees. In the other half there is much rich and fertile land, which bears luxuriant crops, both of corn and grass, and not a little of a middle nature between these extremes. In the parishes, also, N. of Tweed around Kelso, the heavy soil is rather most prevalent, and is, in general, of a good quality. Another considerable portion of it runs along the higher grounds S. of Tweed, in the parishes of Sproufton, Kelso, Roxburgh, and Eckford, some of which is of little value; and there are detached fields of it in other parts of the district. In the bosom, or deeply indented into the sides of these clayey tracts, and especially in the vicinity of Lilliesleaf, are pieces of dry land, of an admirable quality for producing either white or green crops. Of the arable district at least two-thirds may be safely called light and dry.

Sect. V.—*Minerals.*

In several parts of the county, iron stones are found in the soil [*]. There are also some springs weakly impregnated both by it and sulphur [†]; and one of a petrifying nature on the Tweeden [†], which falls into Liddal. There are appearances of petrifaction in other parts; and fragments of agate [†], jasper, and rock crystal, are thrown upon the surface by moles, the plough, and torrents, in many

[*] Speaking of the clayey lands S. of Eildon, Mr Ure says, p. 10. " There " is a certain quantity of iron in its composition from 1 to 6 *per cent.*"

[†] See Stat. Act. of Jedburgh, vol. i. p. 4:—of Crailing, vol. ii. p. 318.— of Castletown, vol. xvi. p. 78.—of Oxnam, vol. xi. p. 319.—of Hahkirk, vol. iii. p. 311.—and Mr Ure's Report, p. 2.

many different places, particularly at *Roberts Linne* *, towards
the confines of Hobkirk parish with Liddesdale. Coal was
discovered about 30 years ago, on the Carter Hill near the
border of Northumberland, and wrought for some time,
but abandoned as of little value. Another, of a better quality, has since been found in the southern extremity of Liddesdale, from which, however, only a very small part of
the county derives any benefit. Through the whole of
that region limestone abounds, but, for want of a demand
and of good roads, little or none is calcined for sale, though
it is of superior quality to what is manufactured farther N.
and N. E. in the neighbourhood of Hawick and Jedburgh.
The poorness of the lime, and the distance from coal, prevent it from being generally burned in other parts of the
county where it has appeared. There is no freestone in
the N. W. or S. E. corners of the county. It seems to run,
with several irregularities, and perhaps some interruptions,
in a N. E. direction, from the farthest point of Liddesdale to
the neighbourhood of Sproustoun, where it is of a fine hard
and durable nature. Different kinds of whinstone appear
every where on the surface, in the beds of brooks, and in
inexhaustible quarries. Vast quantities of shell-marl † lie
scattered through the contiguous parishes of Roberton, Ashkirk, Wilton, Minto, Lilliesleaf, Bowden, Galashiels, and
Selkirk.

---

* They are mostly of an amber colour, with bluish veins, and streaks of
deep red. Some are pure, but full of fractures.

† Mr Ure, p. 47. observes, " It is chiefly the *Mytilus exiguus* (of Lister)
" *Helix nana; H. putris :* this last is by far the most numerous. Mud and
" decayed vegetables are, in different proportions, mixed with the shells,
" many of which are entire. All the varieties are natives of Scotland, and
" are found living in stagnant water, in mosses where marl has been disco-
" vered. They are extremely prolific, a circumstance which accounts for
" their immense number."

Selkirk *. There are alſo large marl pits at Eckford and Ednam; and ſome leſs conſiderable ones in different places. A ſmall quantity of it was lately found on the very banks of Tweed, in the pariſh of Maxton, below a thick ſtratum of coarſe gravel, covered by a light ſoil; and, on the oppo-ſite ſide of that river, at Whittrigg, an angle of Berwick-ſhire, a vaſt maſs of fine marl begins now to be ſold, from which the ſurrounding pariſhes in this county may eventu-ally derive great advantage.

SECT. VI.—*Waters.*

No county in the kingdom can boaſt of more numerous or beautiful rivers and brooks. One of them flows through, and enlivens every little vale. Tweed and Teviot are alone called rivers. The firſt holds a majeſtic courſe along banks, which, in ſeveral places, are ſteep and bold, jutting out at Old Melroſe into a promontory, and forming around Dryburgh a peninſula. It partly bounds and partly inter-ſects the county, receiving on the N. the Gala, which is the boundary with Selkirkſhire and Mid-Lothian for 5 miles; the Leeder, which, for nearly the ſame ſpace, is the boun-dary with Berwickſhire; the Allen (corrupted into El-wand), a paſtoral rivulet, and the Eden, which riſes in Ber-wickſhire, but runs a conſiderable way along the ſkirts and through the lower part of this county. Ettrick, alſo, a boundary of Selkirkſhire for a mile and an half, falls into Tweed on the ſouth. Teviot rolls its pure ſtreams over a pebbled bed, in many delightful windings, through a ſuc-ceſſion of rich, extenſive, and well cultivated vallies, for 34 miles, till it loſes its name in the Tweed, between Rox-burgh Caſtle and Kelſo, one of the moſt enchanting ſpots which can well be conceived. The Ale and Borthwick are the northern branches of Teviot. Both riſe in Selkirk-ſhire,

* In this neighbourhood there is a good deal of *clay* marl.

shire, and are in some places boundaries of the two counties. The Ale flows upwards of 12 miles in this county, through fields of very unequal fertility, many of which have wooded banks, till, emerging from scenery that is truly romantic, it is emptied into Teviot below Ancrum. The Borthwick joins Teviot above Hawick, after passing through a country that is chiefly pastoral, but much improven of late by tillage, and manure, and young plantations. On the S., Teviot is augmented by the Kale, the Oxnam, and the Jed. The first and last issue from the border hills. The Kale, after leaving the mountains, waters, and sometimes overflows, a great part of a spacious and valuable plain of 1200 acres *, adorned on different sides by clumps of full grown trees; while the Jed, rushing along a rocky channel, through narrow and thick wooded vales, washes the bottom of several high precipices, winds around the county town, and terminates another, and still more extensive plain, known by the name of Crailinghaughs, through the middle of which the Oxnam finds its way to Teviot. Nearer to its source, Teviot receives the Rule, the Slittrige, and the Allen, all of which rise on the confines of Liddesdale. In the number and value of its trees, Rule may vie with *Silvan Jed* †, but not in wild and picturesque scenery. Slittrige is not without the beauties of green hills, natural wood, and hollow vales. Allen, like the stream of the same name, N. of Tweed, flows wholly through sheep-walks. Bowmont is another pastoral rivulet, which has its source in the S. E. of this county, and, after a rapid course of nine or ten miles, enters England. But of all the waters in Roxburghshire, few are more indebted to nature, or might be more improven by art, than Hermitage, which rises in the southern declivity of the ridge, from whence Allen and Slittrige go in an opposite direction, and tumbling over a

bottom

---

* See Stat. Acc. of Linton, vol. iii. p. 110.
† Thomson's Autumn.

bottom of rough fhapelefs ftones, amidft green hills, whofe
bafe is generally fkirted with copfewood, lofes itfelf in the
Liddal, and imparts its natural ornament to that larger, but
more naked ftream. The courfe of Liddal is more placid:
it iffues from a flat, not improperly called *Dead Water*, and
comes through a diftrict more marfhy and level. After
their junction, they are increafed by fome confiderable
brooks, and, with a velocity, which has excavated pools of
an uncommon depth, defcend through vallies, capable of
being rendered, by the hands of fkilful cultivators, as productive as they are beautiful, for the fpace of 8 or 9
miles, when they feparate Cumberland from Dumfriesfhire,
and mingling with Efk, are carried into Solway Firth.

In an inland county, whofe loweft point is above 20 miles
from the fea, and 10 from the bigheft tide-mark on the
fides of Tweed, the quantity of falmon is greater than might
be expected. They are chiefly found in Tweed, few of
them in Teviot, and none in the leffer waters, except in the
time of fpawning. A number of a fmaller fize, or, as fome
allege, of a diftinct fpecies, called here *grilfe*, and of fea-
trouts, here called *whitlings*, towards the middle and end of
the fifhing-feafon, vifit Tweed, Teviot, and the larger branches of both. Trouts of different fizes and flavour abound in
every brook; but Ale, Rule, Jed, and Kale, are moft famed
for the number and excellence of their trouts. There are
feveral fmall lakes in the county, fome of which contain a
multitude of perches and pike. Of thefe, the moft remarkable for fize and beauty are Cauldfhiels, on the eftate of
Faldanefide, and Headfhaw, towards the N. W.; and Prim-
fide, or Lochtower, towards the S. E.

CHAP.

CHAP. II.

STATE OF PROPERTY.

SECT. I—*Estates, and their Management.*

WHEN all the lands in Scotland were valued, the rents, payable in victual, seem to have been converted into money at different rates, according to the quality of the grain raised, and the measures used, in different counties. The common conversion for Roxburghshire was, wheat at L. 8; oatmeal, in some places, L. 8, in others, only L. 7; bear, L. 6; and oats, L. 4, all Scotch money, *per* boll. But the rate was much higher in many estates, probably from a mistaken vanity in the proprietors, or a desire of acquiring political importance from the largeness of their rent-rolls. To some such cause, more than to the superior value of the soil, the valuation of this county is greater, in proportion to its extent, than that of any other in Scotland. It amounts to L. 314,663 : 6 : 4 Scotch, of which L. 129,126 : 6 : 7 belongs to 6 peers, L. 128,345 : 7 : 6 belongs to 42 commoners, each of whom has property valued above L. 1000 Scotch; L. 54,097 : 7 : 3 belongs to lesser commoners, including those small proprietors, known by the provincial names of *acrerers, portioners, and feuers*, 18 parcels of whose lands, in different places, are valued in the gross, besides 128

who

who have got their small properties separately valued. The
remaining L. 3094 : 5 : 0 belongs to public bodies. Of the
42 greater commoners, 5 are precluded, by the nature of
their tenures, and 1 from being the eldest son of a peer of
Scotland, from voting for a member of Parliament; 34 are
upon the roll of freeholders, another may enter when he
chuses to apply, and one only is a minor. There are 80
freeholders at present, 12 of whom vote as superiors of lands
not possessed by them, some of them having retained or
purchased that privilege, or obtained a gift of it from their
relations. Besides these, two eldest sons of proprietors are
enrolled, on acquiring from their fathers a right to as much
of the estate as the law requires. It is more worthy of notice, in an agricultural view, that this roll contains the names
of 8 actual farmers, who, by their industry and skill, have
purchased estates.

Property has not, for a long time, undergone any remarkable change. Estates, indeed, of considerable size, have
been sold within the last 40 years; some of them twice, at
such an advanced price, as shews the gradual and rapid increase of the value of land. Stewartfield, near Jedburgh,
was sold in 1768 for L. 7000 Sterling, and again in 1771
at L. 11,500 Sterling; Ednam was sold in 1766 for L. 16,500,
and again in 1787 for L. 31,500 Sterling. Softlaw, near
Kelso, was bought in 1778 for L. 6500 Sterling, and fetched
double that price in 1794. Many other instances might be
produced of a still higher rise in small fields around towns
and villages *. But the small migration of property is evinced by two circumstances. One of them is, that of the
above 42 larger estates belonging to commoners, only 14
have

---

* Crailing indeed was bought in 1766, and sold in 1786, at a very small
additional price; but there were circumstances which render it an unfair
instance of the progressive value of property.

have been in the market during the period mentioned, and that, besides these, only two large estates, belonging to peers, were sold, and another still larger estate than either of them was purchased by a peer from a commoner. The other is, that more than two-thirds of the whole county is possessed, at this moment, by families of seven different surnames, which have had property in it for centuries, as will appear from the following state, which may not prove unintertaining to some of the gentlemen concerned, as well as to strangers:

Surname.	Peers.	Proprietors.	Freeholders.	Valuation.		
Ker,	2	10	6	L. 83869	6	0
Scott,	1	25	6	60989	12	7
Elliot, ●		13	8	24470	3	10
Douglas	1	6	4	23161	3	10
Pringle,		4	3	11191	15	8
Riddel, .		4	3	6225	1	4
Rutherfurd,		6	4	5797	2	0
Total,	4	68	34	L. 217704	5	3

There are several other names of great antiquity in the county, individuals of which still retain the estates of their progenitors to a very considerable amount.

From the best information which I can collect, the average rent of the pasture district will be nearly 3 s. per acre; and supposing 3-5ths of the whole county, or 258,048 acres to belong to it, the amount will be   -   L. 38707 4 0
Deducting, from the remaining 2-5ths, 8000
 acres occupied in wood, pleasure-grounds,
 &c. there will be 164,032 acres of arable
 land at 15 s. per acre,   -   -   123024 8 0

   "Carried forward, L. 161731 12 0

 ● Though the late Lord Heathfield was a native of this county, he never had, and his son, the present Lord, has not any property in it.

    C '

Brought forward,   L. 161731 12 0

There are at leaſt 5290 acres in wood, worth
about L. 300,000, the intereſt of one half of
which may fairly be added to the rent of
the county,   -   -   7500 0 0

And the remaining 2710 acres in pleaſure-
grounds, gardens, &c. cannot be eſtimated
at leſs than L. 1 per acre,   -   2710 0 0

Making the real rent of the whole county, * L. 171941 12 0

The

---

* It becomes me to ſtate the grounds on which this computation proceeds. The bigbeſt rent per acre of any extenſive paſture farm, that has
come to my knowledge, is 5 s. 6 d. and the loweſt is 1 s. 1 d.; the exact
medium between them is 3 s. 3½ d. But the number of acres let above 3 s.
is comparatively ſmall, and their average does not exceed 3 s. 9d ; while a
much greater number of acres, let under 3 s. gives only an average of 2 s.
2 d.; and the medium between theſe averages is 2 s. 11¾. There are, indeed, ſeveral valuable farms, of whoſe real average I am ignorant, and
which are computed at 4 s. But there are other farms, ſtill more extenſive,
concerning which I am equally ignorant, computed at 2 s. or 2s leaſt below 2 s. 4 d. Theſe are the computations of neighbours, who know the
rents, but do not know the exact meaſurements, and judge of theſe by the
number of ſheep kept. Upon the whole, 3 s. per acre cannot be far from
the truth, but is probably rather below than above it.

I am more uncertain about the average of the arable land, and have been
obliged to reſt ſatisfied with a conjecture, formed on ſuch imperfect information as I could obtain. Several intelligent farmers are of opinion that
my average is rather too high. To them I beg leave to ſubmit the following
conſiderations : 1ſt, There are 39 villages in the county, beſides Jedburgh,
Kelſo, and Hawick. Around each of theſe there are from 100 to 200 acres,
which actually yield, or might yield if let, two guineas each. 2dly, There
are many incloſures in old graſs, which are annually let at the ſame rate.
3dly, There are one or two farms under leaſe at L. 2 per acre; ſeveral at
30 s. and 31 s 6 d.; a conſiderable number between 25 s. and 30s.; a ſtill
greater number from 20s. to 25 s.; and large tracks are rented about 15 s.
per acre, and from that to 10 s. 4thly, Though a larger portion of the
arable diſtrict than all theſe joined together, is certainly let ſo very low as
not to exceed 7 s. 6 d. per acre at an average, yet even this will not bring
the

The rent paid for fisheries is not taken into this statement, because houses and pieces of ground are generally set along with them; and, exclusive of these, they do not yield above L. 74 Sterling. As opinions differ concerning the value

the general average below the sum stated. And besides, 3*bly*, There are, within the line of the pasture district, especially on the waters of Kale, Oxnam, Jed, and Rule, some farms almost wholly arable, the rent of which so far exceeds the average of the pasture lands, as to furnish a considerable surplus to increase that of the arable.

The inequalities, however, both in the surface and value of the ground, through every part of the county, render it extremely difficult to fix a general standard with any tolerable degree of precision. There are, indeed, several sheep farms, which have been never or very little ploughed. But there are very few arable farms, which have not a greater or less proportion of coarse or exposed land, fit only for sheep; and most of the pasture farms have a good deal of land in tillage. This has suggested the idea of making three different averages; one for the pasture land at 3 s., but alloting to that district only 2-5ths instead of 3 5ths of the county; a second at 15 s. for the arable land, comprehending one-half of the other 3-5ths, after deducting the 8000 acres, as proposed in the text; and a third for such farms as consist somewhat equally of both, including the remaining half: taking this last average at 6 s. the real rent of the county will be rather less than I have stated it; taking the average at 7 s. it will be rather more. Thus,

2-5ths of the county, or 172,032 acres at 3 s.   -   L. 25804 16   0
Deducting, from the remainder, 8000 acres occupied in wood,

&c. there will be 125,024 acres at 15 s.   -   93768   0   0
And 125,024 acres at 6 s.   -   37507   4   0
Value of wood, garden, and pleasure-ground, as above,   10210   0   0

L. 167190   0   0

Estimating the last 125,024 acres at 7 s. there falls to be
added 125,024 s. or   -   -   -   6251   4   0

L. 173541   4   0

The above computations seem to evince that there can be no material error in the sum assigned as the real rent of the county in the text.

The wood is estimated at a very low rate. From the statistical table annexed, it appears that there are 4682 acres planted. Throwing away 1682 as lately planted, not thriving, and affording no return, there remains 3000.

value of the houfes and little farms attached to the fifheries, this calculation may not be altogether correct.

Of 48 great proprietors *, 18 refide conflantly; 11 occafionally; 7 live in the immediate neighbourhood; and only 12 are abfentees. Moft of the abfentees, and many of the others, have ftewards (here called factors) to receive and difcharge their rents, agree on the terms of leafes, and manage their eftates in other refpects. There are about 10 other gentlemen, who live always in the county in elegance and hofpitality, and feveral, who make it their fummer's refidence. Such as refide, generally farm fome part of their lands, and keep an overfeer or *grieve*, who is equivalent to a bailif in Engla·J, to look after their fervants, and direct the operations of their hufbandry. Some of them, occafionally, retain large tracks in their own poffeffion, to improve and let them at a higher rent. Much was done in this way, with great fuccefs, many years ago, by a few public fpirited and enterprifing proprietors;

Of thefe, 1000 acres contain each 680 trees, from 12 to 20 years old, each tree being only worth 6 d. or L. 18 *per* acre, - L. 18000 0 0

Another 1000 acres contain each 435 trees at 3 s. each, or
L. 65, 5s. - - 65250 0 0

And 1000 acres contain each 221 trees at 15 s. each, or
L. 165, 15 s. - 165750 0 0

There are 608 acres of natural wood, worth at leaft L. 100 .
per acre, - - - 60800 0 0
_____
Making in all, . - L. 309800 0 0

Of which the full intereft, being L. 15,490, falls, ftrictly calculating, to be added to the rent of the county. But I have allowed no lefs than L. 159,800 to be deducted, for defraying all expences of planting, inclofing, and rearing the wood, and the rent of the land occupied by it; and I have only added, to the rent of the county, L. 7500 as the intereft of the remaining L. 150,000. Even this fum yields an annual rent of L. 1 : 8 : 8 for every acre in wood, and furnifhes a ftrong argument for increafing the number of them.—For a fuller account of the particulars in this note, the reader may . confult Chap. IV. Sect. II. and Chap. X.

¶ Viz. 6 peers and 42 commoners.

prietors; and others are now following their footsteps with laudable ardor and perseverance. The small proprietors generally occupy their own possessions, as do the actual farmers, of whom many, besides those on the roll of freeholders, have acquired handsome fortunes. Yet more than 11-12ths of the whole county is let on leases of longer or shorter duration.

Too little attention is paid to the preservation and increase of villages, though they are of great importance to the improvement and cultivation of land. Few of the occupiers of those mentioned in the note labour for hire, except with their horses at the highways, or carrying coals, &c. Of villages, inhabited wholly by cottagers employed in agriculture, there are scarcely half a dozen in the county; and even some of these are falling into decay, like others, whose ruins only remain. Great praise is due to a few, who encourage useful mechanics and labourers to dwell near them; and a village has many attractions and advantages, which are wanting to the solitary cottage.

Sect. II.—*Tenures.*

ALL property holds either of the Crown, or of some subject. In the former case, when of legal extent, it gives a right to vote for a Knight of the shire; but in the latter case, however large, it has not that privilege, and resembles a copyhold in England, with this difference, that the *superior*, or subject of whom it is held, has not equal privileges with a *Lord of the manor*. There are instances of freeholds paying feudal acknowledgments to subjects, some of them to a great amount. This chiefly happens in lands acquired from the Church, of all which the King is *superior*, though the subjects, who first seized or obtained a right to them, afterwards disposed of them at a lower price, under the stipulation

pulation of receiving certain yearly payments in money, victual, or work. No lands, now, are possessed, as they were 30 or 40 years ago, on grants redeemable on certain conditions, known, in the law of Scotland, by the name of *wadsets*. The *few*, or feudal acknowledgment, is sometimes merely nominal, in which case the tenure is called a *blench* or *blanch* holding; and generally it is a small quit-rent, not always demanded, though on particular lands it is very high. It is commonly commuted into money; but in a few places, it is still exacted and paid in personal services, or in the labour of horses. And according to the usual custom in this part of the kingdom, it is doubled, or considerably increased, on the entry of every successor, whether by inheritance or purchase.

CHAP.

CHAP. III.

BUILDINGS.

Sect. I.—*Houses of Proprietors.*

THE houses of proprietors are so numerous, and so different in size and form, that they cannot easily be reduced to distinct classes. A few of them are ancient and princely; others are modern and elegant; some, by judicious alterations and additions, have been rendered handsome and commodious; very many stand in need of being repaired or rebuilt; severals are too insignificant to deserve notice. In situation, magnitude, and grandeur, the house of Fleurs, near Kelso, belonging to the Duke of Roxburgh, holds a distinguished pre-eminence: And there are many neat villas in that neighbourhood, by which its prospects are embellished, and to which it forms a magnificent object. The offices are generally situated near to the house, but out of its view; and, of late, greater pains have been taken, than formerly, to render them ornamental as well as convenient. All the buildings are of hewn or ruble stones, and covered with slates. The smaller proprietors generally build houses for their own residence, of one or two storeys, with clay or lime, and thatched or slated roofs, according to the extent of their properties, their opulence, or their fancies. Attention is shewn to have them substantially done, and to give them a neat appearance.

Sect.

SECT. II.—*Farm-houses, and Offices, and Repairs.*

FEW things are of greater importance in agriculture, than the commodious and comfortable accommodation of farmers, and, happily, it is here much regarded. On farms, where formerly the houses were paltry, or unsuitable, new ones have been built, in a situation, and on a plan, respecting which the tenants have had the chief direction. Where the former houses were in a better style, they have uniformly received such reparations and additions as were found necessary. In every part of the county, they are now mostly of two storeys and a garret-floor, with the addition of a kitchen behind or at one end. Clay built walls, and thatched roofs, though still to be seen, are fast upon the decline; and, if the present spirit continues, will in a few years become a mark of disgrace. In fixing the dimensions, and laying out the apartments of a new house, much depends on the taste of the farmer for elegance or utility. In general, from thirty-six to forty feet in length, and from seventeen to twenty-one feet in breadth, within the walls *, is thought a moderate size; the ground-floor containing an eating-room in one end, and the family bed-room, with a closet behind in the other. The bed is frequently concealed, or thrown into the closet, that this apartment may occasionally serve the purpose of a drawing-room. The second floor, according to the breadth of the house, is divided into four smaller, or two larger bed-rooms with closets, and sometimes into one larger and two lesser ones. Few farmhouses, lately built, are under these dimensions, and several are greatly above them, having a sizeable dining-room and drawing room, four or five bed-rooms, and a kind of business-

* All the dimensions given in this paragraph are within the walls.

nefs-room for the farmer to keep his books, receive and pay money, &c. (one of the greateft conveniencies that he can enjoy), befides a nurfery and apartments for fervants. In the pafture diftrict, where a thin population makes hofpitality more neceffary, the tenants are naturally defirous of having many bed-rooms, however fmall, to accommodate their numerous friends and vifitors; and it is not uncommon to crowd two or more beds into one room. At the fame time, it muft be confeffed and regretted, that, through the whole county, a few farmers ftill prefer the mean habitations, manners, and agriculture of their fathers.

The offices are generally behind the dwelling-houfe, in the form of a fquare, that the cattle and work may be under the mafter's eye; but, in fome places, they are removed to a little diftance, from feeling the fmell to be offenfive, and from a fear of its being noxious. They are moftly built with lime, though few of them are flated. Their common breadth is about fixteen feet; the height of the walls varies from feven to ten feet; and, when the dwelling-houfe forms one fide of the fquare, they confift of two fometimes of three barns, of thirty and even of thirty-four feet in length, on another fide; ftables for ten, twelve, or more horfes, two cow-houfes, here called *byres*, for milch-cows and young cattle, on a third; fheds more or lefs open for feeding from twenty to fifty bullocks, on a fourth. Other fheds for fheltering carts and all other implements of hufbandry from the weather, a chaife-houfe, if the farmer keeps one, as fome of them do, a hen-houfe, a hog-fty, &c. are interfperfed among the other offices, according to circumftances and the nature of the farm. Thefe laft mentioned form a fide of the fquare, when the dwelling-houfe does not. There is commonly a dunghill in the middle, where are fed the lean cattle intended to be grazed during fummer, and fattened the following winter. Above the ftable there is generally

D

a hay-loft, where, or above the cow-house, the unmarried men-servants sleep; and frequently there is a granary above one of the sheds, or above the end of one of the barns. A dairy, pantry, and larder are added to the dwelling-house, in the form either of a wing or of a pent-house. The number and dimensions of offices vary according to the size and nature of farms. Where few or no turnips are raised, less housing is needed for cattle, and an arable farm of 200 or 300 acres does not require such ample accommodation as one of 800 or 1000. The introduction of thrashing machines will probably occasion some alteration in the structure of barns, and lessen the extent of roof, which, in an inland country without canals, must be a considerable saving. In places where the offices were only repaired, they are not unfrequently disposed in an awkward and inconvenient manner; and too little attention has been paid, in former times, to the choice of an elevated and level situation for a stack-yard. The older barns are generally too low in the walls, and admit only of very short joists, here called *balks*, towards the junction of the cupples; whereas it is obvious, that the nearer the joists are to the walls, the building must be so much the stronger. A few have lately been built above cart-houses, stables, &c.; a practice both thrifty and convenient, in an unequal surface, where the ground on one side is frequently level with the second floor. One or two are so spacious, and have such large doors, as to admit a loaded cart, and thus save those stalks which drop from the sheaf, and those grains which start from the ears as the corn is tossed down to the ground.

A similar plan is proposed to be adopted in the construction of feeding sheds; the cattle are to be tied, fronting each other, to two rows of stakes, with a space between the rows where carts may enter and unload. At present turnips are laid down in the open air, covered by bundles

of

of ſtraw in hard froſt, and given to the cattle through holes, oppoſite to their heads, over which boards are ſuſpended on hinges to open and ſhut at pleaſure. At Frogden, above 30 years ago, ſheds were firſt made double, with an open ſpace between them, for carrying away the dung, and another before the heads of the cattle for cleaning the manger, and throwing in turnips. This laſt is always carefully covered with boards, while the cattle are feeding or at reſt. In many places, both where they ſtand along the ſide of the houſe with their heads towards the backwall, and where they ſtand acroſs it, with their heads or tails towards each other, they are fed from behind. The trouble is greater, but they are kept warmer. Milch cows are every where treated in this manner, as warmth is more eſſential to them than to feeding cattle. The ſtables are now moſtly divided into ſeparate ſtalls, though there are ſtill many in which the horſes feed in common, as ſeveral lean carcaſes teſtify. Some farmers are borrowing a practice, from their neighbours in Northumberland, of having workſhops for different artificers employed in ſhoeing their cattle, and in making or mending articles neceſſary for carrying on their work. Their wood, iron, and other materials, are thus wrought under their immediate inſpection; the time and labour are ſaved of ſending their ſervants and horſes to the neareſt village for every trifling job; a ſmall additional wage, or even good fare, will inſure the ready attendance of able workmen; and every thing is gain to a farmer that promotes diſpatch, cuts off from his ſervants all pretence of loitering, and keeps his horſes from unneceſſary travel.

When a farm-houſe and offices are to be new built, the tenant ſometimes receives a ſtipulated ſum, about a year's rent, for executing them on a given plan; but more commonly the landlord pays the materials and workmen, and

the

the tenant carries the one, and furnishes meat and *ser-vice* * to the other. Both methods lie open to objections. In the one case, the tenant may be tempted to make such superficial work, as to last during his lease, and, with some slight reparations, be left barely passable at the end of it. And, in the other case, a great deal of his time, labour, and money, is taken up, which, especially in the beginning of a lease, would be much better employed in improving and cultivating his fields. A preferable way would be for the landlord to do the whole substantially, according to a concerted plan, and charge some additional rent on the tenant. This has been done, in some instances, without any such charge. At present, for the sake of cheapness, the houses are often finished by contract, with those who offer the lowest estimate, and who, to earn a scanty profit, furnish only coarse materials, use them sparingly, and hurry on the job in a careless and slovenly manner. Both dwelling-house and offices are supported, during the currency of a lease, sometimes at the sole expence of the tenant, though more frequently the landlord allows all or some part of the materials.

Reparations and additions, necessary to houses at the entrance to a farm, are made at the charge of the proprietor, with or without the aid of the tenant, according to agreement. Here, as in the former case, a year's rent, or perhaps less, if the buildings are of a moderate size, and in tolerable order, is sometimes accepted by the tenant. But unless the situation be centrical and convenient for the farm, it is the interest of both to have the whole houses removed and rebuilt.

Sect.

* *Service* is a provincial phrase for labourers, to dig away earth from the foundation of a house, prepare mortar, and assist in rearing scaffolds, carrying stones, joists, &c.

Sect. III.—*Cottages.*

Hitherto they are mostly built with clay, and few, if any of them, are slated. Those erected for shepherds are miserable temporary hovels. Their walls are alternate rows of stones and sods, and their roofs are of coarse and slender timber, covered with turf and rushes. A hole in the middle of the roof, surrounded at the top, and a little way down into the house, by a wicker frame, plastered with a mixture of straw, mud, or clay, is the only chimney. A small aperture, with a single pane of glass, and sometimes altogether open, and stuffed at night with old clothes, serves for a window. The same kind of chimney, placed at the gable, with the wicker or a spar-frame, or a thin stone-wall, supported by a strong beam, about four or five feet from the ground, is still used in many of the best cottages, and even in the kitchens of farmers. In general, however, artificers and married labourers are well accommodated. The former have a workshop and kitchen, and often a better apartment. The latter have a kitchen, and a room where grown-up children sleep, provided by their master, if they are at service; or rented in some village, if they are not. The walls are about seven feet high; the windows are of different sizes, from fourteen inches square to four by three feet; the floor is of earth, nicely knead; sometimes of flags or timber. There is a garret above for fire-wood and lumber; the roof is neatly thatched with straw, fern, or broom; and both without and within, every thing has a snug and comfortable appearance. In short, though cottages may be found of every intermediate degree, between the worst and the best of those described, yet every year lessens the number of those that are pitiful, and adds to the number of those that are decent and respectable.

CHAP.

CHAP. IV.

MODE OF OCCUPATION.

SECT. I.—*Size of Farms, and Character of Farmers.*

THE small possessions, which lie around villages, or are scattered through different parts of the county, whether in the hands of proprietors or of tenants, cannot be called farms. The occupiers of them are chiefly mechanics, cadgers, or jobbers * with horses, at different kinds of country work, who find it necessary, for maintaining their cattle, to have a piece of land, which they can labour at their spare hours. Setting these aside, and taking into account only such as are of sufficient magnitude to support a family, the farms in Roxburghshire are of every size, from 50 to 5000 acres, and from L. 30 to L. 1000 of annual rent. The arable farms, in general, run from 150 to 500 acres, and from L. 100 to L. 400 of rent. Some are less, and others greater; but the most extensive of them does not exceed

---

* A considerable number of men, in this county and the neighbourhood, earn a comfortable subsistence, by keeping one or two horses and a cart, and undertaking to make or repair highways, to carry materials for building, coals, lime for manure, goods to or from market, or to plough fields; and they contract to perform these operations by day, by measurement, by weight, or by the lump, according to the nature of the work or things carried. These men are here meant by jobbers.

ceed 1200 acres, and none is rented higher than 1000 guineas. One tenant frequently poſſeſſes two, and ſometimes
three; and there are inſtances of the ſame perſon having
both an arable and a ſheep farm, to obtain the double profit, ariſing from rearing ſheep to a larger ſize, by wintering
them on aftergraſs and turnips, and fattening both them and
their lambs earlier, and better, for the market. With the
breeders of that valuable animal, the command of turnips
is becoming daily a greater object, and may prove an inducement to engage them more deeply in arable huſbandry,
inſtead of accumulating paſture farms. Several of theſe, in
different corners, to the extent of 6000 and even 8000
acres, are rented by one man. A confidential ſervant, who
is commonly married, reſides, with his family, on theſe
led * farms, and takes charge of the work and ſervants in
the maſter's abſence. From 800 to 3000 acres is the moſt
common ſize of a ſheep farm.

The character of farmers, like the ſize of their farms,
admits of much variety. No profeſſion affords more ſcope
for diſplaying abilities; and no county can boaſt of a more
ingenious and reſpectable body of farmers. Many of them
have received a claſſical, and ſome a liberal education.
While the cultivation of their fields, and the ſtate of their
flocks and herds, are pleaſing proofs of active induſtry and
profeſſional knowledge, the ſtyle of their dreſs, and of
their tables, are indications of eaſy circumſtances; and the
general ſtrain of their converſation and manners diſcovers
that frankneſs and candour of mind, which is unfettered by
prejudices of every kind, and equally open to impart or
receive information †. It cannot be expected, that this deſcription

* This is the common name here, and through moſt of Scotland, for
farms on which the tenant does not perſonally reſide.

† See Stat. Acct. of Kelſo, Vol. X. p. 589.

scription is equally applicable to them all. The very reverse of it may rather be confidered as a juft portrait of
feveral tenants, who poffefs pretty large farms, and have
become rich from mere penurioufnefs, yet are ignorant,
vulgar, and unambitious of being diftinguifhed, in point of
drefs, fare, and habits, from their own fervants. Between
thefe extremes, there are, among the farmers, characters of
every intermediate degree. But the happy alteration which
has taken place, both in the fyftem of agriculture, and in
the way of living, is flowly extending its influence to the
narrow-minded and flothful. From the flight trials of a
fearful hand, they are daily making bolder efforts, to break
up, clear from ftones, and enrich with lime and marl, fields
in a flate of nature; to ftraighten crooked ridges, and to
raife turnips and clover. Greater indulgence is fhewn to
land, after being limed. A more liberal rotation of crops
is gaining ground. Grain is more carefully winnowed from
the chaff. Horfes are kept cleaner, and better fed. Finer
linen, and more decent clothes, are worn. The carpet, the
fpit, and the focial bowl, begin to make their appearances
in houfes where they were entire ftrangers. And a defire
is evidently kindling, of mixing more in good company, of
keeping a more plentiful table, and of learning the practices, and fharing the profits of good hufbandry. Befides
thefe fymptoms of improvement, feveral circumftances
combine to promife the gradual extinction of this old-fafhion-
ed clafs. At the expiration of leafes, proprietors of found
underftanding will naturally prefer to them, on equal, and
perhaps on eafier terms, tenants, whofe enlarged ideas afford a fair profpect of bringing the lands into richer cultivation. Farmers of this defcription will even ftretch a
point to outbid men who bring difcredit on their order;
and enjoy, in the competition, all the advantages, which
knowelge, addrefs, and fpirit, have over ignorance, auk-
wardnefs,

wardnefs and timidity. The rapid progrefs of improvements has fo greatly raifed the rent of land, that, without enterprife and fkilful management, no farmer can profper. And the moft rigid parfimony cannot fave from ruin thofe, who trudge in the beaten track of their fathers.

While neceffity quickens the induftry and invention of fome, others inherit thefe qualities from nature. Several farmers in Roxburghfhire, originally fervants, or bred to fome other profeffion, have rifen to eminence by the dint of fuperior talents and merit, and contend for the palm of good hufbandry with thofe who were trained up to it from their youth. Among the higher claffes of farmers, a fpirit of laudable emulation has gone forth, to keep their fields in proper order, and to raife thofe kinds, and that fucceffion of crops, by which their lands may be cultivated to the beft advantage. From their frequent intercourfe with each other, and with ftrangers, and from the books which they purchafe, or perufe from thofe public libraries, of which many of them are members, they have accefs to become acquainted with the moft approved practices in the line of their bufinefs through the kingdom, and have difcernment to avail themfelves of every hint, whereby their farms may be further improven, and the fcience of agriculture may be brought to higher perfection. They are likewife entitled to much praife for the plainnefs and good faith of their dealings. Bargains are not made with lefs chicane or higgling, or fulfilled with more honour, by the firft houfes in the kingdom. Thofe exceffes of the bottle, both in alehoufes and at home, which formerly characterized them, and led to the neglect of neceffary bufinefs, have now given place to the more rational and temperate ufe of that cheering enjoyment. They are ftill extremely focial when they meet, and hofpitable to ftrangers; but feldom indulge in thefe pleafures to fuch a degree, as to divert their attention from their more important concerns.

E

SECT.

Sect. II.—*Rent.*

ALL farms, till very lately, were let by the lump: This
is still the case in the pasture district; but some of the arable
farms are taken by measurement. A few small spots are
occupied in nurseries, gardens, and orchards, at the rate
of L. 5 *per* acre. Some fields around the principal villages
are rented at L. 4, and several at L. 3 *per* acre. There are
not fewer than 300 acres at these high rates. The quantity, which fetches from L. 2 to L. 3 *per* acre, cannot be estimated with any certainty. It is not less than 5000 acres,
and will not probably exceed 10,000. The highest rent,
given for a farm of any considerable extent, is two guineas
per acre. From 20 s. to 25 s. is very common for farms of
300 or 400 acres. A few farms, much larger, fetch 20
or 21 s. *per* acre. But very great tracts do not yield 7 s.
6 d. and cannot be expected to double that rent, unless improven by the proprietor, at an expence which no tenant
can bear *. Pasture farms are let from 1 s. 1 d. to 5 s. 6 d.
per acre; and considering the different qualities of soils and
climates, it is easy to conceive that the highest rented may
be the most eligible bargain. Their value is chiefly enhan-
ced, by the luxuriance and dryness of the soil, the quantity
of sheltered pasture which they afford in severe winters,
and the proportion of land capable of producing natural or
artificial grasses for hay. Their value is lessened, by the
height and exposure of their situation, their extent of barren

* From some remarks made on Mr Ure's report, as well as from the opinion of several well-informed people in the county, I was inclined to state
the average rent of pasture-lands at 3 s. 6 d. and of arable-land at 16 s. 6 d.
per acre, till I found, upon an extensive inquiry, that the average which I
have given, though rather low, is nearer the truth. But there can be little
doubt, that, in a very few years, when the present leases expire, many of
which were granted a long time ago, the average will rise at least one
fourth above what it is at present.

ren furface, and the penury and coarfenefs of the food which they furnifh.

To draw, in rent, any part of their produce, would occafion perpetual difputes between the landlord and tenants, and would diminifh the value of the remainder. Sheep, wool, and cheefe, would fell at a lower price, after being thus divided. Though the fame objection does not lie againft drawing the rents of corn-farms in kind, yet here too there are infurmountable difficulties. For, not to mention the wrangles which might arife concerning the quality of the grains, and various other particulars, the diftance from markets, and the expence of a long land-carriage, would put the proprietors to no fmall inconvenience in difpofing of their victual. Purchafers would not fend for it to the fpot where it is thrafhed, without a great difcount. And to devolve on tenants the burden of delivering it at the diftance of 24 or perhaps 30 miles, would be a cruel addition to the heavieft of all the local grievances which they fuffer. For thefe fubftantial reafons, all rents are paid in money; and perfonal fervices, though ftill exacted, are on the eve of abolition. Tenants, on arable farms, inftead of having time to drive coals or other articles to their landlords, are fometimes obliged to hire the carriage of fuel and manures for themfelves. And fheep-farmers keep no more horfes than are neceffary, for bringing home their winter's provifion of peats, turf, and coals, and for managing the patches of arable-land which are attached to their farms. A certain number of tame-fowls, and in fome places of frefh-water fifh, is generally a part of the annual-rent, but feldom exacted in kind *. In fhort, both mafter and
tenants

* I am forry to be informed, that perfonal fervices are ftill exacted in kind, both from tenants and vaffals, by one very confiderable proprietor;
and

tenants find it their mutual interests to convert all payments into a specified sum of money; by which they become alternately losers or gainers, according to the rise or fall of markets.

Sect. III.—*Tithes.*

ONE or two clergymen have a right to some tithes, but have been in use, time immemorial, to accept a small sum in lieu of them. . This is a loss to them, but a material advantage both to the proprietors and tenants of the grounds, who are thereby freed from a vexatious obstacle to useful improvements *.

Sect. IV.—*Poor-Rates.*

THERE are 979 paupers maintained constantly, by an assessment of L. 2776 yearly, the interest of L. 2148 sunk in different parishes, and the weekly collections at the church-doors, which may amount to L. 400, making in all L. 3283, 8 s. of yearly expenditure; of which, if L. 300 is allowed for cases of incidental necessity, there will remain a mere trifle over an average of L. 3 Sterling each for the settled pensioners, who receive their allowances weekly, month-ly,

and that he positively refuses to accept a reasonable commutation for them. Nor will he consent to exchange a single inch of land, for the accommodation of his own, or of neighbouring tenants; perhaps from a desire of transmitting the limits of his property in the precise state in which he found them. I forbear to comment on these prejudices; and I am not without fear of being accused of credulity, for believing that they exist at the close of the eighteenth century.

* Since writing the above, I learn that a clergyman has actually drawn, in 1796, the tithes of lamb, wool, green or new pulled lint, and natural hay, in kind, from one part of his parish, and has farmed the tithes of these articles in another part.

ly, or quarterly, according to the practice of different parishes. The assessments are levied, in terms of the law, in equal shares from the proprietors and tenants, and every year are increasing. The above statement, taken chiefly from the Statistical Accounts of the different parishes, collected and published by Sir John Sinclair, so far as they furnish information, and from the kind communications of private friends, where these Statistical Accounts are defective, reaches no further than 1793; since which time, the prices of provisions are doubled, and the poors-rates are raised at least one-third. Their introduction, though attended with several advantages, is nevertheless to be regretted. It was formerly the fashion for people, of all ranks, to attend public worship, and to give liberally to the poor. The weekly collections were committed to the care of the kirk-session, a set of grave and active men, who, without any emolument, industriously sought out and relieved the modest objects of charity. By the prudence and frugality of their management, the wants of the needy were supplied, and a small fund was amassed, in many parishes, to be lent on interest until a time of extraordinary scarcity should arrive. These men still continue to act with the same disinterestedness and attention; but the absence of some proprietors from the county, the desertion of public worship by others, the scanty contributions of those who attend, because of their being subjected to an assessment, and the natural effect of this general conduct to contract the *public* bounty of the truly charitable, together with the practice, in several places, of demanding one-half of the trifle that is collected to augment the parochial funds, leave very little in their power to manage or bestow. From this change two serious evils arise. One of them is, that the poor no longer receive supply, with backwardness and gratitude, a charity from the administrators of public bounty, but claim

it

it boldly as their legal right; and in expectation of it, relax their diligence and œconomy: And the other is, that the numerous class of servants and day-labourers, many of whom are in easy circumstances, cease to contribute their mites, from an idea, that any little thing which they could spare would not serve the poor, but go into the pockets of the landholders and their tenants. Yet, in the present state of society, when religion is in so little request among the higher ranks, and they, who still respect its ordinances, are divided into so many sects, the poor-rates have the advantage of subjecting all men equally, according to their possessions, to the necessary burden of supporting the indigent. If there be an alarming prospect of this burden's becoming annually heavier, let the rich and the great reflect, that the best preventive is, their regularly attending the national church, and encouraging others by their example to enlarge the weekly collections. Such a conduct might have the double effect of lowering the assessments, and of acquiring such a kindly influence over the poor, as would foster their natural shame to apply for charity, except in the most urgent necessity, and quicken their efforts to provide against it. A law might be made obliging sectaries to maintain their own poor, or add their collections to the parish funds: but it would be oppressive, as they pay their share of assessments in the different parishes to which they belong; and it would serve no other purpose, than affording a plausible pretence to the opulent among them to withhold their contributions, and putting a cruel constraint on the poor to adhere or return to the established church. Yet, while matters continue as they are at present, the number of poor, and the funds for their support, must yearly increase.

SECT.

Sect. V.—*Leafes.*

THERE is a difference in the duration and conditions of leafes in the pasture and arable districts. In pasture farms, they are generally from seven to fifteen years; a few are nineteen and twenty-one; and the tenants are subjected to no restrictions, except with respect to the quantity of ground to be sown with grain. Here, the only improvement being a kind of open drains, which are made at a trifling expence, and need to be repaired annually, or completely renewed every fifth or sixth year, the length of a leafe is of less consequence. But in arable farms, where a great deal of money must be laid out for several years successively before a suitable return can be expected, and where a constant supply of manure, and the frequent recurrence of crops rather meliorating than profitable, are requisite to preserve the lands in good condition, leafes are given for nineteen or twenty-one years. The stipulations in them vary, according to the fancies of different landlords, the objects they have in contemplation with respect to the farms, or their opinion of the tenants. In some entailed estates, a little more rent will purchase an exemption from all limitations. In general, however, strict provision is made to prevent the lands from being impoverished by severe cropping towards the end of leafes. The common restrictions, insisted upon with this view, are, that a certain portion of the farm shall be left in grass, in fallow, or in a green meliorating crop, according to the nature of the land; that the straw raised shall be consumed on the farm, except the last crop; that all the dung made shall either be laid on the land, or belong to the succeeding tenant; that, for the last three, five, or seven years, two white crops shall not be taken successively from the same field, except perhaps when first broken up from

old

old grafs, or richly manured; and, that even in thefe excepted cafes, not more than two fhall be raifed. All thefe
conditions may feldom, if ever, be found in a fingle leafe;
but there are few leafes, in which one or more of them are
not required.

The inclofure of lands occafions fpecialties in leafes. Fences have fometimes, though very rarely, been made, during
the currency of a leafe, at the expence of tenants, on their
being reimburfed at the end of it, or receiving then the
real value of the fences, according to the appraifement of
arbiters. In this cafe, they take care to keep the fences in
proper order, that they may draw the larger fum. Fences
have likewife been made by landlords, under the direction
of the tenants, and on condition of their paying a certain
intereft on the money expended, and upholding the fences.
In this cafe, they have been frequently neglected. Both
thefe methods have lately given place to a third, which is
found to be more effectual for preferving the fences, and
lefs burdenfome to the parties concerned. Fences are now
often made, and always upheld, at leaft for the firft feven
years of a leafe, at the mutual expence of the mafter and
tenant; the former laying out the money, and charging
one-half of it on the latter, who willingly pays it, to be
freed from the trouble of attending to them, and employ-
ing his fervants in repairing every breach or gap. When
there is wood upon their farms, tenants come under ftrict
obligations to preferve it: but, when it is fo young as to
ftand in need of being inclofed, the proprietor commonly
takes the charge of repairing the fences.

Tenants are ufually, though not always, debarred from
fubfetting their farms; and are obliged to uphold and leave
the houfes upon them in a habitable condition. The entrance to farms, both in the pafture and arable diftricts, is
generally at Whitfunday; and to fuch parts of them as are
under

under corn, at the feparation of the crop. Rents are commonly paid, in equal halves, twice in the year. The firft half year's rent becomes due at the Martinmas after the tenant's entry, and the fecond at the Whitfunday; but they are rarely exacted till the Candlemas or Lammas following. In many corn-farms, thefe half-yearly payments do not take place till the tenant has reaped a crop. There may be a few inftances of leafes commencing at Martinmas, and of rents being paid only once a-year. Leafes for one or two lives were more common formerly than they are at prefent. Perhaps there are not more than three or four of them in the whole county. The more reprehenfible practice of letting long leafes at a low rent for a fum of money, though much on the decline, has not entirely ceafed. Several farms were fome years ago, and a few are ftill, poffeffed without leafes *. There may be other fingularities in them, all of which it is impoffible to mention.

Sect. VI.—Expence and Profit.

Not being myfelf an actual farmer, and thinking it rather indelicate to trouble thofe friends, for information on this fubject, to whofe liberal communications I am fo much indebted in other refpects, I can only give a general fketch, from conjecture, of the expence and profits of an arable and pafture farm, at the average rent of the county.

1. Of an arable farm of 400 acres, the rent at 15 s. per acre, is   -   -   -   L. 300 0 0

Carried forward,   L. 300 0 0

* In Chapter XVI. I have taken the liberty to offer fome obfervations on the fubject of leafes.

F

Brought forward,	L. 300	0	0

1. To 9 work and 1 saddle-horse, at
   L. 20,   -   L. 200 0 0
2. To 40 black cattle, of all
   ages, at L. 6,   -   240 0 0
3. To 8 single carts, at L. 6, 10s. 52 0 0
4. To 5* ploughs and 5 pair of
   harrows,   -   -   16 10 0
5. To † cart and plough harness, 16 16 0
6. Thrashing-mill and fans,   40 0 0
7. A variety of small articles, 10 0 0

                    L. 575 6 0

2. Interest on that sum, at 10 per cent,   57.10 0
   1. To 20 black cattle, bought at
      Whitsunday, for the pas-
      ture and after-grass, at L. 8
      each,   -   L. 160 0 0
   2. To 20 ditto, bought at Lam-
      mas, for grass and turnips,
      at L. 10 each,   -   200 0 0

                    L. 360 0 0

3. Interest on this sum, at 5 per cent.   18 0 0
4. To 12¾ bolls of seed-wheat, at L. 1, 16s.
   for 25 acres,   -   -   22 10 0
5. To 30 bolls seed-barley, at L. 1, 5s. for
   50 acres,   -   -   -   37 10 0

                    Carried forward,   L. 435 10 0

* Valuing the ploughs only at a guinea, and the harrows at L. 1, 4 s.
per pair.

† This article varies so greatly, according to its quality, that it is very
difficult to hit upon a proper medium. I think it rather under-rated.

Brought forward,   L. 435 10 0

6. To 36 bolls feed-oats, at L. 1, for 50 acres,   36 0 0

7. To 12½ bolls feed-pease, at L. 1, 10 s. for
25 acres,   -   -   18 15 0

8. To clover, 5¼ cwt. at L. 4, 4 s. per cwt.
and 50 bushels rye-grass, at 4 s.   -   33 2 0

9. To turnip-feed for 46 acres, at 6 d. per lb.
and potatoes for 4 acres, at 10 firlots per
acre, and 2 s. per firlot,   -   5 3 0

10. To wages and maintenance of 4 men-servants, at L. 18 each; and of 2 boys, at
L. 14 each,   -   -   100 0 0

11. To wages and maintenance of 3 maid-ser-
vants, at L. 12 each,   -   36 0 0

12. Extra-labour at gathering stones and weeds,
hoeing turnips and potatoes, hay and corn-
harvest, &c. 250 acres, at 6 s. each,   75 0 0

13. Maintenance of 10 horses, at L. 13, 10 s.   135 0 0

14. Taxes, shoeing horses, cleaning ditches, repairing fences, and pocket-expences, at
L. 1, 5 s. per week,   -   65 0 0

15. Interest at 7½ per cent. on money sunk on
household-furniture,   -   15 0 0

Gross yearly expenditure,   L. 954 10 0

PRODUCE.

1. To 25 acres of wheat, at 4 bolls per acre,
or 8 from the feed, being 100 bolls, at
L. 1, 12 s. or L. 6, 8 s. per acre,   160 0 0

2. To 50 acres of barley, at 4 bolls per acre,
or 6½ from the feed, being 200 bolls, at
L. 1, 1 s. or L. 4, 4 s. per acre,   L. 210 0 0

Carried forward,   L. 370 0 0

Brought forward, L. 370 0 0

3. To 50 acres of oats, at 5 bolls *per* acre, or
very near 7 from the feed, being 250
bolls, at 18 s. or L. 4, 10 s. *per* acre,   225 0 0

4. To 25 acres of peas, at 3 bolls *per* acre, or
6 from the feed, being 75 bolls, at L. 1,
10 s. or L. 4, 10 s. *per* acre,   -   112 10 0

5. To 50 acres clover, at 150 ftones *per* acre,
and 4¼ d. *per* ftone, or L. 2 : 16 : 3 *per*
acre,   -   140 12 6

6. To 46 acres of turnips, at L. 2, 10 s. *per* acre,   135 0 0

7. To 4 acres of potatoes, at L. 10 *per* acre,   40 0 0

8. To 150 acres pafture, at L. 1 : 2 : 6,   168 5 0

Grofs annual produce,   L. 1191 7 6

Deduct 10 *per cent.* for loffes by vermin, weather, and bad debts, and alfo for accidents
happening to horfes, cattle while feeding,
&c. &c.   -   -   119 2 0

Real produce,   L. 1072 5 6

Deduct expenditure,   -   -   954 10 0

The farmer's yearly profit,   L. 117 15 6

This profit is certainly much fmaller than what is due to
his induftry and rifk. But it may be increafed by his prudence in guarding againft thofe loffes and accidents, for
which he is allowed no lefs than 10 *per cent.* of the whole
grofs annual produce. It is impoffible, indeed, to protect
hay from being injured by inclement weather, or corn from
being deftroyed both by it and vermin, or cattle from being
choked with turnips, or perifhing by eating wet clover;
yet much may be faved by activity and diligence, which
would be loft by indolence and inattention; and, by dealing
always

always for ready money, or with safe hands for a moderate profit, he may avoid the danger of suffering from bad debtors. Besides, I have only calculated the actual value of his hay, pasture, and turnips, supposing them to be sold or let, without taking into the account either the second growth of clover, or the profit which he makes by using them himself. Whatever gain graziers would make by renting his pasture fields, at L. 1 : 2 : 6, or his turnips, at L. 2, 10 s. per acre, goes into his own pocket, if he feeds cattle upon them. Nor is it immaterial to observe, that, on every arable farm in this county of the extent supposed, a greater or less quantity of sheep is now kept, from which some additional profit is derived. But to have brought all these articles into my computations, would have rendered them too complex. It may be proper, likewise, to mention, that I have reckoned upon a horse, a plough, and a pair of harrows, more than are absolutely necessary for carrying on his work, from an idea, that it is good management to have a spare horse, for bye-jobs, or for preventing the least stop in case any of the labouring ones should chance to be disabled, and also some spare implements, in case any of these commonly used should fail.

A PASTURE FARM of 2600 Acres will maintain 2000 Sheep.

The rent of it will be at 3 s. per acre,	L. 390	0	0
Prime cost of 2000 sheep of all kinds, - L. 1800 0 0			
Interest thereon at 5 per cent. -	90	0	0
Salving, at 4¼ d. each sheep, -	37	10	0
Wages, &c. of 3 shepherds, at L. 20 each,	60	0	0
Drains, and annual expences, -	15	0	0
Gross annual expenditure,	L. 592	10	0

After

After making allowance for casualties, the produce of the sales will be,

Lambs, great and small, 200, at 6 s. each,	L. 60	0	0
Young wethers, 260, at L. 1 each, -	260	0	0
Ewes, 260, at 15 s. each, - -	195	0	0
1890 fleeces, at 2 s. 6 d. each, -	236	5	0
Annual produce,	L. 751	5	0
Deduct amount of expenditure,	592	10	0
The farmer's yearly profit,	L. 158	15	0

An actual sheep-farmer has favoured me with the following statement, which I have taken the liberty of abridging and arranging in a more concise order.

The flock on a breeding farm, where the farmer sells his wethers at 2¼ years old, to be put on turnips, supposing the herds to be paid in money, and the farm to winter 2000 sheep, will at Whitsunday yearly be nearly as under :

1000 ewes, at 20 s. -	L. 1000	0	0
600 ewes and wether-hogs, (a year old), 13 s. 6 d.	405	0	0
280 dinmonts, (wethers, two years old), 16 s.	224	0	0
20 old tups, at 40 s. -	40	0	0
1900 *	L. 1669	0	0
Interest on this sum, at 5 per cent. -	L. 83	10	0
The rent as formerly, " - -	390	0	0
Salving as formerly, " - -	37	10	0
Carried forward,	L. 511	0	0

* In this number, the lambs of the season, then following their mothers, are not included.

		Brought forward,	L. 511	0	0
Herds as formerly,	-	-	60	0	0
Drains as formerly,	-	-	15	0	0
Grass during summer for 33 score, or 660 lambs,	16	10	0

L. 602 10 0

In this way of stocking the farm, all the sheep are clipped, except such as die. There will, therefore, be sold nearly 20 packs of wool, at L. 11 *per* pack, L. 220 0 0
Of small lambs, at 5 s. each, he will sell in the month of July 140, - - 35 0 0
In the month of October, he will sell of ewes 280, at 15 s. - - 210 0 0
And at the same time, of weathers, 280, at 17 s. 238 0 0
In such a farm, the ewes being generally milked, their produce in that way, with a few tups sold, the skins of sheep and lambs which die, and the wool plucked [*] from uddens, will yield about - 50 0 0

	Gross annual produce,	L. 753	0	0
	Deduct the annual expenditure,	602	10	0

The profit nearly as formerly; is L. 150 10 0

To this calculation, much more respect is due than to the other. In explanation of it, I beg leave to observe, that 2000 sheep are made up, to be kept during winter, as under:
At Whitsunday, there were on the farm precisely, of all ages, - - - 1900
Sold of ewes, - - 280
—— of wethers, - 280
560

Remain only, 1340
Supplied by 33 score or 660 lambs, 660
2000

[*] See this practice explained in Chapter XIII. Sect. 2.

It is manifest that thefe profits, both on an arable and a fheep farm, are too fmall, to enable a tenant to live comfortably, to maintain and educate a family, and to exercife hofpitality. From whence it feems to follow, either that he muft obferve rigid parfimony, or that he muft poffefs more farms than one. But by judicious management, he may keep his flock and implements in good prefervation, and thus add, to his yearly income, the whole or greateft part of the intereft charged on their value. Befides, it is not uncommon to have two or more farms, or one of greater extent than thofe from which the above computations are made.

The preceding calculations are founded upon a medium between the former low and the prefent high prices. Some years ago, the farmer's profit was much lefs. At prefent, it is much greater. In proportion as it increafes, the rent of land will rife.

CHAP,

CHAP. V.

IMPLEMENTS.

THE Scotch plough, with a long flout beam, and a long narrow point, though ftill ufed in ftiff clay land, efpecially when it is to be broken up from grafs, and even in light foil, when the furrow is interrupted by ftones, has in general given place to the Rotheram plough, improven by Small. The former is thought by fome to expofe a larger furface to the atmofphere, by which the foil, when harrowed, admits of a finer pulverization; but the latter is allowed to make a neater furrow, as well as to loofen and turn up more earth from the bottom. It is commonly made exactly according to Mr Small's model *, with this difference, that the beam is two, and fometimes even four inches longer. The moulds (or mould-boards as they are termed) of caft metal, recommended by the Dalkeith Society of Farmers, are much ufed; and the head or peak, inftead of being covered with plates of iron, is not unfrequently made wholly of it, or of caft metal. The *fbath*

too

* See his Book on the Subject, printed at Edinburgh. 8vo. 1784.

too or *sheath* ⁕, including the head or peak, is sometimes one entire piece of cast metal. Opinions differ with respect to the structure of the muzzle. All ploughs have a rod of iron, doubled so as to embrace the beam either perpendicularly or horizontally, with four or five holes in that part of it which crosses the point of the beam, in one or other of which the harness is fixed. This *bridle*, as it is here called, moves upon a strong pin piercing the beam, about four or five inches from its point in some ploughs, and in others about fifteen or sixteen inches. In the former case, the bridle is placed horizontally, and has a long tail, by means of which, the depth of the furrow can be regulated. In the latter case, a piece of wood, with four or five holes in it, is fixed to the end of the beam, sometimes in a horizontal direction, to regulate the width, and sometimes in a perpendicular direction, to regulate the depth of the furrow, by means of the bridle, which is always placed the opposite way from the piece of wood. This structure is preferred, as making the draught more steady. And some use a chain, partly to strengthen the beam, and partly to assist the movement of the plough, in very stiff soil, by the shake which it occasions.

The plough is drawn by a strong stretcher, commonly called a *two-horse-tree*, with an iron staple in the middle, and a hook in it to go into one of the holes in the bridle, and with two iron ends, in each of which there is a hole to receive a smaller hook coming from the middle of two lesser stretchers, or *single-horse-trees*, to whose extremities the ropes were formerly tied, and now the chains are fastened,

⁕ I do not know the proper English name for this part of a plough. It is called *sheath* in a great part both of England and Scotland, and by some classic writers on agriculture. The annexed Plate will enable the reader to understand the part of the plough that is meant.

ed; which reach from both fides of the collars of two horfes placed abreaft.

The common harrows are chiefly ufed, but are made in
a neat and fubftantial manner. The thick bars are not
weakened by large round holes, to admit ftout rods, but
are pierced by narrow oblong flits, into which thinner bars
are nicely and firmly mortifed. To prevent one from
juftling above another, they are joined together, fometimes
by a ftrong ftick, each end of which moves upon a pivot,
and fometimes by a ring fliding on two iron-rods fixed on
the approximating bars of each harrow; but the moft common contrivance is, two or three pieces of wood, placed
erect or obliquely on the extremity of the foremoft or left-
hand harrow, and alfo of the middle one when three are
drawn together. The improved harrows by Mr Low at
Woodend, a plate whereof he has given in his " General
" View of the Agriculture of Berwickfhire," have made
their way into the lower part of this county, and have received ftill further improvement from Mr Dawfon at Frogden.
He draws them by the ends inftead of the middle of the
ftretcher: He places the two hinges exactly on the fame line
of draught; and he ftrengthens the principal bars, by the addition of a few diagonal ones. Two chains, fixed both to the
harrows and the ftretcher, meet at two and a half feet from
the harrows, and are faftened to the *two-horfe-tree* already
defcribed. The harrows are in the form of a rhomb, devi-
ating from the fquare as far as is neceffary to make the teeth
or tines cut the ground at equal diftances from each other.
Harrows, when fquare, or of an improper rhomb, may neverthelefs be made to go over a larger furface, and to cut it
at more equal diftances, by lengthening one chain, and
shortening

shortening the other, till the line of draught is brought to the degree of obliquity required [*].

Few or no waggons are now to be found in the county. Nor are two-horse carts so numerous as they were some years ago. There can be little doubt that they would be every where superseded by single horse ones, did not the frequent and steep pulls, in the public roads, along which heavy carriages pass, and in several parts of many farms, require two horses. The dimensions of both vary so very much in length, breadth, and depth, as not to be easily reducible to an average standard. The single-horse carts, in general, are about 16 cubic feet, and hold about 16 Winchester bushels of marl or lime in shells, or 10 cwt. of coals. The two-horse carts are about 25 or 26 cubic-feet, and for every such foot hold a Winchester bushel of marl, or of lime in shells, or 16 cwt. of coals. Both kinds carry more on particular occasions, but are then heaped, or perhaps are of larger dimensions. The body is always strengthened by iron-stays, tightened by screws. The height of the wheels is from 4 feet 2 inches to 4 feet 6 inches. Iron axles are much used; and they are commonly cased in wood, to render their concussion less hurtful to the horses. There are many timber ones; and they would be still more general, were it not for the danger and inconvenience of their failing in long journies with heavy carriages. Some are of timber, with iron ends having long tails, bolts, and screws. There is a common cart at Riddel, with an additional wheel before to ease the horse's back. Frames are often put above the common carts for carrying hay, corn,

or

[*] A plate of a plough, and of Mr Dawson's harrow, is annexed. From the last, the reader may see, that it makes no fewer than 36 ruts at equal distances.

or ftraw, adding about five or five and a half feet to their length, and about three or perhaps three and a half feet to their breadth. But long-bodied carts ftill continue to be made for thefe purpofes, generally, but not always, with a kind of wings projecting quite over the wheels, fupported in the middle by a board fet acrofs the top of the cart, and at each end by ftout rods refting on crofs bars, which, with that view, jut out from the bottom of the body: fuch a cart is commonly about ten feet long, by feven feet in breadth. It carries a larger load than a frame, and can be more fafely conducted through fields that are fidelong and uneven: But it is more bulky and incommodious in the fhed, and cannot be laid up or brought forth fo quickly, and with fo little trouble.

Both Cook and Perkin's patent machines, for fowing different grains in rows, have been tried in this county. They are fo conftructed, as to make the rows at any diftance from 9 to 36 inches. I faw a field of barley, which had been fown with the one, and a field of wheat, which had been fown with the other, in drills nine inches afunder. Both were upon a declining furface, and both looked well. Though apparently thinner than what were fown broadcaft on part of the fame fields, yet the ears were longer, and the grains in them were larger [*]. There are other machines for fowing

---

[*] Mr Church at Mofftower, having feen in England a drill-roller, with iron-rings at the diftance of nine or ten inches from each other to make gentle ruts in the ground, into which the feed, when fown broadcaft, naturally flides, or is fhoved by the harrow, thought the fame purpofe might be as well anfwered by making very flight furrows with a fmall plough, and follows this method fuccefsfully, efpecially where the land is likely to produce weeds. When thefe fpring up, they can be more eafily pulled by the hand, or cut with a hoe, by the corn growing in rows; and when the crop is luxuriant, all appearance of drills is loft long before the approach of harveft.

fowing turnips, on ridges previoufly formed by laying together two furrows with a common plough. Thefe are of
different forms, moftly drawn by horfes, though fome are
drawn, and others pufhed forward by men. All of them
have a fmall coulter to make a flight furrow, or rather rut,
on the fummit of the ridge, into which the feed drops through
a narrow pipe or funnel, immediately behind the coulter.
A very light roller precedes the coulter, to fmooth the fummit of the ridge, and is fo long as to go over the one laft
fown, and cover or gently prefs down the feed. Some of them
have a little barrel, moving on an axis, with holes through
which the feed falls, and others have a kind of cannifter, from
which it is fhaken, into the funnel or upper end of the
pipe. They generally go upon two flender wheels, from
two to three feet afunder, according to the diftance at which
farmers chufe to make their ridges. But, where the top of
the ridge is tolerably fmooth, many prefer one wooden
wheel, about two and a half or three feet in diameter, and
three inches broad in the rim, to go along the very fummit
before the coulter, and another wheel, lefs and lighter, to
follow it. In this machine the barrel is always ufed, and
turned round, by a pinion, or elfe by a band connected
with the foremoft wheel. A very fmall and light plough,
with moulds on each fide to fhift at pleafure, is drawn by
one horfe between the rows of potatoes or turnips after
they advance a certain length, to fupprefs weeds, and to
ftir and lay up frefh earth, from time to time, around the
plants.

A portable inflrument, for hoeing drilled crops, was made,
by the direction of an ingenious young farmer in this county, from a defcription which he read of it in a publication
by an Agricultural Society at Bath. When it is carried to
or from the field, the beam folds back between the handles.

ties. When ufed, one man draws it by the beam, and another directs it by the handles. Inftead of a coulter and fhare, it has only a hoe, which cuts the weeds immediately below the furface; and a larger or fmaller hoe can be put in it, according to the width of the drills. In fields free from ftones and well dreffed, it is very effectual and expeditious.

Brake-harrows, with huge teeth *, fome of them very heavy, are ufed on ground, that is newly broken up, or full of clods, or overrun with inveterate weeds. Rollers, alfo, both of wood and ftone, abound every where, and are of very different fizes and weights. It is difficult to manage a ftrong clay foil without the aid of both thefe inftruments. Mallets, too, are neceffary to make a fine mould for barley, efpecially when clover is fown among it. There is little occafion now for brake-harrows on the light foil, as it is, in general,

---

* It may be proper to mention, that formerly the teeth, both of brake and common harrows, were fquare pieces of iron, tapering and fharp at the point, fixed diagonally, fo that one corner of them might always cut the ground. They were alfo driven carlefily into the wooden frame, and when they loofened, were either driven further, or made firm by wedges. They are now frequently made fomewhat triangular, with two longer and one fhorter fide. The fharp angle, between the two longer fides, is placed foremoft; and they are neatly faftened in the timber by fcrews fixed to their heads. But I have not heard that any harrows, in this county, are made without piercing the timber, although, many years ago, the late Sir David Kinloch fhewed me a pair, with the teeth in eight plates or rods of iron, each of which plates was very little fhorter than the wooden bar, commonly here called a bull or bill, funk into the bottom or lower part of it, and firmly bound to it by iron girds or hoops. When any of the teeth were blunted, or hurt in any manner, the plate or rod, to which it belonged, was carried to the fmithy in a man's hand, inftead of a horfe being employed to bring the harrow or pair of harrows, as is done at prefent. The timbers, too, if properly rounded at top, and carefully painted, by not being pierced, are lefs liable to accidents or decay, and may laft during the currency of an ordinary leafe.

general, brought into excellent order; but, even on that foil, it is found to be of much advantage to roll barley, wheat, and fometimes oats, immediately after they are fown; and wheat, oats, and clover, when in the blade, in fpring. The lot defigned for potatoes and turnips is likewife frequently rolled.

Sir John Buchanan Riddel has the merit of introducing a kind of inftrument or *plough*, which cuts and removes about a foot fquare of earth, and, with fix horfes and five men, will drain a greater extent of furface in a day, than 100 men. Some farmers, who have tried it, allow that it will anfwer extremely well, where the ground is not too fteep, or too deep for horfes in the yoke. He likewife conftructed a fnow-plough, from one belonging to the Honourable Mr Baillie, by joining fome coarfe boards, fomewhat in the form of a wedge, with which, when drawn by fix horfes, during the fevere lying fnow in the beginning of 1795, he opened a road ten feet wide, and brought marl to 180 acres of land, at the rate of thirty carts *per* acre.

The common fcythes are employed in mowing hay, but corns are cut with the fickle. Both are put upon the cart and ftack, with a common two-pronged fork. A fork with three or more ftout and long prongs, and a handle three feet long, fills dung into the cart *, and fpreads it on the field. Lime and marl are fpread with a fhovel. Both the Englifh and Dutch hoes are ufed in cleaning potatoes, turnips, and other drilled crops. Stones are loofened, broken, and removed from the earth by picks, large hammers, and levers both of wood and iron. Even gunpowder is fometimes

* Dung is pulled out of the cart by an inftrument, called a *marl-hough*, whofe handle is about four and a half feet long, with two prongs nearly at right angles to it, but bent a little backwards towards the points.

times made an implement of hufbandry. Docks are taken up with a fpade contrived for the purpofe. Other weeds, efpecially thiftles, are cut with a weed-hook. Hedges are pruned and dreffed by bills and fhears. There are one or two machines for chopping ftraw, and mafhing corn. A fpade is preferred to the knife for cutting hay.

Milk veffels are fometimes fcooped out of a piece of folid wood, and nicely turned and fmoothed; but more commonly are made of oaken ftaves: Earthen cans are alfo ufed. Churns are of various forms; each miftrefs or dairy-maid preferring that kind, which, fhe thinks, requires leaft labour, and is moft eafily cleaned. Cheefe-preffes are conftructed on the principles both of the lever and the fcrew; the laft feems to prevail moft, efpecially in pafture-farms, where cheefe is chiefly made.

In the end of the year 1795, there were only ten thrafhing-machines in the county. They are now multiplying fo faft, that about 20 more were erected during the courfe of the year 1796, and there will probably be 36 or 40 at work before this account can come from the prefs. Thofe firft made, either were driven by water, or required four horfes, and coft about L. 80. Though they did great execution, thrafhing about 25 and even 30 bolls in a day, yet their weight and clumfinefs have induced farmers to try lighter ones, pulled by two horfes, which are found to fwitch from 15 to 20 bolls very completely in 10 hours, and coft only about L. 40. When fans are attached to either, there is an additional charge of L. 5 more. Thofe lately made have all rakes for removing the ftraw. It is alleged, that, by their circular motion and fevere draught, horfes are ftupified, become lefs eager of food, and more unfit for their ufual work. It is alfo alleged, that, in rainy feafons when the corn is a little fpoiled and the ftraw moift,

H they

they perform the work very imperfectly ". But thefe allegations are denied and ridiculed by all who have made the trial, and do not feem to gain much credit. Thrafhing machines are the moft neceffary, and bid fair to be the leaft unpopular innovation in hufbandry. Few men are dextrous at handling a flail; and ftill fewer are willing to ufe it when they can get any other employment. Moft labourers would rather work without doors, even in drizzly weather, and on marfhy lands, than in a barn. Nor do they, without taking unufual time and care, beat the grain fo thoroughly from the ftraw, as a well-made machine does. Their wages and maintenance have been ftated at † L. 18 each yearly. Allowing one of them to earn that fum at the flail, either by day's work, or by the piece, a machine muft be a great faving, as it will thrafh as much in 26 days as he can thrafh in a year, while the number of hands required by each is precifely equal. For the grain thrafhed by a man, fuppofing it to be $1\frac{1}{4}$ of a boll each day, cannot be properly winnowed without the work of five people, for five or fix hours every week, which is fully more than 26 days in the year; and, with the affiftance of the fame number for 26 days, a machine will thrafh and clean 15 bolls each day, or 390 bolls in a year. Now $1\frac{1}{4}$ of a boll, (or $6\frac{1}{4}$ Linlithgow ftandard barley firlots) of all the common grains, is rather a large average for an ordinary thrafher, while 15 bolls are the leaft quantity expected from an ordinary machine, drawn by two horfes. It has alfo the additional advantages of being fet to work on bad days, when little elfe can be done, and at any other time, when the prefence of the farmer prevents all abftraction of grain,

or

" Thefe allegations are mentioned in Mr Ure's Report, and in fome marginal remarks on it.

† See Chapter IV. Sect. 6, on Expence and Profit.

or when it is his interest to have a large quantity of it in the market. It is certainly true, that both for feed and for grinding, the generality of grain, after coming through the machine, stands in need of being riddled, and carefully dressed by the common fan; but it is equally true, that grain, designed for these purposes, for the most part, gets an extraordinary dressing when thrashed by the flail: and, when corn is moist, too luxuriant in the straw, or not perfectly ripened and filled, the quantity thrashed by each is proportionally less: When there is any difference, it is in favour of the machine.

This county can boast, not indeed of inventing *fans,* but of being the first in Scotland where they were made and used. It is pretty generally agreed, that one Rogers, a farmer on the estate of Cavers near Hawick, about the year 1733, or at least before the 1737, either saw a model or a description of one which had been brought from Holland [*], and that from it, having a mechanical turn, he first made and afterwards improved those, which gradually came to be used in all the neighbouring counties, and which have since received further improvement from his descendents, who fell about 60 of them every year at L. 3 or 3 guineas each. They are remarkably simple in their construction, and answer the purpose extremely well; but corn must be put always twice, and often thrice through them, before it is fully cleaned. An improvement upon them has been attempted by one Moodie at Lilliefleaf, which is much extolled by several farmers. He has introduced and happily combined some properties of other fans, by which the moving

[*] One report states, that he accidentally saw one lying as useless in a granary at Leith: Another report states, That he got the model or description from Mr Douglas of Cavers, who had been in Holland. See Mr Culley's View of the Agriculture of Northumberland, p. 49. Mr Ure, p. 52 and Stat. Acct. of Hawick, Vol. VIII. p. 525.

ving powers can be more eafily regulated, increafed, or di-
minifhed, and the grain, at one operation, can be both feparated from the chaff and lighter feeds, and completely
riddled from loofe ftraws, and all other coarfe refufe. The
expence is double, the machinery is more complex, and
one operation is not always fufficient; but the ingenuity
of the ftructure deferves praife, and may furnifh ufeful hints
to fuch as are employed in attaching fans to thrafhing-
machines.

CHAP.

CHAP. VI.

INCLOSING, FENCES, GATES.

A GREAT deal of this county is inclosed. In the pasture district, a fence, either temporary or permanent, is generally thrown around the ground in tillage, and likewife around grafs-fields intended for hay, or for sheep that are weakly, difeafed, or fet apart from the flock for any particular purpofe. A ftone-wall, alfo, about five feet high, frequently feparates thofe parts of contiguous farms which are moft expofed to inroads from each other's cattle. Of the arable diftrict, at leaft two-thirds are divided into inclofures of very different fizes and forms. This was occafioned, partly by the irregular limits of fome eftates, which the owners were unwilling and could not be compelled to alter, and partly by the eagernefs of little proprietors to inclofe the lots which fell to their fhare, upon the divifion of commons and of fields belonging in alternate ridges to many individuals, without attempting, by judicious exchanges with their neighbours, to render their poffeffions more compact and agreeable to the eye. The inclofures, however,

are

are mostly quadrangular and shapely, and contain from 5 to 60 acres, as best suits the nature of the ground, the conveniency of the farms, or the particular views of proprietors. A few near villages may be left, and some lawns around princely feats may be larger, than these dimensions.

In a county, where stones abound, and lime is dear, it is natural to build walls without cement. They were formerly coped with two layers of turf, the lower one inverted; and are so still in many places: But to set the turfs on edge, to condense them together with a spade, and to cut them even both on the top and sides, makes a neater and more durable cop. A few large stones, placed loosely on the top above a kind of projecting cop, with apertures to admit light *, deter both black-cattle and sheep from attempting to break through. When well built with good stones, these walls will last a good while †. Thorn-hedges, however, are rather a more prevalent fence. Two ditches, each from 3 to 5 feet wide, and from 2 to 3 feet deep, are dug about 8 or 10 feet from each other. The earth taken out of them is laid above two rows of thorns planted in the intervening space. Pales and a hedge-row are placed on the top. Experience has shewn that, without double pales, this fence is useless. Cattle climb up either side, trample upon the thorns, nip the young trees, and break down the pales. A single ditch and row of thorns make a quicker and better fence, at one-half of the expence, except

* Here called *Galloway-dikes*, walls of that kind being common in Galloway.

† A wall of dry stones, originally six or seven feet high, with a coping of stones, but now lower, and covered in some places with turfs, surrounds about 450 or 500 acres, formerly called the *great deer park of Hallydean*, has stood at least above two centuries, and is still a tolerable fence. Stat. Acct. of Bowden, Vol. XVI. p. 241,—2.

cept the pales. This fence has several advantages. It occupies only six, seven, or at most eight feet, instead of fourteen or even eighteen feet; it is more easily kept in order;
the pales can be fixed, so as to escape all injury themselves,
and to protect the thorns from the feet and teeth of cattle;
and there are no trees to withdraw nourishment from the
thorns, or obstruct their growth, by overshadowing them,
and by collecting rain and dew into huge drops, which
thereby are either withheld from them, or fall upon them
with destructive weight. The ditch slopes gradually on both
sides, and is very narrow at the bottom. The turfs taken
from the surface are placed inverted, sometimes about five
or six inches back from the lip or edge of the ditch, and
sometimes immediately upon it. In the one case, thorns
are planted on them; in the other, five or six inches backward, and at the distance of three or four inches from each
other, and their roots are carefully covered over with good
earth. The stuff dug from the bottom of the ditch, of whatever kind it be, is thrown upon the top of the mound above
the good earth which covers the thorns. Thorns are now
planted five, six, and even seven inches from each other,
and, in some places, are protected by walls of sod, upright
on one side with earth laid to the other. Making a single
ditch, till very lately, cost only from 5 d. to 8 d. or perhaps 9 d. the rood of 6 yards, according to the ease or difficulty of working the soil. At the same period, stone-
walls, 4¼ feet high, were built for 1 s. 4 d. the rood of
6 yards, when the stones were brought to the spot; when
furnished and carried by the undertakers, the price depends
on their quality, their distance, and the roads. The ditch
now costs from 7 d. to 1 s. and the wall 1 s. 8 d.

Hedges, when first planted, were disliked and neglected
by farmers, a. cumbering the ground, and harbouring birds
to eat the produce, and flies to torment the cattle while
feeding.

feeding. They certainly take up more room than stone-walls, and shelter destructive birds and insects. But, by breaking the force of high-winds, they prevent the corn from being shaken, while by admitting and softening the circulating air, and reflecting in no small degree the rays of the sun, they create an artificial warmth, which, though it may not improve the quality of the grain, and may retard corn and hay, after they are cut, from being so soon ready for the stack, is nevertheless highly favourable to the luxuriant growth both of straw and grass for the sickle, and of a thick sward of rich pasture for cattle. Besides, the disadvantages attending them might be lessened, if they were judiciously managed. By putting a tolerable depth of earth and a little dung or marl below them, by inter-twisting their straggling twigs carefully along the stems close by the ground, like wicker-work, every year while they are very young, by weeding them at least twice every year, and, as they grow up, by training and pruning them into the shape of a narrow-inverted wedge, they would occupy less space, they would become so close as scarcely to admit a sparrow, especially if trimmed just as the corns begin to fill, and they would be less liable to be hurt by cattle. This seems now to be perfectly understood, and will no doubt be attended to by farmers, when their inclosures are in tillage, as they are in possession of the necessary instruments.

Thorns, of late, have been planted on the top or at the back of low walls, about 2½ or 3 feet high. Having a good depth of earth below them, there is little fear of their thriving; and some labour will be saved, as the wall will not crumble down annually like the sides of a ditch. But it is very difficult to keep them clean, as the roots of noxious weeds cannot be disentangled from the stones, and continually send forth fresh shoots. The thorns, too, in a little time

time, by the force of their roots, may puſh away the wall, and cattle will ſoon enlarge the gap, if it is not immediately repaired.

Fences, of alternate layers of ſtone and turf, and of earthen mounds with whins on the top, are now moſtly diſuſed. Temporary ſheep-folds are ſtill incloſed by ſods, placed above one another uprightly, to the height of four or five feet. In particular ſituations, alſo, where thorns will not grow *, and ſtones cannot be found, ſuch fences, ſometimes backed with earth, with ſlender and ſhort ſtakes ſtuck into their ſummits, are thrown around plantations of young trees. They need frequent inſpection and reparations, but are preferable to rails or pales, through which young cattle creep, and which old cattle are apt to break down.

Embankments fall to be mentioned more properly here than in any other part of the plan preſcribed by the Board. They are of two kinds; one, to reſtrain waters from encroaching upon the ſoil, the other to prevent them from overflowing fields, and deſtroying or carrying off the crops. To accompliſh the firſt purpoſe, ſtrong buttreſſes have been erected of huge ſtones, ſometimes laid looſely together, and ſometimes built in wooden frames; bruſh-wood has been cloſely interwoven together, and faſtened by ſtakes driven through it into the ground; and ſmall ſtones have been gathered from the ſurface of land in graſs or tillage, and tumbled careleſsly down by ſides of waters, not unfrequently
                                                                    mixed

* In Stat. Acct. of Kinloch, Vol. XVII. p. 475,—6, there is mention of fences made of larches, where thorns will not grow. They are planted in two rows, at the diſtance of eighteen or twenty inches from each other in the rows, and thoſe in the one row are always placed oppoſite to the open ſpace in the other. I have heard that a fence of this kind is now rearing near Hawick.

I

mixed with different weeds, whose tough and fibrous roots find nutriment from the particles of earth which adhere to the stones, and serve for a cement to the bank which they form. The buttresses generally fail, for obvious reasons: they do not leave sufficient room for the water to pass easily when in a flood: they are too perpendicular: these two circumstances, together with their weight, expose them to be undermined; and they are constructed with smooth stones, which cannot cohere without mortar, and are apt to be removed by the current. The brush-wood and the land-stones answer much better, but do not always succeed, from want of attention to two circumstances; the water is too much hemmed in, and thereby acquires accumulated force; or they are not sufficiently sloped, and present a direct instead of an oblique resistance, by which the stream is led, both to press upon them with greater violence, and to form an eddy and excavation below them. Bulwarks, unskilfully reared against Tweed in the rich plains of Melrose, have repeatedly been thrown down by inundations. While those, made in a more unpromising situation by the late Mr Turnbull of Know, near 40 years ago, with a more judicious attention to divert the force of the river Teviot, continue at this day to save a valuable tract of low land from devastation.

Embankments, to preserve lands from being overflown, are chiefly found in Liddesdale. A mound of earth, on a broad base, with sloping sides, covered with green sods, is raised above the highest flood-mark, at such a distance from the water as to allow it an ample range. The space, between the water and the bank, is always in grass, and, when kept free of brush-wood, affords admirable pasture. The field, within the bank, secured from inundation, may be brought to a state of high cultivation. Concerning such embankments, I have only to observe, that it is of the

greatest

greateſt conſequence to make the baſe hroad, and the ſide
towards the cultivated field very much ſloped; as thereby
the water is not ſo likely to make an impreſſion, and ſhould
it, on an extraordinary occaſion, riſe above the top of the
mound, it would deſcend ſo gradually and gently as not to
hurt the ground.

Gates are of various forms; of one leaf, or of two, of
four and five horizontal bars and a diagonal one, or of two
or three horizontal bars, and a number of upright ones,
ſometimes of equal, and ſometimes of unequal height. The
diagonal bar is generally higheſt towards the poſt or pillar
on which the gate is hung, with a view of leſſening its
weight, and aſſiſting its movement. Both theſe effects are
more effectually produced by a ſimple and obvious improvement, lately made by Mr John Eaſton *, overſeer to Mr
Bell

---

* To him I am indebted for the annexed draught of this gate, and of the
plough. In addition to his improvement, it has occured to me, that the fide-
poſts, on which gates hang, might be made as ſtrong and more durable, by
an alteration in the manner of fixing them. They are generally driven or
built into the ground, with their broad fide towards the gate. This is thought
to give them great advantage in ſuſtaining the weight of gates and the ſudden ſhock of loaded carriages, eſpecially when their tops are made faſt to
the pillars or walls behind by a ſtrong iron-hook or piece of wood. But it
is well known that all timber, ſtuck or built into ground, is apt to rot
where it touches the ſurface, and that even Lord Dundonald's tar, the beſt
preſervative hitherto diſcovered, cannot long ſave it. Poſts are not only liable to fail, but to loofen, and to be drawn aſide or forward, by the weight
of gates. To remedy theſe diſadvantages, I propoſe to make poſts of oaken
planks, four and a half or five feet long, ſeven inches broad, and three inches
thick, to round their two outer corners about an inch, to build them edge-
wiſe into the pillar or wall, except the inch that is rounded, and to reſt them
on long and ſolid ſtones, raiſed above the ſurface of the ground, having oun
end fixed below the building, and the other projecting ſo far beyond the poſt
as to receive the pivot on which the gate turns. A piece of tough wood,
likewiſe, ſhould be dove-tailed into the poſts both at bottom and top, ſo as

to

Bell at Langlee. His gates move upon a pivot brought forward to the inside of the back-post; that post is made very maffy; the bars are made to taper from it; and the fore-post is made light. By thus increasing the weight behind, and leffening it before, the gate is nearly balanced, lefs apt to fway or loofen the post or pillar on which it hangs, and its motion becomes fmooth and eafy. At Riddell, the upper bar of the gates is strengthened by a flight covering of iron against the preffure of cattle. Others prefer wooden fpikes for that purpofe.

to be entirely covered by the building, the piece at the top should flope downward, and both should run back three or four feet into the pillars or walls. The pillars or walls, alfo, should be at least thirty-two inches if not three feet thick, and will be lefs expofed to damage from carriages, if made circular, where they embrace the posts. Mafons object to this plan, becaufe a circular building is never fo strong as a fquare one, and becaufe the posts, in fome degree, divide and weaken the pillars or walls. Instead of posts, therefore, they prefer long blocks of hard wood, or freestones, built into the pillars or walls, into which may be fixed the tails of the hinges, or of the rings to encircle the pivots. But both blocks and freestones are liable to be loofened and diflodged by any violent fhove or tug upon the gate. Whereas posts, placed in the manner I have defcribed, notwithstanding the acknowledged inconvenience of weakening the pillars or walls, poffefs the double advantage, of being farther removed from the danger, and of connecting the whole building together, and making all the parts fupport each other, fo as either to refift every fhock, or to fall in a mafs. A fingle freestone or flag, of fufficient length, and without any fracture, fixed erect in the ground, and connected with the wall, would be still stronger, but cannot always be got, and cannot be raifed, tranfported, and fet up, without much trouble and many hands. Far from infinuating that there may not be many contrivances preferable to the one I have fuggested, I may be allowed to affert that it is at least better than thrusting wooden posts into the earth.

CHAP.

CHAP. VII.

ARABLE LAND.

Sect. I.—*Tillage.*

THE plough, which has been already defcribed, is always drawn by two horfes or two oxen a-breaft, and managed by one man, except where new ground is to be broken up, overrun with roots of brufh-wood, or full of earth-bound-ftones; in which cafes, an additional horfe or ox, or perhaps two, with a boy to drive them, are fometimes, but not generally, employed. Moft of the horfes are fo thoroughly trained, as to obey the voice, and feldom to need either the whip or the rein. Many of the ploughmen are exceedingly expert; and take pleafure in keeping their horfes in good condition and difcipline, and in making complete work *.

In

* When Mr Dawfon at Frogden firft introduced the drill-hufbandry, he had great difficulty to teach a ploughman to manage two horfes without a driver, and to make ftraight furrows. Mr James Macdougall, now tenant

in

In clay lands, there are still some crooked, broad, and elevated ridges, which the tenants allege it would not be their interest to alter, both on account of the prodigious labour, and also because thereby some of the best soil would be buried, while a good deal of cold and barren earth would come upon the surface, which could not be meliorated without long time, and a great expence of manure. But there is no part of Roxburghshire where this plea can be admitted, if the lease be of moderate length. Ridges have been lowered, straightened, and lessened, on clayey lands of very different qualities, to the great benefit of the farmers; especially when in tillage, the luxuriance of the crops on the deep land thrown into the old furrows, fully compensating for the deficiency of it on the new and bare soil on the tops or middle of the former ridges; but the case is otherwise when the land is in grass *, the produce being generally poor; and there is every reason to expect equal advantage, from extending this practice to the few monuments, which remain, of the unskilful husbandry of former times.

In such a diversity of soils, it may be natural to expect that the ridges shall be of very unequal form and breadth. In flat lands retentive of moisture, they are often as narrow as 9 and even 7 feet, raised up a few inches in the middle, and sloping gently towards each side. That size is sometimes found to be most commodious on similar lands, though there is a sufficient descent for the water. They run, in general, from that breadth to 18 feet, according to the degree

of

in the parish of Linton in Tweeddale, was the first who learned to plough in this manner; and from him, the practice spread through this county, and the neighbouring ones of Northumberland, Berwickshire, East Lothian, and Tweeddale.

* There are instances of their produce in grass being better than in corn.

of ftiffnefs in the foil, and the declivity of the furface. Where-
ever there is the leaft mixture of clay, they have always a
little rife and a regular defcent, that no furface-water may
ftagnate upon them. Wheat and clover require a form that
will throw off the water, and bear the frofts of winter. The
fame nicety is not fo neceffary in other crops: In fuch
cafes, the dimenfion and fhape of ridges depend on the
judgment and experience of the farmer.

In light lands where the bottom is dry, it is often an object of attention to have as little appearance of ridges as poffible. They are made indeed for the convenience of being
more accurately fown; but the fmall diftinctions between
them are nearly filled up in the harrowing. The favourite
breadth feems to be 14 feet, and from that to 16 feet, as
being fully reached by two eafy cafts of the hand. As the
fower fteps up one fide and down another, no part of the
ridge runs the rifk of being miffed, and the feed, falling moft
copioufly on the middle where the two cafts meet, will ftill
be fufficiently thick, though fome of it fhall be trailed by
the harrows into the furrows, or devoured by birds. But
there is no general rule, either about the breadth of ridges,
or manner of fowing. They are fometimes fo narrow as to
be fown at one caft, and fometimes fo very broad as to require three cafts, or even more. In laying down fhallow
land into grafs, it is of advantage to have no ridges, that the
whole may be of equal depth. When the pofition of fields
permits, ridges are laid N. and S., that the crops may be
equally ripened, by fharing alike the influence of the fun.

Good ploughing is thought to confift, in turning over the
furrow fo as to occupy a middle pofition between lying flat
on the ground and ftanding perpendicular to it, in clearing
out the bottom, in keeping the top level on light land, and
in lowering every fucceeding furrow a little where the foil
inclines

inclines towards clay. A furrow of 9 inches, and of a proportional depth, is taken before winter on land that is meant to be ploughed again in spring; but 7 or 8 inches is a sufficient breadth for furrows intended to receive the seed, and they are made very shallow. In ploughing declivities, judicious farmers take care that their horses shall not be incumbered, at the same time, both by the steepness and weight of the furrow. It is always made to fall from the plough when the horses ascend the bank.

The manner of treating lands before winter, which are not to be sown till spring, is determined by their nature, their state, and the crop which they are next to bear. Fields, in good order and neatly ridged, are often not ploughed for pease till seed-time, though that grain is also sown on land that has been ploughed in winter. For oats, one ploughing only is generally given, as early as possible, and at any rate some weeks before they are sown. Light lands, intended for barley, potatoes, or turnips, are always ploughed before winter; and the former divisions, sometimes too the shapes of the ridges, are carefully altered: Two other ploughings are given in spring; but of late barley has been sown on the winter's ploughing with great success. The management of clay lands depends altogether on the season; when ploughed before winter, every precaution is taken, of which the nature and disposition of different fields admit, to lay them in a position where they are least liable to be injured by water.

SECT. II.—*Fallowing.*

Fallowing here is only practised in the clayey district, as a preparation for wheat, and is carefully attended to in the proper season for cleaning and pulverising the soil. The

number

number of ploughings is more or lefs as appears neceffary:
One of them (if not two) is always acrofs the ufual ridges, and
there are at leaft three fometimes five, befides. The land is harrowed both with a brake and with common harrows, once and
often twice, between every ploughing; and frequently it is
broken by a heavy roller and mallets. Thofe roots of weeds,
which the fun and weather do not deftroy, are gathered, and
either carried off or burnt. Dung is laid on at the rate
of 24 double carts of 1500 or 1600 cwt. each, or 30 fingle
carts of 1200 cwt. each, or 18 or 20 tons *per* acre, fometimes
more. and inftantly ploughed down. This operation, as well
as that of fowing the wheat, depends on the feafon, but the
whole is always over if poffible in September, though fometimes neceffarily delayed till October.

Upon the entry to leafes of light lands, it is fometimes neceffary to fallow fields, which cannot be put in order for
turnips; but this feldom or never happens after the firft
year.

Sect. III.—*Rotation of Crops.*

Agriculture, efpecially by the more enlightened farmers, is conducted rather upon general principles, than by a
regular rotation. While they keep their lands clean and in
good condition by a judicious intermixture of white and
green crops, they are frequently determined, in the choice of
the particular grains to be fown on different lots, by the feafon, the greater demand for one grain than another, and the
peculiar aptitude of their foil to produce one fpecies of grain
more furely, more abundantly, or of a better quality than
any other. The long continuance of the fnow, in fpring
1795, obliged many farmers to fow barley on fields intended for fpring wheat. The high price of wheat has indu-
K   ced

ced them to devote a greater quantity of ground to it in 1796, than ever was known. In some lands, barley is found to be such an uncertain and unprofitable crop, that oats or wheat are substituted in its stead. In other places, pease grow and ripen so slowly as to become very precarious, and are given up. Oats in many, and wheat in a few farms, are the only white crops from which any certain returns may be expected. One part of a farm, too, when of a soil materially better or worse than the rest of it, is necessarily subjected to a very different management. Fields, that are ticklish or difficult to labour, when once well dressed and thrown into grass, are suffered to remain in pasture for a series of years. Turnips are seldom raised on clay soil, not because they do not thrive well, but because the land is equally hurt by the carts when carrying them off, and by the paddling of sheep when eating them, and thereby cakes so much as not to be easily pulverised for the ensuing crop, whether, of wheat or of barely and grass-seeds. On some lands of this description, a severe rotation, which was once more general, still continues to be followed, viz. 1. Fallow with dung; 2. Wheat; 3. Pease; 4. Barley; 5. Oats. In general, however, it is giving place to the following more judicious rotations, one or other of which is adopted by farmers according to their command of dung. 1. Fallow with dung; 2. Wheat; 3. Pease; 4. Barley with Clover; 5. Clover; and 6. Oats: or 1. Fallow; 2. Wheat; 3. Clover, to lie two or three years, and then oats: or 1. Fallow; 2. Wheat; 3. Pease; 4. Barley, with Clover to lie two or three years, and then oats.

The following rotation has been tried, but is not approved of by good farmers: 1. Fallow with dung; 2. Wheat; 3. Pease; 4. Oats with clover; 5. Clover; 6. Oats or Wheat. Grass-seeds are often sown along with the clover, and the land pastured, especially where dung cannot conveniently be applied every fifth or sixth year. When dung

can

can be obtained, two of these crops are omitted, and the fallow recurs every fourth year. After land has been completely cleaned and enriched with manure, the fallow is sometimes thought unnecessary, and a small alteration is made in the rotation: 1. Wheat; 2. Pease; 3. Barley or Oats; 4. Clover; the dung being laid on with the pease, or ploughed down on the face of the clover. Where there is a small mixture of blackish sand with the clay, a rotation, omitting peas altogether, has been followed with success: viz. 1. Fallow with dung; 2. Wheat; 3. Barley with Clover, and a little rye-grass; 4. Hay; 5. Oats, and then fallow as before *. When the climate is too cold, or the soil would be too much hurt by wheat, it is changed into oats; and grass-seeds are sown along with the clover, that the land may rest a few years in pasture. Clover is rarely allowed to remain two seasons, as the frost generally makes the clay throw out its roots the second winter: There are instances of its being sown among wheat, and succeeded by oats: Nor is this practice thought improper in land, where barley does not thrive, or where want of dung makes a six years rotation necessary, viz. 1. Fallow with dung; 2. Wheat with Clover; 3. Clover; 4. Oats; 5. Pease; 6. Oats. Here, too, after the land is put into fine order, clover might come profitably in place of the fallow as a preparation for the wheat, and the pease might be dunged. It seems, however, to be generally admitted, that barley, if it can be produced, makes the best nurse for clover; and, where it cannot, experience alone must determine, in what soil and in what circumstances, the preference should be given to wheat or to oats. Beans are not cultivated to such

an

* This rotation is not thought consistent with good husbandry by many farmers in the county.

an extent as to become a regular crop in any rotation. Some vetches and tares are raised every year, to be given to the horfes, generally in the fame field with the peafe.

There is one farm in the county, of a rich deep loam, with fome mixture of clay, fome parts of which carry wheat regularly every fecond year, and turnips or clover every intermediate year. All the crops are generally good; and there can be little doubt, that the fame rotation would anfwer other farms, if enough of dung could be procured.

It is in light lands, chiefly, that a regular rotation is difregarded The dung is invariably laid on the field, where turnips or potatoes are to be raifed. They are fucceeded, in different places, by wheat, oats, and barley. Clover is generally, but not always the next crop. Peafe fometimes, and fometimes barley with clover, come after wheat or oats. But two white crops, in clofe fucceffion, are rarely taken by judicious farmers, except on very rich and deep land, or in fome very peculiar circumftances. Clover fields, after producing one crop, are ploughed fometimes for wheat, but more generally for oats, and after two crops, are always fown with oats. There are fome inftances of potatoes having been planted after clover, and yielding an aftonifhing increafe. A practice begins to obtain of mixing different kinds of clover and graffes in the fame field, and furrendering it to fheep, for a fucceffion of years, without being once cut. This is thought more beneficial to the land, and brings nearly as much profit as hay, with lefs trouble. Lands long in grafs are commonly broken up for oats; and produce two crops of them fucceffively, without being materially hurt, efpecially if dreffed for turnips, with a competent dofe of dung, the following feafon. The old

ruinous

ruinous fyftem of raifing oats till the ground was quite exhaufted, and then leaving it to reft, is univerfally abandoned; yet fome portion of its harfh fpirit ftill directs the hufbandry of thofe farmers, who, after enriching their land
with lime or marl, feem to have no other object than to
impoverifh it again as faft as poffible by a fevere courfe of
white crops, without any intermiffion, or help from dung.
With them, to be contented, on land newly limed or marled, with two crops of oats, one of peafe, and one of barley, would be unexampled moderation. Their more common rotation is, 1. and 2. Oats; 3. Peafe; 4. Barley;
5. Oats; 6. Turnips, with a fcanty dreffing of dung; and
7. Barley or oats with clover. Prejudices, however,
though fortified by ignorance and lazinefs, give way, by
degrees, to a fenfe of intereft. Land is found to be more
productive by gentle treatment; and the more luxriant
crops and larger profits of good farming are daily recommending it more and more to general imitation. The following rotations may be confidered as fpecimens of good
hufbandry, and they admit of being varied, according to
circumftances. They have all been tried with fuccefs in
this county. One of them is, 1. Turnips; 2. Barley and
Clover; 3. Clover; 4. Oats; 5. Peafe; 6. Barley, with
pafture-graffes; the field to remain in pafture two or more
years, and to be broken up with one or two crops of oats,
fo as to make a rotation of ten years before the turnips and
dung are repeated, and thereby allow fufficient time, and
the whole force and manure, to improve and enrich every
part even of an extenfive farm. Another is, 1. Turnips;
2. Barley with Clover; 3. Hay; 4. and 5. Pafture; and
6. Oats. This rotation may be varied both with refpect
to length and crops. It may be fhortened one or two years,
by having the land only one feafon in pafture after the hay.

or by taking oats without pasturing it at all; and there can be no doubt of this being the simplest and best rotation, when land can be dunged again the following summer for turnips. In a rich soil, too, wheat may be taken in place of the barley, or of the oats after a single crop of clover. In either case, grasses have succeeded very well among the wheat, especially for pasture: But, if dung can be obtained, it is reckoned the best management to have, 1. Turnips; 2. Barley; 3. Clover; and 4. Oats or Wheat, according to the quality and state of the fields. In short, farmers study to put their ground in good order, and always follow that rotation, which is found by experience to be least exhausting to the soil, and best suited to suppress weeds.

Beans, tares, vetches, cabbages, carrots, Swedish turnips, flax, and rye, though sometimes raised in pretty considerable quantities, do not enter, as far as I know, into any regular rotation or system of cropping in this county.

SECT. IV.—*Crops commonly cultivated, &c.*

THE quantity of arable land in the county, after the deduction of what may be occupied by woods, gardens, &c. has been stated at 164,032 acres. On these, according to one computation, the distribution of crops is as follows:

Grass, natural and sown,			$\frac{9}{20}$ or	73,812
Oats,	–	–	$\frac{1}{4}$ or	41,008
Barley,	–	–	$\frac{1}{10}$ or	16,404
Wheat,	–	–	$\frac{1}{20}$ or	8,202
Pease,	–	–	$\frac{1}{20}$ or	8,202
Turnips,	–	–	$\frac{1}{10}$ or	16,404

164,032

But

But this diftribution cannot be exact, whether it refers to
the prefent or to a former period. At prefent, there are
fewer acres in grafs and peafe, and more in wheat and turnips, than it allots. And, till very lately, the proportion
of land, in oats, was much greater, and in barley, wheat,
and turnips, fmaller, than is here reprefented. About ten
or twelve years ago, the diftribution might be nearly thus:

Grafs, natural and fown,			$\frac{45}{100}$	or	73,812
Oats,	–	–	$\frac{31}{100}$	or	50,030
Barley,	–	–	$\frac{11}{100}$	or	14,763
Wheat,	–	–	$\frac{7}{100}$	or	5,741
Peafe,	–	–	$\frac{10}{100}$	or	8,203
Turnips,	–	–	$\frac{14}{100}$	or	11,483
					164,032

Since that time, the quantity of ground in oats has dimi-
nifhed, while the quantity in wheat and turnips has confiderably increafed. In the year 1796, there is perhaps lefs
land in grafs and peafe, than for many years paft. The following may not be far from the truth.

Grafs, natural and fown,			$\frac{40}{100}$	or	65,610
Oats,	–	–	$\frac{40}{100}$	or	41,008
Barley,	–	–	$\frac{10}{100}$	or	16,404
* Wheat,	–	–	$\frac{12}{100}$	or	9,842
Peafe,	–	–	$\frac{8}{100}$	or	6,562
Turnips,	–	–	$\frac{10}{100}$	or	24,606
					164,032

In

* Several intelligent farmers allege, with no fmall probability, that the
quantity of land in wheat is double to that in peafe. Though I am not fully
convinced that they are right, yet perhaps $\frac{11}{100}$ of wheat, and $\frac{7}{100}$ peas, may
be nearer the truth, than what is ftated above.

In all thefe computations, beans, tares, and vetches are included under the article of peafe; rye under wheat; flax under oats; and potatoes, cabbages, ruta-baga, carrots, &c. under turnips; and they proceed entirely on conjectures, formed from comparing the opinions of farmers in different parts of the county. It was impoffible for an individual to obtain more authentic and precife information, without fuch a minute inquiry into the meafurement of the fields, fown with the different grains, as would have been very troublefome and tedious, and as might not have been thought very civil.

Wheat, in the opinion of the beft farmers about 40 years ago, could only be produced on fome favoured fpots. The culture of it is now extended over the whole arable diftrict, and has even been attempted in cold and expofed fituations, where a profitable return could not be reafonably expected. Two kinds are moftly ufed, known by the names of the red and the white. The former is the hardieft, and yields both the fureft and largeft crop; but the latter brings the higheft price. There are feveral varieties of both. A fpecies of the white, called the White Kent, is moft efteemed; though the Effex bids fair to become a dangerous rival. It is fmall, round, and gives a great deal of flower. In the beft foils, all thefe degenerate, if the produce of the fame feed be fown from year to year: for which reafon, farmers fupply themfelves with feed, either directly from the S. of England every third or fourth year, or every fecond year from the produce of what was brought moft recently from it by their neighbours. It is the general, but not the invariable practice, to fprinkle the feed copioufly with ftale urine, or elfe to fteep it in that liquid, or in a ftrong pickle of falt and water, and afterwards, in both cafes, to duft it with quick-lime, till it becomes fufficiently dry to feparate eafily

when

when fown. The ftale urine and lime have been found, by long experience, to protect the crop in a great meafure from fmut; though it is not always an effectual prefervative, and has this difadvantage, that the grain, if not immediately fown, is in danger of being rendered ufelefs. The changeable weather makes farmers afraid of letting flip a favourable opportunity of fowing their wheat, by waiting till it is thus pickled, and fometimes they are obliged to fow what is pickled, in very improper weather, left it fhould be loft. Hence a confiderable quantity is annually fown, without this falutary precaution, and occafions the fmut in wheat. The falt and water is chiefly ufeful to free the feed from fuch grains as are faulty and light enough to float. It likewife quickens the fpringing of it, and gives vigour to the young fhoots. Wheat is generally fown broadcaft on ridges neatly ploughed with a furrow of feven or eight inches, and carefully harrowed; fometimes the field is previoufly harrowed and rolled, when the wheat is fown and covered by a narrow and very flight furrow. In both cafes, the land, after all thefe operations are over, receives a furrow more or lefs deep to carry off the furface water. By this concluding furrow, it is often divided into diftinct and equal ridges, and fometimes interfected in fuch a manner as beft fuits the declivity. When wheat comes after peafe, potatoes, turnips, or a fingle crop of clover, the land is only once ploughed; but when it fucceeds grafs or clover two years old or upward, the land gets three or even four ploughings. On fallow and after clover, it is always fown in September, if poffible, or early in October; and after all other crops, as foon as the land can be prepared. In fpring, it is generally rolled on light land, as a defence againft being loofened at the root by winds, or parched by drought; and, on heavy land, it is frequently both rolled and harrowed, that the foil may more eafily admit moif-

L   ture,

ture, and, in cafe of being foaked with rain, may not fo readily be bound together by dry weather. Few put lefs than $\frac{1}{12}$, or more than $\frac{1}{7}$ of a boll upon an acre. When fown by a drill-machine in rows, nine inches afunder, even one firlot is more than fufficient. The grain can be hoed and weeded by the hand, till it fprings up into the ear, and afterwards the rows are hardly difcernible. Two Englifh acres were dibbled in November 1795, and required little more than a firlot of feed. In holes about $2\frac{1}{2}$ or 3 inches deep, and diftant from each other four or five inches, two or three grains were dropped, and inflantly covered. In fimilar holes, at the diftance of eight or nine inches, about eight or nine grains were put and covered. In all other refpefts, the field was equally managed, harrowed and hoed; coft in all for labour of dibbling and hoeing, L. 1, 8 s. 2 d. and produced $10\frac{1}{4}$ bolls. That part of it, where the holes were at the greateft diftance, and contained the greateft number of grains, yielded the beft crop; had the other part been equal to it, the produce would have been a third more. The flraw was uncommonly ftrong, the ears long, and the grain large. Dibbling is tried this feafon on a larger fcale.

Big, or rough bear, a coarfe fpecies of barley with fix irreguiar rows in a fhort ear, was, in former times, raifed on the beft land newly dunged and over-run with annual weeds. The produce was fcanty, and the grain of an in-ferior quality. It is ftill fown in hilly diftrifts, where other barley would not come fo early to maturity, and has been fo much improven, by judicious attention, as to weigh in different places 21 ftone per boll, and fometimes ftill more. In all the richer parts of this fine county, it has given place to the long-eared barley of two rows, and fifteen or fixteen

grains

grains in each [*], which is found to be a more certain and productive crop. This kind probably came originally from France, Flanders, or England. From the latter place, supplies have been annually procured for a very long time; and it degenerates here in weight, colour and shape. When brought from Lincolnshire, it is fair, plump, and weighs about 27 stone *per* boll. After being once sown here, it has been found to weigh from 25 to 26 stone, but in three or four seasons it gradually falls to 23 or 23½ stone, which may be considered as the common weight of good barley in the county. Though the colour depends, a good deal, on the season, the soil, and preceding crop, yet, in the most favourable circumstances, the produce is seldom, if ever, so bright and pure and sleek, as its English progenitor. Polish barley, (called also Thanet) having in the ear six rows, each containing about ten or eleven small and round grains, has also been tried, and thrives well; but its comparative properties cannot yet be ascertained. Battledore, or spratt barley, likewise, has made its way into the western parts of this county from Selkirkshire [†], whither it was brought some years ago from the county of York. On light lands, barley is sown after turnips, potatoes, or peas; on heavy lands, generally after peas; very rarely after a white crop on any soil, and as rarely after clover or pasture. The seed is not pickled like wheat: And the ground is so thoroughly cleaned, pulverised, and dressed by the plough, harrows, roller, and mallet when necessary, that no other culture or attention is given to the crop while growing, except to preserve it from cattle and birds, and to pull any dock or thistle, which may have been left in the field, or mixed with the seeds of clover and grass, sown alongst with the barley. Seed-time commences early in April, when the land

is

[*] Thirty grains have sometimes been found in a row.

[†] See Agricultural Account of that County, Chap. VII. Sect. 4.

is in fine condition, but is delayed till May when there are clods to be broken, or weeds to be deſtroyed.

Oats, though they ſcarcely cover one-half of the ſpace that they once did, are ſtill the ſtaple grain of the county. The following ſeven diſtinct kinds are chiefly cultivated.

1. *Church's oats*, which, Mr Culley calls " a ſpecies of " the Poliſh *," and Mr Ure † aſſerts " differ conſiderably " from them," are deſcribed by both, as ſhort, plump, large, early, requiring a rich ſoil, and giving a great increaſe, both from the ſeed and in meal. They weigh about three ſtone, and yield in meal about two ſtone *per* boll, more than the common average of any other oats. They were propagated from a ſmall handful, which Mr James Church at Moſstower near Eckford, got in 1776. From his being the firſt who raiſed them, they go by his name ; and from their not degenerating after being ſown on different fields for ſome years ſucceſſively, they have gradually riſen into great eſtimation, though they are apt to ſuffer from high winds.

2. *Dutch oats* made their appearance about the ſame period. They are nearly as early, and ſtill more eaſily hurt by winds than Church's, not ſo large or thin in the huſk ; and conſequently, though the ſame quantity may grow on an acre, they will fall ſhort in meal about three or four ſtone *per* boll. They are ſtill uſed with ſucceſs on low and ſheltered land, which is not of ſufficient ſtrength to bear the other.

3. *Red*

* Northumberland Agricultural Survey, p. 33.

† Roxburghſhire Agricultural Survey, p. 30.

3. *Red oats* were introduced a few years ago from Pee-bles-shire. Mr Dawson at Frogden procured a boll of them, and finding them early and productive for two succesive seasons, recommended and sold them to his neighbours. They are small, have a thin hulk, and have a very faint of red, prosper on high and cold land, are soon ready, stand the force of winds better than any other oats, and give a very good return in meal. They have not much straw; and, in some places, it is not good; in other places it is greatly liked. In hilly districts, these oats will proba-bly be much used. But even there the preference is al-ready disputed by the

4. *Black oats*, which Mr Potts of Penchrise got from the west of England, and has cultivated, for several seasons, in that high exposure, nearly 1200 feet above the sea, with so great success, as to obtain 8½ stone of meal from the boll. They have since been tried in many other places in a simi-lar climate, and have answered equally well. Their hulk is black, their grain is rather long, but firm and hard, they grow with vigour and luxuriancy, ripen soon, bid defiance to all weather, and their straw makes excellent fodder, though on some soils it is rather hard and sapless.

5. *The common white oats*, however, though later than any of these, and more liable to sustain loss from winds than the two last mentioned, bid fair to maintain their su-periority through the county at large, as being admirably suited to every variety of soil and climate. Church's oats, which they resemble in shape and colour, and to which alone they yield in size, and weight of produce, can only be raised on the best soils. The other oats are far inferior to them in these respects, and they excel all the oats hither-to known in quantity and value of straw. They are said to be natives of the county; and they are produced of an excellent quality in many parts of it, especially at *Blainslie*

its

its northern point. The foil there is fhallow, has a fmall mixture of moor, is inclinable to clay, on a cold bottom, with an expofure towards the N. E. But the lands have a gentle declivity, the fubftratum is not altogether impervious by water, and no wild oats mix with the crop. The harveft is three weeks later there than in the greateft part of the arable diftrict. And as white oats, in thefe unpromifing circumftances, arrive at fuch perfection as to be fent annually to diftant parts both of Scotland and England, this is decifive of their coming to maturity in any place, whofe foil and climate are not more unfavourable than thofe of Blainflie.

6. But neither this kind, nor any of the early oats, anfwer well on the ftrong clay foil in the arable diftrict. A fpecies of *Gray Oats*, alfo a native of the county, generally fucceeds much better, and yields a better increafe. The ftraw of thefe gray oats is not fo ftrong, and is fomewhat inclinable to the colour of filver; their chaff is white; they have every quality of good oats, but are very late of coming to maturity.

7. *Angus oats*, both white and gray, are fown here, the latter efpecially are very common, and on light land, when tolerably deep and rich, feldom fail to yield a prodigious increafe. Their fhape is not unlike that of the white oats, but their hulk is thicker and not fo fair; their ftraw has more branches, but is fcarcely fo rank, more brittle, and not fo much relifhed by cattle; they ripen more flowly by eight or ten days; and the fame quantity will not give as much meal. Yet they are fuch a certain crop, and fo extremely prolific, that in a favourable foil and climate, the farmer's profit *per* acre is greater on them, than on any other kind of oats; on which account, they are now frequently fubftituted for the *gray* laft mentioned.

For

For all thefe different kinds of oats, the land is only once ploughed, unlefs where it has never before been in tillage, or on fome very particular occafions. The time of fowing them depends wholly on the feafon. It fometimes begins in February, but more frequently in March, and generally ends, when it can be effected, on the firft week of April, though both Dutch and Red oats may be fafely fown later in any part of the county. The quantity allowed to an acre varies from $\frac{1}{12}$ to $\frac{1}{10}$ of a boll : Perhaps $\frac{1}{12}$ may not be far from the average. More is required of Church's and the Dutch oats than of any other, as they do not fend forth many ftalks. Much always depends on the nature and ftate of the lands. Thin foils are commonly rolled, that they may be in lefs danger from drought. Other foils, alfo, are fometimes fubjected to that operation. Thiftles and other weeds, which might incommode the reapers, or over-run the ground, are cut or pulled, when they appear among oats or any other grain.

Peas are fown of two kinds : One of them is called *hot feed*, or early peas, the other is called *cold feed* or late peas. The former are fmaller, fpeckled, may be fown as late as May, feldom grow long in the ftraw, and, except in that cafe, are always early ready. The latter are larger, have few or no fpecks, require to be fown in March, or even fooner, yield abundance of ftraw, but fill and ripen fo flowly, that they are often not reaped fo early as the other. The early kind is chiefly fown n foil that s fhallow and fharp, and it is only once ploughed, unlefs it is dunged, limed or marled. The late kind is fown on heavy land, after two ploughings, or on deep and dry land after one. Of the former, about $\frac{1}{11}$ or $\frac{1}{12}$ of a boll, is fown upon an acre. Of the latter fomewhat more.

All

All thefe grains, as well as the fmall quantity of rye and
beans which are raifed, are cut *, with a common hook or
fickle, by reapers hired, in a few places, by the day, but
more generally during the whole harveft.   Men formerly
got 10 d. and women 8 d. *per* day, or the one got 20 s. and
the other 16 s. *per* feafon ; but the hire rofe to 1 s. a-day,
or 24 s. the feafon for men, and 10 d. a-day or 20 s. for
women ; and is at prefent much higher.   Whatever their
wages are, they are all fed by their employer, and get
commonly a mefs of oatmeal *porridge* or hafty pudding
and milk to breakfaft, 20 ounces of coarfe wheaten bread,
and a bottle of fmall beer to dinner, and either the fame
mefs they had at breakfaft, or bread made of peafe and
barley, with a little milk, to fupper.   They cut, at an average, from 144 to 168 fheaves each in a day, making bands,
and laying the corn neatly into them, or from 12 to 14
ftooks or fhocks, each confifting of 12 fheaves : wheat has
fometimes 14 fheaves. Stooks are made, by placing fheaves
on their ends, with the grain aloft, in rows of five each,
two and two always fupporting each other, with an opening between the rows, and between each fheaf, and two
fheaves, floping downwards with the grain undermoft, covering their tops.   One man binds the fheaves, cut by fix
reapers, and fets up the ftooks.   After ftanding from ten
days to three weeks, according to the weather, the nature
of the grain, and the expofure of the field, the corn is fork-
ed into a cart, carried into the yard, and built into round
fxacks

---

* There are fome inftances of different white crops being cut with the
fickle, by the farm-fervants, and alfo by piece-work, at the rate of 2 s. 6 d.
per acre, and from 2 s. 6 d. to 3 s. more for gathering, binding, and ftooking
the corn. There are alfo fome inftances of fields being cut with hooks, by
meafurement, at 5 s. 6 d. and 6 s. 6 d. *per* acre, according to their ftate.
But both thefe practices are rare, though the fcythe is creeping flowly into
more general ufe.

ftacks, from 24 to 40 feet in circumference, with bodies quite ftraight or gently fwelling towards the middle, fo as to throw off the drop in cafe of rain, and tops tapering in to a point. The ftacks are carefully thatched with ftraw, tightly faftened with ropes. When thrafhed by the flail, the labourer is fometimes paid in grain, receiving the 25th part of what he has thrafhed, or the market price of it in money; fometimes, he gets 4 d. or 5 d. per boll, and his meat, 8 d. or 10 d. without meat, the rate depending fomething on the kind and quality of the grain; and fometimes he works for the ordinary day's wages of the neighbourhood. But there is at prefent every appearance of thrafhing machines fuperfeding the flails.

The produce of the different grains, per acre, will be nearly as follows, on the very beft lands, on the pooreft lands, and at a medium:

		Beft lands.		Worft lands.		Average.
Wheat,	-	6 bolls,	-	2 bolls,	-	4 bolls.
Barley,	-	6	-	3	-	4½
Oats,	-	6	-	2½	-	4¼
Peas,	-	4	-	1½	-	2¼

It is impoffible to afcertain, on any grounds except mere conjecture, the annual exports of grain from this county; but it may be fafely affirmed, that about one-half of the whole produce is carried out of it, chiefly in corn, though much alfo in meal. There are about eighty mills for all forts of grain, either in the county or on the very confines of it, and moft of them have fufficient employment. Several farmers, efpecially in the northern parts of the county, grind a good deal of oats, and fend the meal to Dalkeith, where it generally finds a ready fale; and from the neighbourhood of which they bring home coals or lime: And many millers and fome fmall tenants make

M

a decent livelihood, by buying grain of different kinds, manufacturing it into flour, meal, or pot-barley, and carrying these to different quarters where there is a demand. Langholm and Peebles, till very lately, received large supplies of grain from this county. Berwick is at present the principal market. Dealers from that town and neighbourhood attend some of the fairs, and the weekly markets at Kelso, to purchase grain. A good deal of wheat, and of wheat flour manufactured at Hawick, is still carried to Langholm, and the neighbourhood of Carlisle and Dumfries; from which return-carriages are brought of slates, coals, and lime.

Turnips. There is reason to believe that attempts were made, not without success, near 30 years ago, by farmers in different parts of the county [*], to raise some small fields of turnips, both in broadcast and in drills. But the practice was not followed by others, nor persevered in long by themselves. Mr William Dawson, who had made himself complete master of the best modes of English husbandry, by a residence of several years in those counties where it is carried to greatest perfection, after his return to Scotland, tried, among other improvements, to introduce the culture of turnips in drills, upon a large scale, about the year 1755; but the farm, which he then possessed, not proving friendly to their production, he wisely suspended the further prosecution of his attempt, till he entered upon his present

[*] Particularly by Dr John Rutherford at Melrose, Mr Turner at Linthaughlee, near Jedburgh; and Mr George Cranstoun, then at Crailing. Among these, the palm of priority is disputable. The last, who died very lately, related, that he and Mr John Hood, then at Nisbet in Berwickshire, but now in this county, had fields of turnips, about the period mentioned, but were obliged to drop that crop, as neither themselves nor their servants understood the management of it properly, and as the turnips were mostly stolen by idle and curious people, before they attained their full growth.

present farm of Frogden near Kelso about 1759. Finding here a propitious soil, he refumed his original purpose with fuch fpirit, as to have annually from 80 to 100 acres of turnips. The celerity with which his cattle became fat for the market, the excellent condition of thofe which he reared and kept, the large quantity of dung which was produced, and the luxuriance of the crops which fucceeded the turnips, foon made profelytes of his immediate neigh- bours, and recommended his new method gradually to ge- neral imitation. But fo flow has been its progrefs, that, during twenty years, it fcarcely fpread as many miles, and, at this moment, after the experience of thirty-fix years, it only begins to be practifed in fome diftant parts of the coun- ty.

Mr Dawfon at firft made his drills at the diftance of three feet from each other, which, in land wretchedly managed, and full of weeds, was not improper. But, after cleaning his fields, he found fo great a width unneceffary, and both he and the other cultivators of turnips have now reduced it to thirty or twenty-feven inches; fome perhaps make it ftill lefs. The general rule for preparing the land is, to clean level and pulverife it, to form the ridges ftraight, to allow the water a fufficient defcent, and to preferve as much na- tural fap as poffible. Hence the number of ploughings muft vary according to the ftate of the ground. In fome cafes, not fewer than eight have been found neceffary to reduce it to form, and to deftroy the weeds; but, where it is in tolerable order, four are fufficient, viz. one before winter, one acrofs about the middle of April, a third in May in the fame direction with the firft, and a fourth to form the drills, or more properly ridges, in June, or as foon thereafter as circumftances permit. The land is generally harrowed before it is ploughed acrofs, and always after both that and the fubfequent ploughing; and the roots of

such

such weeds, as do not perish by these repeated operations, are carefully gathered, and carried off or burnt. After the ridges are formed, dung is laid down in small heaps in every third furrow, instantly spread along the bottom of it, and the one on each side, and quickly covered by a common plough; the tops of these new-made ridges are a little flattened by a light roller; and the seed is deposited directly above the dung, by one of the machines, and in the manner, already described *. It is of great importance to have all this done speedily, to prevent the moisture both of the dung and of the earth from evaporating. The best time for sowing them is from the 8th to the end of June, though very good crops have been obtained, when they were sown much later. There is sometimes occasion to sow them a second time, if the tender plants, on their first appearance, are destroyed by frost, snails, caterpillars, or a small fly; but these evils have never hitherto been generally or severely felt. A little quick lime, carefully strowed on the tops of the drills when newly sown, is a great preservative against the fly and snails. When the land has been much impoverished, 24 cart-loads of dung and even more are given to it, each load being at an average about 1500 or 1600 cwt.; but, after land has once been put in good order, 16 or 18 of these cart-loads are thought sufficient. The quantity of seed sown on an acre may be from 1 to 2 lib. By springing up thickly, plants shelter each other both against frost and insects, till they get their fourth leaf. They are then very attentively thinned, and hoed by the hand, and those which are most vigorous are left at the distance of nine or ten inches, or even one foot asunder. Two remarkably thriving plants sometimes stand nearer to each other, with a space of fourteen or fifteen inches on either

ther

* See Chapter V. on Implements.

ther fide. Some horfe-hoe their turnips firft, to render the hand-hoeing eafier and more expeditious:—but the other plan is preferable, becaufe the weeds and fuperfluous turnips, being drawn by the hoe into the hollows, are afterwards covered by the plough, and converted into manure. This plough is very light, only from five to fix inches wide behind, and has a mould on each fide, which can be extended or contracted as occafion requires. One mould only is ufed, when the earth is taken away from the plants, and turned into the hollows above the weeds, four, five, and even eight days after the hand-hoeing, as the weather happens to be more or lefs favourable, and as the turnips take firm root, and grow erect; but both are needed to replace the earth about ten or twelve days after it was taken away; and, in the intervening time between the two ploughings, the turnips are hand-hoed a fecond time, and made ftill thinner in thofe places where formerly they were left too clofe together. A third hand-hoeing is fometimes neceffary, where the land has been much out of order; and, even in the beft managed fields, the earth is laid up twice to the roots of plants, from a belief that, by ftirring it thus frequently, they are refrefhed and nourifhed. Sometimes, too, the earth is taken away a fecond time when the land is not fufficiently cleaned. To hoe an acre properly the firft time, requires from three to fix women for a day; the fecond time only half the number. A plough, in taking away the earth, will go over more than two acres in a day, and, in laying it back, will manage four. It is, in a few places, followed by one or two attentive hands, to difencumber the weaker or later plants from the earth that fometimes bears them down, efpecially where the intervals between the ridges are narrow.

Three kinds of turnip-feeds are commonly mixed, and fown on the fame field. The white or globular, efpecially the

the early Norfolk, spring up and grow most rapidly, arrive soonest at maturity, and have the sweetest relish, but do not stand severe frost so well as the others. The green, though broad on the top, and not very hard, resist every viciffitude of weather. And the red, from their oblong shape and firmness, must be hardy and heavier than the other two in proportion to their bulk. Judicious farmers begin to perceive the propriety of sowing them separately; that the white may occupy the field which is to be first cleared for wheat, and the others may afford a regular succeffion of green food to the cattle, till removed to make way for barley. If the present spirit continues for feeding sheep and raising spring wheat, the early Norfolk, here called the *globe* turnip, will come more into use, as there is no doubt of its being the heavlest crop in the early part of the feafon. One or two have meafured forty inches in circumference, and weighed above 30 lib., but in general few exceed a stone, and their common fize is from four to ten lib. The green and red kinds are not fo large, though feveral of them reach 18 or 20 lib., and they run not unfrequently from 4 to 6 or 7 lib. through a whole field. Suppofing them to weigh only 4 lib. each, and to stand a foot afunder, the produce of an acre, at this rate, would be upwards of 34 tons, and would feed two bullocks for fixteen weeks, at 3 cwt. each every day. But 24 tons is a large enough average for an acre of tolerable turnips, and 2¼ cwt. is a fufficient allowance for a middle-fized bullock. Hence an acre of pretty good turnips will ferve two of them for 12 or 13 weeks, and two fuch acres will fatten three of them to 45 stone in four months, increafing their allowance to 3 cwt. each *per* day: And the turnips, at ¼ d. *per* stone, will fetch about L. 8 *per* acre.

Turnips are given both to cattle and sheep, to rear them to a larger fize, to keep them in good condition, and to

fatten

fatten them for the market. For cattle, they are always drawn and carted home. Their leaves, here called *shaws*, and a few of the smaller ones are given to calves, and yearlings in the straw-yard, or an open shed; their bulbs to milch-cows, and feeding cattle in the stall. For young sheep, and those intended to be kept, they are likewise drawn generally, but not always, and carried to the pasture-field. But sheep, fed for the butcher, are inclosed in hurdles or nets, on a portion of the field on which the turnips grow, and after clearing it, are removed to another. This method both saves labour, and enriches the land by the dung and urine of the sheep. As soon as they have eat the whole length of the field, either along or across the rows, that part is instantly ploughed. Many fields are sold by farmers, to be consumed in these ways, both by cattle and sheep. To be ensured of a moderate profit, without any risk, and, at the same time, to retain the full benefit of the dung, they willingly undertake the trouble of attending and feeding the cattle, and of removing the nets or hurdles of the sheep. They are sometimes paid by the measurement of their fields, and sometimes by the number of weeks that the cattle or sheep are fed; receiving, from L. 3 to L. 4 for an acre of tolerable turnips, from 2 s. 8 d. to 4 s. *per* week, for feeding cattle, according to their size, and from 4 s. 6 d. to 6 s. *per* week for a score of sheep. A practice obtains, in some places, of alternately carrying off a few drills to be used in the stalls, and of leaving a few to be eat in the field; which may be useful, when done early, to allow late crops more air and time to increase in size, and to furnish some additional dung equally to a whole field which had got rather a short allowance at seed-time; for the space that is cleared, is as much benefited by the sheep, as that where their food stands. It is thought that,

in

in many cafes, a field, if wholly eat by fheep, would yield too luxuriant a crop the enfuing feafon, and, if wholly drawn and carted to the ftall, might not be fufficiently productive. Both thefe extremes are avoided, by carrying off and leaving drills alternately.

The great profit arifing from fattening fheep on turnips for fale, the advantage derived, by the reft of the flock, from eating that valuable root for fome weeks in fpring while grafs is fcarce, and the fuperior crops produced on fields where turnips are thus confumed, muft engage farmers both to extend ftill further the culture of turnips, and to allot a greater proportion of them to animals, which, without any controverfy, are the ftaple commodity of the county. A confiderable variation will, thereby, be occafioned in the prefent agricultural fyftem. From the dung of cattle fed on one crop of turnips, the next is chiefly raifed. In proportion as fheep are fed on the field, this fource is leffened; and, to fupply fuch a material want, turnips muft be raifed by the force of lime, marle, compoft dunghills, and the lefs quantity of dung produced by fewer cattle on a more fcanty portion of green food during winter. The crop will probably be lefs valuable, and may not be fafely repeated; except after a longer interval than is ufual at prefent; but the ground, by the fheep, will be put into excellent order for yielding all the other crops in the courfe of an ordinary rotation; and, from the greater abundance of fodder thus obtained, the quantity of dung will receive a confiderable addition.

Potatoes, about forty years ago, were not raifed in the fields *, except on narrow beds, in deep marfhy fpots. The
beds

* A gentleman, now dead, remembered, that fome years before the 1745, he was admitted as a great favour into a garden to fee potatoes growing.

beds were covered with inverted turfs dug from the trenches around them. The sets were laid upon the turfs, and covered with such earth as the bottoms of the trenches afforded. The species of them then chiefly used was of a deep red colour, and seems now to have wholly vanished. The *kidney* potatoe began to be introduced soon after the red, and was cultivated in the same manner, significantly called *lazy-beds*. I cannot pretend to ascertain, by whom, and at what time, they were first planted in regular drills, as at present, but I remember that in 1768 it was thought a novelty, in some parts of the county, to drop them after the plough, and that, to make the most of the ground, they were put into every furrow. I have reason to believe that the common white kind, now mostly raised, was first brought from Airshire by Dr Macknight * in the 1770. It is a species of the kidney, and now comes annually, in considerable quantities, from Langholm as a salutary and profitable change of seed. Various other potatoes, both of the early and late kind, have since been tried, of all which, next to the common white, the one in greatest esteem is the *red-neb*, which I suspect to be the same known in England by the *pink-eye*. It is large, prolific, and well-flavoured, but becomes rather strong-tasted and unpleasant in spring. About the year 1774 or 1775, potatoes were very generally planted only in every third furrow made by the plough, and at the distance of nine or ten inches from each other in the row. As they grew up, the plough could go between the rows, and gradually raise them into ridges. Many still retain this practice, as the best defence against crows, and as producing the surest and heaviest crop. But, in general, the land is prepared, the ridges are formed, and dung is spread for

N   them,

* When he was translated from Maybole to Jedburgh. He is now minister of Edinburgh.

them, in the same manner as for turnips. It is no objection
to dung that it is coarse; the sets are placed directly upon
it, and covered pretty deeply with earth, by a round of the
plough, to protect them from being reached by frost, or dug
up by the crows. The desire of saving seed no longer
tempts people to hazard the failure of a crop by making
the sets too small, and great care is taken to cut them so as
to leave in each an eye from which the sprout issues. The
best season for planting them is unquestionably the two last
weeks of April; when planted earlier, their tender shoots,
on piercing the surface, are apt to be nipt by frosts; and,
when planted later, there is a risk of their not arriving at
maturity. About three weeks after they are planted, the
field is harrowed across the rows, to tear up and drag into
the hollows such weeds as were not formerly destroyed, and
to favour the growth of the potatoes. They are afterwards
hand-hoed and horse-hoed like turnips as often as appears
necessary, and are taken up, in the three[*] last weeks of October, sometimes by the common three-pronged dung-fork,
but more frequently by the plough. Every digger with a
fork has two gatherers; and a plough requires at least fixteen people to shake the potatoes from the earth, to gather,
and to carry them to the cart, or to heaps on the field. They
are carted in the evening to some covered shed or barn, where
they remain several days, and are carefully turned over.
The spoiled and small ones are picked out for cattle or
swine; and the rest, after being sufficiently dried, are carried to the pit or house where they are to remain during
winter. In dry ground, a pit is dug a foot or eighteen inches
deep, a thin layer of straw is spread along the sides and
bottom.

[*] Early potatoes are seldom planted, except in gardens or in some detached spots, and are taken up, as they become fit for use, from the end of
July to the middle of September.

bottom of it, the potatoes are piled up in the form of a roof, and covered, first with a thicker layer of straw, and afterwards with the sods and earth which came out of the pit, smoothed with a spade, and made to slope very much. Where the substratum is not dry, the potatoes are laid upon the surface, piled up and covered in the manner already described; and the earth, laid above them, is taken from a trench thrown around the heap to carry off surface-water. But most people have houses, where they can be stored in safety, by laying dry-sand or saw-dust on the floor, stuffing the sides of them well with straw, and covering them with it or the chaff of oats.

The quantity planted upon an acre is about two bolls, and the average produce is about eighteen or twenty returns of the seed, or from 36 to 40 bolls per acre [*]. I have heard of 40 returns, and I know that from 25 to 28 is not uncommon. But the crop sometimes fails altogether, and often does not exceed twelve or fifteen returns. In dry soil properly dunged and managed, the average, which is stated above, may always be confidently expected. But

clay

---

[*] The potatoe boll is the same with the one used in the county for oats and barley, is about $\frac{14}{100}$ larger than the standard boll of Scotland, and is equal to 7 bushels, 3 pecks, 11 pints and a fraction of English standard measure. In the Mid Lothian Report, (p. 108.) 30 bolls Scotch standard measure is thought a large enough average per acre. But the soil of Roxburghshire is much better adapted to the culture of this root than that of Mid-Lothian, and gives larger returns; though they are still inferior to those of Lancashire. The common average there of 200 bushels, each weighing 90 lb. is 18,000 lb. = 1285 stone, 10 lb. Whereas 36 Teviot bolls, about 30 stone each, is only 1080 stone; and 40 bolls, at 30 stone each, is only 1200 stone. The highest average there of 300 bushels is 27,000 lb. = 1928 stone = 64¼ Teviot bolls, about 30 stone per boll. A greater weight, than even this, has been produced in Roxburghshire, though very rarely. Setting aside the few acres, which are mismanaged for want of skill, neglect, and greed, the average given would be rather too low. Including these, it cannot be far from the truth.

clay lands do not yield so large an increase, or such mellow potatoes. The number of acres occupied by this root may be about 1300 or 1400. A population of 32,000 will consume the produce of 1050 acres, supposing each acre to yield 36 bolls, each boll to weigh thirty stone English, and each person to eat two pound English, for 250 days in the year. The produce of other 300 acres will fully supply all that is given to cattle, or used for seed.

The curl was little known here till very lately. It is generally ascribed to some weakness, either in the land or the plant; and that weakness may be brought on, by neglecting to clean, enrich, and cultivate the land, by allowing the seed to be spoiled by improper moisture, heat, or pressure, exhausted by too great sprouts, or affected by frost, before it is taken up the preceding season, or while spread on the ground or a floor to dry, or during winter, while in the pit or house, or after it is cut into sets, or even after it is planted *. But it is certain that this disease is also occasioned, by planting, on contiguous fields and similar soils, the same seed for years successively, or by repeating the crop too often on the same spot, though the seed has been changed. After making many inquiries, I have only heard of two instances of the curl appearing among potatoes planted on ground where they never had been planted before; and I heard of no instance of potatoes being touched by it, when the seed was raised on *lazy-beds*, or was within

in

---

* A tradesman left some potatoes to be planted, in his absence, by two labourers. They took coarse dung, picked out the best sets, and planted part of the field. On his return, he planted the sets, which they had left, on the remainder of the field, with finer dung, a few days afterwards. What the labourers planted were mostly curled; what he planted were entirely free from curl; and he suspects the coarse dung, by keeping the earth too open, admitted the frost to check the tender sprouts.

in five or six generations of coming from the *apple* or fruit upon the stem. There are frequent instances of rows, planted with the seed raised on the farm, being infected by the curl, while it did not appear in the least on other rows, close beside them, planted with seed from a different soil and climate. And there can be no doubt that a repetition of the crop on the same spot will both lessen its quantity and hurt its quality.

A species of coarse potatoe, called *yam*, is raised principally for horses, and is said to be more prolific, and to grow on poorer land than the finer kinds. It might also be an object with farmers, especially near villages, to give it to milch-cows, as it would save their other green food, and does not much affect the taste of either milk or butter.

Sect. V.—*Crops, not commonly cultivated.*

THERE are other crops raised annually in Roxburghshire, but not to a great extent, such as rye, beans, flax, tares, and rutabaga.

Rye is generally sown from October to January on poor and light lands, which can bear no other crop. Being a smaller grain than wheat, less seed is requisite for the acre, and the produce is seldom above three or four bolls. As it is found to impoverish the ground, to yield a poor return, and to fetch only a low price, the culture of it is mostly given up, except on single ridges around corn-fields near dwelling-houses, to defend other crops from poultry, and to furnish thatch for stacks or houses, for which its straw is admirably adapted.

Beans,

Beans, too, thrive well, but are so liable to be hurt by frost and rain in a variable harvest, and so severe upon the land, that few of them are sown; and for these few there is no sure and ready market. These are insuperable objections to the extensive cultivation of beans. If the drill-husbandry shall be more generally adopted, there may be a probability of their becoming a regular crop in the rotation of several farms, as then, they may be sown more early, kept more easily clean, cut down sooner, and force themselves into more general consumpt. When safely stacked, no crop is more profitable. They are sown alone in rows, at the same distance from each other as those for turnips are; and the land is dressed in the same manner, with this difference, that, when the season permits, it is ploughed across and formed into drills or ridges before winter, to be ready for receiving the dung and seed early in spring. Like turnips, they are weeded, and hoed by the hand, and with a horse as occasion requires. They commonly succeed a white crop; the acre gets $\frac{4}{7}$ and even $\frac{10}{7}$ of seed, and sometimes yields about six bolls. They are likewise sown broadcast, mixed with peas, sometimes in equal proportions, but more frequently $\frac{4}{7}$ of a boll of beans are given to $\frac{1}{7}$ of a boll of peas for an acre. Their produce, when mixed, is so uncertain, that it cannot be reckoned more than four bolls on the acre. There may be about 60 acres of them raised annually, or perhaps near 70 in some seasons.

· Flax may occupy nearly the same number of acres. It is sown towards the end of April or beginning of May, generally after fallow or turnip, at the rate of six or eight pecks, or from $1\frac{1}{4}$ to 2 firlots *per* acre, carefully weeded by the hand, and pulled in August, though often allowed to stand till September, that the bolls may ripen for seed or

for

for the mill. From 16 to 25 ftones of fcutched or fwitched
lint have been produced on the acre; but the average will
fcarcely exceed 20 ftone; and of feed, may be about 26
pecks or 6¼ firlots. The land, in a great part of this county, is not adapted for producing good crops of it; and, even
where it grows moft luxuriantly, fcarcely enough is raifed
for home confumption, becaufe, in an inland county, whofe
ftaple is wool, it can neither find a ready market, nor be
manufactured to advantage, and becaufe, though an excellent nurfe for clover from its being well weeded and foon
pulled, yet it is found to exhauft the foil. Befides, the operations of ftripping off the bolls and winnowing the feed, of
fteeping, fpreading, gathering, and dreffing the lint, are all
of them fo unpleafant, and fome of them fo offenfive, that
they are much difliked by fervants. Though fewer fields
may be raifed of lint than of beans, yet, as a fmall quantity of the former is fown almoft on every farm, for the family ufe of the tenant or his cottagers, an equal extent of
ground may be affigned to each. There are two lint-mills
in the county, which have pretty good employment, though
a great proportion of the flax raifed is fcutched at home.

A few tares are frequently fown on corners of peas-
fields, to be cut green for horfes. What they do not ufe is
kept for feed; but the quantity raifed annually is trifling.

Swedifh turnips, or rutabaga, are on the decline. They
have been tried for five or fix feafons, both on a fmall and
a large fcale, and were uniformly found to be hard, heavy
in proportion to their bulk, much relifhed by cattle, proof
againft every feverity of feafon, and very fweet and nutritive even after coming into flower. But their roots extract
much nourifhment from the ground, their ftalks grow too
upright,

upright, and their leaves do not fpread, to catch moifture
from the atmofphere, to prevent exhalation, and to fupprefs
weeds. They are likewife expofed to fuffer much from
hares during winter; and, when taken up and ftacked before it begins, they have not that richnefs and nutritive quality which they acquire from frofts. It is likewife remarked, that, though they can be eafily tranfplanted, they do
not attain the fame fize, as when allowed to remain where
they were fown. They are fown in the end of April or
in May, and treated, in all other refpects, in the fame way
with turnips.

Other crops are occafionally but not conftantly cultivated. Great numbers of cabbage-plants are raifed annually, and fold in the neighbouring counties of Dumfries, Lanark, and Peebles. They are found to thrive remarkably
well here in the open fields; and, though not fo profitable
as potatoes or turnips, are fo ufeful for milch-cows in the
end of autumn and beginning of winter, when the fecond
growth of clover fails, and before the turnips are fully ready, and affect fo little the tafte of the milk, that it is fur-
prifing they are not more attended to. A few rows of them
only are fometimes to be feen in the potatoe or turnip-fields,
or in fome fmall detached fpots. They are planted from
the middle of March to the beginning of June in rows from
2 to 2½ feet afunder, and at the diftance of 14 or 18 inches
from each other in the rows, and managed like a crop of
potatoes or turnips.

A few carrots have, at different times, been raifed for
horfes, milch-cows, and for fale. They were firft tried in
the field about 24 years ago, and the trial has been frequently repeated in many places, not without confiderable fuccefs. But the culture of them cannot become very general
or

or extensive in this county, because few spots are proper for
their growth, and these few can often, if not always, be
more profitably employed; there are many risks and much
trouble in rearing them; if they were placed in rows at
such a distance as to admit of being horse-hoed, the weight
of the crop would be so much diminished, as to render it
comparatively of little value; and to hand-hoe, weed, and
dig them up, would be so expensive, as to reduce the profit to a mere trifle. They are known to be nutritive
for both horses and cattle, and to give butter a beautiful
colour and rich taste; but even these advantages cannot
compensate for the minute and constant attention which
they require, and which, in a large scale of farming, it is
impossible to bestow.

Buck-wheat has been sown for five or six years at Green-
wells near Melrose, and, though the soil is very unsuitable,
it has thriven well, yielding one season fourteen fold. The
seed raised there, when sown the following season, gave as
good a return as what was brought directly from England.
It was, for the first time, tried in 1796 at Riddel on some
exposed heathy ground, newly broke. Though sown too
late in the season, and checked by a severe frost in the end
of May, or beginning of June, yet some of it came up
vigorously and flowered, but could not be said to produce a
crop.

Tobacco, during the American war, was cultivated to a
considerable extent in the neighbourhood of Kelso and Jedburgh, and in some other spots. Its produce was so great,
that thirteen acres at Crailing fetched L. 104 Sterl. or L. 8
Sterl. per acre, at the low rate of 4 d. per lib. and would
have brought more than three times as much, had not an
act of Parliament obliged the cultivator to dispose of it to

O   Government

Government at that price. This county loft about L. 1500 Sterling by that act, which paffed while the tobacco was growing; yet it excited not as much murmuring and cla-mour among the fufferers, as have been elfewhere repeatedly raifed, with lefs reafon, againft other acts in no refpects fo arbitrary and oppreffive.

Rhubarb, teafels, woad, and other fimilar plants, are not raifed in the field.

CHAP.

CHAP. VIII.

GRASS.

SECT. I.—*Natural Meadows and Pastures.*

IT has already been stated, that about ⅓ or 188,048 acres of this county are conftantly in pafture. Of thefe, the quantity faved for hay is very fmall, and fo difperfed up and down in fpots of different fizes and figures, that no probable conjecture can be formed of its extent. The hay, in general, is coarfe, foft, and not eafily made ; though a good deal of it, efpecially by the fides of waters, has a finer and firmer ftalk, is fweet, and much relifhed by cattle and fheep. A larger quantity is cut in Liddefdale than in the reft of the county, and given to black cattle during winter. The natural hay confifts chiefly of *Anthoxanthum odoratum,* fweet fcented vernal grafs ; *Holcus lanatus,* meadow foft grafs : *Poa pratenfis,* fmooth meadow grafs ; *Dactylis glomerata,* tough cockfsfoot grafs : *Alopecurus pratenfis,* meadow

meadow foxtail-grafs: *Aira cæfpitofa*, hair-grafs ; *Avena flavefcens*, oat-grafs. But the moft common of all, efpe-cially in the higher parts of the county, are different fpe-cies of *Carex*, here called *pry*, and by Ainfworth interpret-ed fheer-grafs; and *juncus*, comprehending various plants, dif-fering from though not unlike a finer kind of rufhes, all of which are known pretty generally through the fouth of Scotland by the name of *fprats* *.

The fheep are allowed to pafture the hay-fields till the middle or end of April; and, on that account, it is not rea-dy for the fcythe till the end of Auguft, which increafes the difficulty of getting it into a proper ftate for keeping in a ftack. Could farmers be perfuaded to remove their fheep' fome weeks earlier, their hay would be of a better quality, fooner ripe, and made at an eafier rate. But they muft be left to judge whether they would fuffer more by depriving their fheep of the beft pafture at a fcarce time of year, than they would gain by bettering their hay, and leffening the expence of labour.

Early in fpring, fheep, in marfhy diftricts, feed much upon the *eriophorum vaginatum*, called by the farmers and their fhepherds *mofs*: The roots as well as the leaves are nutritive, and fheep pull, fcratch, and even dig them up with avidity. The *Poa annua* grows every where by the fides of roads and walls where the foil is dry and firm, comes early, and remains long. Their paftures alfo abound

with

---

* There is a good deal of bent-grafs in different places, but it is never made-into hay, becaufe it is fo tough, hard, and elaftic, that, except in very dewy mornings, or wet weather, it eludes the ftroke of the fcythe, and be-caufe the fheep are remarkably fond of it for two or three months while it is green, but cannot eat it when fit for being made into hay. In fome fpots, where it grows very luxuriantly, a fhift is made to cut a little of it and dry it for litter to black cattle. Rufhes, alfo, are ufed for the fame purpofe. Stacks and fhepherds-cots are in fome places thatched with them and with *fprats.*

with *festuca ovina*, sheep's fescue; *cynosurus cristatus*, crested dogtail; several species of *Agrostis* or bent-grass, and a variety of other common herbage. The *Digitalis purpurea*, or foxglove, is likewise found, especially on those pastures which lie on red granite.

Sect. II.—*Artificial Grasses.*

The quantity of land, annually sown with artificial grasses, corresponds pretty nearly to what was in turnips the preceding year. For though turnips are sometimes succeeded by oats, wheat, and even by barley without grasses, yet grasses are as often sown among barley or oats coming after pease.

Red clover, intended for hay, is generally, if not always, sown among barley, at the rate of 10 or 12 lib. per acre on light, and 14 or 16 lib. on heavy land, with 1 bushel of foreign or two bushels of home-raised rye-grass seed. When mixed with yellow clover, 6 or at most 8 lib. on light, and 10 or 12 lib. on heavy land, are sufficient for an acre, from 4 to 6 lib. of the latter being added. For pasture, red, white, and yellow clover are sometimes sown with wheat and oats, as well as with barley, in equal proportions, at the rate of 12 or 15 lib. on light, and from 15 to 20 lib. on heavy soils. But, for the most part, a greater proportion is given of the red than of the other two. The yellow is often omitted, and 8 lib. of red sown with 4 lib. of white to the acre. The quantity of rye-grass is generally the same. Rib-grass, too, is frequently added, though only in small quantities, both it and white clover being congenial to the soil almost of the whole county, and growing spontaneously, or spreading fast from very little seed. All these are

commonly

commonly fown together in the months of April and May,
and the field immediately rolled. When they accompany
barley, the ftones are gathered inftantly, and carried off the
field ; but that operation is delayed till the following fpring,
when they are fown among grain already fprung up. The
ground fometimes gets a fecond rolling before winter, and
always one in the enfuing fpring, unlefs other labour more
prefling comes in the way. A good deal of land, in high
condition, thus fown with graffes, inftead of being mown
as formerly, is paftured by fheep from the beginning of the
very firft feafon. The quantity, alfo, cut green for cattle
and work-horfes, is annually increafing. The fecond crop,
efpecially, when two are taken in a feafon, is devoted to
this purpofe, but cattle are more frequently turned out to
be fattened upon it. Yet more hay is made now, than before thefe practices became fo prevalent. Lefs than 150
ftone *per* acre is reckoned a poor, 200 ftone a good, and
250 ftone a great crop. The average may run from 180
to 200 ftone ; and it fells at 4 d. or thereabouts from the field-
ricks. In ftacks the price varies very much according to
local fituation, or occafional neceffity. The vicinity of a
populous town, deep fnow lying for feveral weeks, or a
troop of horfe ftationed in a place during winter, never
fail to increafe its value. Horfes, being hard wrought, require more nutritive fuftenance than ftraw, and eat hay at
leaft four months every year. It is frequently given to
cattle when weakly, delicate, and unhealthy, to cows newly calved, to oxen employed in the draught, and even to
feeding cattle during a violent froft, when turnips are lefs
palatable and not fo eafily pulled, or late in fpring when
green food fails, to keep them from falling off, till good beef
becomes fcarce. Many of the neighbouring gentlemen confume more hay than they raife. Farmers find purchafers
in them and the inhabitants of contiguous villages for any

furplus

furplus they can fpare. Several of them keep large ftacks from year to year, left a fevere winter fhould oblige them to feed their fheep. And fuch as have no fheep, are then fure of a ready market, and a high price.

A fpecies of burnet grows wild in Liddefdale, and is much liked by cattle, which may induce the gentlemen and far-mers there to attempt the cultivation of it. Lucerne has alfo been tried on a fmall fcale by two or three proprie-tors; but moft of them have rooted it up: And, as far as I can learn, it remains now only on one fmall corner. It cannot be expected, that a plant, which grows fo flowly, and requires to be retained fo long in the ground, will ever become a favourite with tenants on the ordinary length f leafes.

Sect. III.—*Hay Harveft.*

There are many ways of working hay in this county, but the fimpleft and leaft expenfive daily gains ground. It is cut with a fcythe, but, inftead of being inftantly put into fmall cocks, or toiled loofely about the field, as was once the cafe, it is fuffered to remain in the fwath for two days or three, according to the ftate of the weather, and then turned fo carefully as to difcompofe its natural order and regularity as little as poffible. After another day, or two at moft, in dry weather, it may be turned again in the forenoon, or let alone as circumftances require, and put up in fmall ricks in the evening, to ftand for fix or eight days, or perhaps longer, and then ftacked. In the fwath, it re-fifts rain much better than in any other form, preferves its

colour,

colour, retains its flavour, and, by being made ready more slowly, is both a weightier and more nutritive crop [a].

Natural or meadow hay, being of a softer and more flexible nature, and cut later in the season, is more apt to be compressed together by damps and showers, and not so easily put into a state of preservation. It is often carried from the place where it grows to some dry knoll, more exposed to the sun and winds, where it is spread out every morning, and collected every evening into large cocks. In the best weather, it requires near a fortnight's labour; and in rainy seasons, much more. As it only grows in irregular patches, seldom if ever in large fields that have been measured apart, and is not sold or weighed, the average produce of an acre can only be stated, by conjecture, at 150 stone.

Hay-stacks are sometimes built round, with a conical top, but more commonly in an oblong form, shaped and drawn together above like a house. They are thatched with straw or rushes, neatly bound down by ropes of straw or hay, crossing each other diagonally, and making the whole covering of one piece, which will resist the force of every blast during winter.

SECT.

---

[a] See some very pertinent observations on this subject, in the Improved General View of Agriculture in Mid Lothian, p. 116, 7. To these observations, I heartily subscribe, with this exception, or perhaps rather explanation, that, whatever be the state of the hay, whether it has escaped from rain, or has been drenched, whether it has remained in the swath, or has been turned over, on the morning of the day on which it is put in ricks, it should be narrowly examined, and those parts of it, which are wettest or fullest of natural sap, should be exposed for an hour or two to the sun and the wind.

Sect. IV.—*Feeding.*

Some farmers fatten a few sheep on the common pasture, or in inclosures near their houses. And they all endeavour to put the ewes, lambs, and wethers, which are intended for the market, in as good condition as possible. Many of them, and several gentlemen, purchase, in spring, ewes great with young, to go on their richest fields, use at home, or sell the lambs as soon as they are sufficiently fat, and feed off the mothers in three or four months thereafter. They also buy a few wethers, either in spring or autumn, to be fattened on grass or turnips, according to circumstances. It is computed that three ewes and lambs will consume nearly as much as four wethers. An acre of good land will feed three large or five small ewes and lambs. Three Dishley ewes and four lambs, supposing one of them to have twins, and allowing the mother to be sold fat at the same price paid for her when great with young, will yield 55 s. 6 d. *per* acre; the lamb being valued at 10 s. 6 d. and the fleece at 4 s. 6 d. Four Cheviot ewes and lambs, computing their lambs at 8 s. and their fleeces at 2 s. 6 d. each, will only bring 2 guineas *per* acre. And 5 black-faced ewes and lambs, estimating the lambs at 6 s. and their fleeces at 1 s. 6 d. each, will produce L. 1 : 17 : 6 *per* acre; but these last being kindly feeders, both their lambs and they themselves will be sooner ready for the table, and leave the pasture to be otherwise occupied; and being delicate mutton, the mother will fetch a higher price than the other sheep, in proportion to her weight. Greater profits than these are sometimes, and should always be obtained, as land, capable of fattening three Dishley or five black faced ewes and lambs, would let at 30 s. *per* acre. The profit on wethers is scarcely so much, but there is less risk and trouble in feeding them; they are sooner made fat; and can be replaced, in

P   August

August or September, by others, who, after advancing a little on the pasture, are more easily fed-off on turnips. Many, both of them and of the black-faced ewes, are kept by families for their own tables.

A number of small and lean cattle are generally purchased by some gentlemen and farmers, at the northern markets, or on their road to England in the months of October and November, to consume their straw during winter, and to be fed on grass and aftermath the ensuing season. Such of them, as are not then fit for the market, are put on turnips. Many half-fed cattle are likewise picked up, in the months of July and August, to be fattened on the second growth of clover.

Butchers frequently rent inclosures, especially near towns, to receive their purchases of cattle, sheep, and lambs, until the best of them are wanted in the market, and the rest become ready for the shambles. Hence such pastures are sometimes overstocked, and scarcely afford food enough to prevent the animals from falling away; and, at other times, are so much saved, as to improve very quickly such as are not fully fed. Conveniency is more regarded than gain.

CHAP.

CHAP. IX.

GARDENS AND ORCHARDS.

THERE being no large towns in Roxburghshire, and the population being small in proportion to its extent, there can be little demand for the productions of the garden, and few raise articles for sale. All the gentlemen and farmers, and most of the principal inhabitants of the towns and villages, have gardens of their own, from which their tables are furnished with the common vegetables and fruits. The climate, in the lower part of the county, is favourable to the culture of such as are more choice and rare. The nicer kinds of apples, pears, and plums, apricots, peaches, and nectarines, are brought to maturity on open walls, built commonly of stone and lime, and sometimes lined with brick. In some places, they are assisted by flues. There are many hot-houses, and common hot-beds for melons, grapes, pine-apples, and different kinds of exotic plants and flowers. Attempts have been made to raise all these in the higher parts of the county, not with-

out

out fuccefs, though want of climate did not allow many of
them to attain the fame perfection in ripenefs and flavour.
The more common fruits are every where produced of an
excellent quality. Cherries, early apples, and pears, fome
coarfe forts of plums, goofeberries, ftrawberries, rafpber-
ries, and currants of different kinds, are all found in very
high and bleak fituations, where fome vegetables for the
kitchen do not thrive; onions, artichokes, brocoli, and
other articles, are either too nice in their choice of foil, or
too weak, to ftand the feverity of the climate. Abundance of onions, however, are raifed in moft parts of the
county, and fold in the markets at a reafonable rate, to
feafon the homely difhes of the poor. Every cottager
has a garden, in which little is planted except potatoes, and
fometimes a few cabbages for fummer, and, for winter, green
or open *kail*, a hardy plant, not unlike the *cole* in England,
which is feldom hurt by the fevereft froft. Of late a few
beans and turnips have been introduced, but they are greedily devoured by children before they are fit for ufe. Some
farmers are, in this refpect, in the fame fituation with their
cottagers; but many of them, and a great number of fmall
proprietors and artificers, have neat and curious gardens,
carefully and fkilfully managed, producing not only the beft
kinds of common vegetables in great profufion, but many
uncommon plants and flowers, both for beauty and for
ufe *.

There

* Rhubarb has been raifed of a large fize, and admirable quality, and
teafels which have anfwered as well for fmoothing the furface of cloth, as
thofe brought from England. Woad too is cultivated. Mofs-rofes are very
common. The double-leaved yellow rofe is alfo fometimes feen. There
are feveral other plants, equally valuable or beautiful, whofe names I do not
recollect.

There are feveral fmall orchards, moftly belonging to gentlemen, who do not fell the fruit. A few, at Jedburgh, Kelfo, Melrofe, and Gattonfide, are let to gardeners, or retained by the proprietors, who, for the fruit, undergrowth, and grafs, may draw annually from L. 6 to L. 10 *per* acre. Jedburgh has long been famous for pears. The beft kinds there are the Lammas or Crawford, the Auchan, and the Longueville. The two laft, efpecially, are much valued, and in great demand over a large track of country. There are feveral other pears of good kinds, and fome very bad ones. In fome feafons their produce is incredibly great. A variety of apples, moftly for the kitchen, are likewife raifed there, and a good many indifferent plums. All thefe fruits, except the Auchan and Longueville pears, grow in the other orchards, and are carried to a confiderable diftance. Goofeberries, ftrawberries, currants, and plums, being unfit for a long carriage, are fold in the neighbourhood at a low price. At Melrofe and Jedburgh, there are fome very old trees, fupported by props, and ftill very prolific *. They were probably planted by the priefts belonging to thefe Abbeys, and fhew that, among the other qualities afcribed to them, they were not inattentive to good fruits.

It has, of late, become very common for gentlemen to keep fmall nurferies for fupplying themfelves with plants of thorns and foreft-trees. There are likewife feveral nurferies, in which every kind of fhrub, large and fmall fruit

and

* Wonderful ftories are told of their fertility A fingle tree of the thorle pear at Melrofe, has for thefe 50 years paft yielded the intereft of the money paid for the garden where it ftands, and for a houfe let at L. 7 Sterling yearly. Another tree there has carried fruit to the amount of L. 3 Sterling annually at an average for the fame period. In the 1793, two trees there brought to perfection about 60,000 pears, which were fold for 3 guineas. Thefe facts are well authenticated.

and foreſt trees, is raiſed for ſale. The whole ground, occupied in this way, does not exceed 120 acres, yet produces
enough to anſwer all the demands of this county, and many commiſſions from diſtant parts. A large ſhare of it belongs to Meſſrs Dickſons, in the neighbourhood of Hawick,
whoſe plants have an extenſive ſale through all the north of
England and ſouth of Scotland.

CHAP.

CHAP. X.

WOODS and PLANTATIONS.

ACCORDING to the beft information which I could obtain, there cannot be fewer than 5290 * acres in
wood, natural and planted, in Roxburghfhire. The amount,
in feveral parifhes, being flated upon conjecture, perfect accuracy cannot be expected. But, if every error was recti-
fied by an exact furvey, I am confident the number of
acres on the whole would rather be more than lefs. There
is lefs danger of miftakes in computing the quantity of
planted than of natural wood. The one is regular and
compact, all its trees are of the fame age, and a probable
conjecture may be formed of its extent from the number
of them which it contains. The other is fo irregular and
fcattered, and its trees are of fuch unequal age and growth,
that conjectures can ftand on no certain bafis, and muft be
altogether vague. The only fafe way is to keep within the
mark, which many may think I have done much too far,
in ftating the whole natural wood in this large county only at 608 acres. The number planted is nearly 4682. In
neither of thefe are included, hedge-rows, ftraggling trees
in lawns and fields, and tufts around villages and farm-hou-
fes;

* See the Statiftical Table annexed, Chap. XV. Sect. 8.

fes; although all thefe are moftly hard-wood, and many of them would bring a great price. In feveral places, and particularly at Ancrum, a number of trees were felled of a large fize about 30 years ago. I cannot learn their meafurement or folid contents, but I am affured, that one afh was fold for L. 25 Sterling, and proved an excellent bargain; and that there are, at this moment, on that eftate, feveral trees, whofe circumference is from 10 to 13 ft. and whofe trunk is from 7 to 15 ft. in length. An afh, on a neighbouring eftate, which was bought in 1796 for feven guineas, meafured 10 ft. round, and contained 174 ft. of wood. Many trees, equally large and valuable, ftill remain, in different and diftant parts of the county, untouched by the ufe or the weather. From poverty of foil, injudicious management, or fome accidental circumftances, feveral hundred acres, planted fome time ago chiefly with Scotch firs, have totally failed; and nearly as many, lately planted, do not promife well. But, in general, every tree, which thrives in other parts of Scotland, may be found here healthy and vigorous. Of thofe commonly cultivated, the beech, the plane, and the lime, are the moft luxuriant and beautiful, and the afh and Scotch fir are the moft profitable. For though oak and elm are as valuable as afh, and much more fo than fir, they do not grow fo quickly, are not fo foon ready for ufe, and do not produce fo much from the acre. There is no ftage of their growth after they are 12 years old, in which afh and fir are not fit for fome ufeful purpofe. Old afhes, oaks and elms, fell at 1 s. 6 d. and 2 s. per ft.; beech and plane, from 10 d. to 1 s. 2 d.; and firs, from 7 d. to 1 s. A fpecies of willow, known by the name of red faugh or fallow, is efteemed next in value to afh, oak and elm, and brings 1 s. 6 d. or 1 s. 8 d. Thefe variations in the prices are occafioned, partly by local fituation, but chiefly by the age and quality of the trees. Birch

and

and alder are not fold by meafurement. The timber of other trees is feldom ufed, except for fome very particular purpofes. A number of larches are coming forward in different places, and may, in a few years, be applied to many purpofes, for which, at prefent, recourfe is had to foreign fir. It is brought from Berwick and Leith, where the prime coft of it, in time of peace, was about 1 s. 2 d. and 1 s. 4 d. *per* ft. and now is 1 s. 8 d. and 1 s. 10 d.: the carriage being nearly a halfpenny *per* ft. for every four miles, the foot of it may amount, in fome diftant parts of the county, to no lefs than 2 s. 5 d. This enormous price has induced fome gentlemen lately to make a fair trial of fir, produced in the county, for the joifts and roofs of their houfes. There are already inftances of its remaining perfectly found in roofs above 40 years; and the planks, now on fale, are older, larger and better, than thofe formerly ufed. Some trees at 1 s. *per* ft. have fetched about 50 s. each; and the average of thofe fold in a feafon will be 24 ft. in length, 7 inches in the fide, and about 8 ft. of wood *. Towards the beginning of this century, the celebrated Sir William Bennet, Sir   Elliot of Stobs, Mr Douglas of Cavers, Mr Elliot of Wells, and Mr Bennet of Cheflers, made large plantations of this ufeful tree, from which their defcendants have reaped great advantage. Thefe are now moftly cut down; but others, planted only a few years after them, are now on fale at Wells (on Rule water) and Stewartfield, from 7 d. to 1 s. *per* ft. according to their fize and quality: And there is every appearance of twenty or thirty acres being equally ready every year

Q   for

---

* Very many of thefe contain from 15 to 18 ft. of wood; but the average is brought thus low by the number of fmaller trees, which are cut yearly, to give larger ones more room.

for half a century, unlefs want of cafh fhall tempt fome proprietors of eftates entailed on diftant connections, or fome young fucceffors to eftates which they cannot fell, to employ the axe too freely, and cut down large parcels before they attain full maturity. Some planks, carried in 1795 from Wells to the extremity of Liddefdale, were of fo large a fize, fo good a quality, and fufceptible of fo fine a polifh, as fully to equal a great deal of what is brought from the north of Europe. This fact deferves to be mentioned, both as it may fet other gentlemen upon fimilar experiments, and as it may encourage them to plant firs on many thoufand acres which cannot be turned to fuch good account. Perhaps, indeed, there never was lefs occafion, than at the prefent moment, for a hint of this nature. A great deal of land has been lately planted, and in a manner, too, that bids fairer for fuccefs than any that was formerly followed. The belts, efpecially in expofed fituations, are made very broad; the ground is ploughed, and in fome cafes manured; the foil, where fhallow, is deepened immediately below the trees; it is annually dug around them; and fometimes it carries potatoes, turnips, cabbages, or kaill. The plants, by thefe operations, are refrefhed and nourifhed; thofe that are weakly or have been hurt may be helped; and thofe that perifh may be replaced *. A good many willows, likewife, of different kinds, now occupy feveral marfhy fpots. There is little doubt of their growing; and, if they are managed as fkilfully as in the fenny diftricts of England, the profits arifing from them may probably extend

* I have remarked, in traverfing this county, that the moft vigorous and fulleft-grown firs, are always found above rocks of lime, free or whinftone, and that firs, on a bottom of clay, till, and even gravel, are apt to pine and decay about the age of twenty or twenty-five years, and fome earlier.

tend their culture to other lands of a fimilar nature, which cannot be fo profitably employed. There are numerous fhrubberies, fome of them on a large fcale, and furnifhed with many foreign fhrubs as well as with all thofe which the ifland produces. Several farmers and tradefmen have great delight in rearing them, and by affiduity and care bring fome rare ones to high perfection *.

* Since writing the above, I obferved a plantation of hard-wood, furround-ed by a belt of firs and larches, and interfected by rows of them at the dif-tance of 25 or 30 yards from each other. Both were thriving.

CHAP.

CHAP. XI.

WASTES.

IT is difficult to annex any precise meaning to this expression, when applied to lands in Scotland. In former times, there were several commons, in which the cattle, belonging to different proprietors, went promiscuously under one *herd* or keeper. The arable land, also, was possessed in alternate ridges, separated by broad *balks*, on which the large stones were laid when the indolent husbandmen could take that trouble, and was pastured by the cattle, after being freed from the crop. The best part of it was dunged every third year, when barley was raised; the other crops were oats and peas. The worst or most exposed part of it carried oats for years successively, till it was exhausted, and left to the cattle. Lands, thus aukwardly possessed, and wretchedly managed, might not improperly be called *wastes;* and though acts of Parliament passed, so early as the 1695, for dividing them, at the instance of any proprietor having interest, yet no advantage was taken of such beneficial laws, till the year 1738 or 1739, that the lands of Smailholm

holm were parcelled out among the several proprietors, in
proportion to the *valuation*, or rate, by which they paid the
land-tax. At that time, a mighty clamour was excited, and
renewed on every subsequent division of a common, that the
poor were spoiled and oppressed, and the country was ruined,
to enlarge the possessions of the great. This cry became
louder, when several small farms, lying contiguous, were
thrown together, to make one or two compact and commodious farms, on which tenants could subsist more comfortably
at an advanced rent, by having it in their power, to make
inclosures of a competent size *, to do more work with the
same number of hands and cattle, and consequently to draw
much more profit from the same extent of ground. Through
the influence of these popular prejudices, the division of commons and blended property went slowly on for some years;
but a sense of private interest, and of general good, by degrees, has broken these absurd fetters, and there has not been
a single common in the whole county these 20 years. Large
farms have likewise become more general, and where they
do not swell to a very immoderate size, are no longer regarded with an evil eye. It is not incurious to observe, that,
in general, they are kept in much better order than smaller
ones,

---

* The multitude of diminutive and aukward inclosures in the north of
England, particularly in Yorkshire, Derbyshire, Lancashire, &c. can only
be accounted for, by supposing, that they once belonged to as many small
proprietors, or were rented by successive generations of small tenants, who,
looking on them as a kind of inheritance, threw around them walls built
with the stones picked up from their surface, or planted some defenceless
thorns to be trodden down by cattle or sportsmen, chiefly with a view of as-
certaining the boundaries of detached spots, possessed by different individuals, in different corners of the same manor, without reflecting that, if the
property or possessions of each were laid together by fair exchanges, or an
equal apportionment of rent, their inclosures would be more sizeable and
commodious.

ones, for which substantial reasons can be assigned. Possessors of large farms have more force to make sudden and vigorous exertions, by which every part of their work can be expeditiously done in the proper season; and their farms are primary, while small farms are only secondary objects of concern. Men naturally bestow most attention where their interest is most at stake. They, whose subsistence and profit wholly depend on the product of the ground, will cultivate it to the best advantage, while cadgers and mechanics, who have other more gainful employments, are apt to neglect their fields *.

A considerable part of this county still is, and probably will always be, in a state of nature, because there is no way of rendering it more productive, except at an expence which its amplest returns could never repay. This remark applies to most of the pasture district, which can only be improven by drains. To lime or marl its surface, would cost much more than the price at which it would sell in a market, and yet would not double its present rent. Belonging to distinct proprietors, being admirably adapted for sheep, and fully stocked with them; and even the morasses which cannot be pastured, yielding fuel, or manure, or both, it can in no sense be called *waste*. That harsh name, however, may be justly given to a small tract of heathy land near the county-town, the whole soil of which, in the course of centuries, has been completely stript off in turfs for fuel. Before good roads opened up ready access to coal, the inhabitants of Jedburgh and its neighbourhood used chiefly peats and turfs; and to supply them with the latter, the tenants around literally maintained their families, and paid their rents, by selling

ing

* On this principle, I must plead for indulgence to the defects in this work. Other pursuits demanded the largest share of my time and thoughts, and obliged me to make it the amusement of my leisure hours.

ling the foil, till they reduced the ground to the moſt de-
plorable and irremediable ſterility.   No feed will vegetate;
no plant can live ! Still nearer to that town, there is a larger
extent of admirable foil for turnip huſbandry lying utterly
neglected.   When I add, that the tenants have leaſes of a tolerable length, at an eaſy rent, and the example of worſe
land around them in excellent culture, what forer reproach
can be caſt upon them ?

CHAP.

CHAP. XII.

IMPROVEMENTS.

Sect. I.—*Draining.*

A Great deal, both of the pasture and arable district, is drained. In the former, the drains are mostly open, from 16 inches to 2 ft. wide, and about 1 ft. or 14 inches deep, and made to run along declivities in such directions as will catch and carry off the greatest quantity of water. They cost about 1 d. each rood, and often only 1¼ d. the two roods of 6 yards each. In most lands 2 men will dig from 50 to 72 roods in a day; and, where they cannot do so much, they charge more for the rood. By these drains, land, which formerly retained and collected water, and produced nothing but rushes and unwholesome food, is converted into safe and valuable pasture, especially in winter, yielding sweet and nutritive grasses, and affording both meat and shelter during snow, when it is not remarkably deep

and

and hardened by a severe froft fucceeding a fhort and gentle thaw. Natural hay, too, is much improven in quality and increafed in quantity by fuch drains, when they furround, or interfect, in a judicious manner, the fwamps or meadows where it grows. A little attention to remove the ftones and clods which tumble into them, the ftraggling ftraws, leaves and mofs, which are blown into them by the wind, and the earth which in froft crumbles down from their fides; will preferve them a long while in good order; but, if this precaution be neglected, they will ftand in need of being renewed in a very few years *.

A large portion of the arable diftrict is fo dry that no drains are neceffary : and other parts are fufficiently drained by the plough, and the ditches thrown around inclo-fures when they are planned with fkill. Marfhy fpots, in corn-fields, are fometimes made perfectly dry, by finking a pit, till a ftratum of fand or gravel appears, and then filling it up with loofe ftones. A furrow, a flight open drain, or even a covered one, according to the fituation of the fields, conveys the water from the fprings to the pit. In forming ridges, great care is taken to give the water an eafy defcent ; and a furrow is often drawn acrofs them to facilitate its paffage. When fprings, or furface-water, cannot be carried off by thefe fimple means, drains are cut of dif-ferent dimenfions, and filled up in a different manner, ac-

R   cording

---

* A farmer in this county, on reading an account of the manner in which fome fenny lands in England are drained, thinks a fimilar attempt might be attended with fuccefs on marfhy fheep-walks. By cutting and removing three rows of fods, each fod being precifely thirty inches long, ten broad, and fix deep. By digging the fpace below the middle row to the depth of nine or ten inches more, and by replacing the fods acrofs the cut or drain, through which, under this covering, the water may flow, marfhes might be drain-ed, and their whole furface preferved for the fheep. The experiment cer-tainly deferves a fair trial.

cording to the nature of the ground, and the materials
which can be got. The main drain, which receives all the
water from the leſſer ones, is often ſo wide as 4 ft. and about
3½ ft. deep, ſometimes both broader and deeper, eſpecially
when a large extent of wet land is drained, or when it
pierces pieces of riſing grounds. The rood of ſix yards
coſts, on ſtony or hard land, about 1 s. 4 d. or 1 s. 6 d. on
eaſy-wrought land, from 8 d. to 1 s. But, except in very
particular caſes, this drain is only about 30 inches, or at moſt
3 ft. wide, from 26 to 36 inches deep, and from 1 ft. to 20
inches broad at the bottom, and is made for 9 d. or perhaps
1 s. on hard, and as low as 4½ d. on ſoft land. The branches
are generally about 2 ft. wide at the top, and 14 or even
18 inches at the bottom, the depth depending very much
on particular circumſtances, but being always ſufficient to
admit eight or ten inches of ſoil over the materials with
which the drains are filled. They coſt from 2 d. to 8 d.
the rood, according to the nature of the ground. It is of
importance to catch the ſprings; and, for this purpoſe, it
is neceſſary to dig below the ſoil, and in ſome caſes below
the ſtratum on which it is incumbent. It is likewiſe of
importance to keep the bottom as broad as poſſible; and
the ſides as perpendicular as can be done without danger of
their giving way, that the water may have more room to
find a vent, after depoſiting the mud and ſand which it forces along. Hence their depth, and their width both at top
and bottom, may ſometimes exceed the above dimenſions,
and the expence of making them be proportionably increaſed. Their ſides are frequently lined with flat ſtones ſet on
their edges, which prevent the earth from mouldering
down, and leave ſpace enough for the water to drip into
the drain. Main drains, and even ſome croſs-drains, are
often built like ſewers, to the height of 8, 10, and perhaps
14 inches, and from 12 to 18 inches wide, both height and
width

width being proportioned to the quantity of water computed to pafs. They are then covered, firft with flags or
coarfe ftones of fufficient length, next with fmall ftones, and
laftly with inverted turfs, ftraw, rufhes, quickweeds or
brufhwood, to prevent the earth that is laid above from
finking into the drain in the courfe of ploughing. But a
more common method is to pick out the largeft and round-
eft ftones, and lay them in rows along the middle and fides
of the drain, at fuch a diftance as to allow feveral paffages
of two or more inches between the rows, through one or
other of which the water may always run. The ftones
approaching neareft to that fize are laid, immediately above
thefe, fo as to leave fimilar interftices, in cafe all the lower
ones fhould, in procefs of time, be choked with mud. The
fmaller ftones are then thrown in, and covered with invert-
en turfs, &c. as already defcribed. Equal attention is not
paid to the leffer drains. They are commonly filled with
ftones, tumbled into them out of the cart, but covered in
the fame careful manner.

Among other improvements, Mr Dawfon, not having
ftones for fome drains on his farm at Frogden, had recourfe
to an admirable expedient, which he had feen in Effex, for
fupplying that want. With implements contrived for the
purpofe, he made the drains wide at the top, of the neceffary depth, and very narrow at the bottom. He then filled them with broom, placing the bare ftalks undermoft,
to leave ample fpace for the water, and compreffing their
bufhy tops above, to prefent a clofe and firm covering,
through which the earth can penetrate but a very little
way. Some of them have lafted upwards of 30 years,
without any appearance of failure.

After all the numerous and expenfive drains which have
been made, much ftill remains to be done in this way, both
in the pafture and arable diftrict.

SECT.

Sect. II.—*Paring and Burning.*

Some years ago, huge crops were raised by paring and burning, to the great emolument of the tenants, but much to the prejudice of their farms and their successors. The perniciousness of the practice is evinced by its being generally abandoned. It is, however, the opinion of intelligent farmers, that there are many fields in Roxburghshire, of a deep soil, and at a distance from other manure, where paring and burning would be a substantial improvement, if they were, at the same time, properly drained, cleared from stones, neatly ridged, and gently cropped. But as it reduces to ashes some of the best soil, and has hurt ten acres for every one it has benefited, it should be prohibited or subjected to severe restrictions in all leases.

Sect. III.—*Manuring.*

The manures, chiefly used in this county, are dung, marl, lime, and compost.

All the animals about a farm-yard are plentifully supplied with litter, to retain their dung and urine; the stables and cow-houses are regularly cleaned every day, those where feeding cattle are kept much oftener, hog-stys and hen-houses twice or thrice in a week; and what is gathered there, the ashes produced in the dwelling-house, and the rubbish of thatched houses, are generally all carried to the same dunghill. If the thatched houses have been inhabited, their roofs saturated with soot make excellent muck, This mass is, sometimes, allowed to remain untouched un-

til

til it is laid upon the land, fometimes, is turned over in the
court or place where it was formed, and fometimes, is removed to the field appropriated for it, to remain there in
a heap and to be turned over as often as may be neceffary
until it is ufed. While in the court it is trodden by cattle.
Some farmers, fenfible that this retards the fermentation,
either carry it away foon, or convert their court into a
ftraw-yard for feeding young cattle, and find fome fpot
near their offices for a dunghill, to which cattle have not
accefs. In many places, particularly in towns and villages, the ftreets and roads are fcoured, and the mud and
filth collected from them are thrown upon the dunghills.
Nor is it unufual, when a dunghill is placed in a field, to
intermix with it thin layers of a good foil. In both cafes,
however, and efpecially in the former, the feeds and roots
of noxious weeds are apt to harbour in the dung, and fpring
up in the land. With the exception of a few inftances,
where poor land has got an immenfe or rich land a trifling
dofe, the average rate of this dung, given through the county to an acre, may be from 20 to 24 carts, of 15 or
16 cwt. each, or from 16 to 20 tons. Such a cart-load when
bought fetches about 2 s. But very little dung is fold. Moft
of the villagers and cottagers are defirous of having, each
his own pittance laid on a feparate lot of land, on which
they plant potatoes, or perhaps fow lint : And generally
fome farmer accommodates them for the fake of getting his
land well dunged, and of their giving him fome work in
harveft. The common terms are, that the farmer does all
parts of the work where horfes are required ; and that the
people furnifh their own feed, perform all the manual labour, and have the whole produce. This plan deferves
commendation for its humanity in providing the poor with
food at an eafy rate ; but the farmer lofes the advantage of
mixing their various kinds of dung into one heap with
that

that raifed by himfelf, and runs the rifk of having not a
few ridges miferably neglected, and of feeing, in the following feafon, a patched field, with fome fpots too luxuriant, fome almoft parched, and fome full of weeds. according to the different qualities of the dung, and the different degrees of culture beftowed on the preceding crop,

When cattle are well littered, and fully fed with turnips, about 12 of them will yield a cart of dung in 24
hours; but that quantity will fcarcely be produced by 16
or even 18 kept on ftraw, with a fmall allowance of turnips to preferve them frefh and fleek. An acre of very
good turnips, with an adequate proportion of ftraw, will
make upwards of 16 cart-load of dung; but 10 will be a
large enough average for all the acres in the county. Thus
nearly the produce of two acres will be requifite to dung
one the enfuing feafon. Manure, for the reft of the lot in
turnips and potatoes, is furnifhed, by the horfes and other
cattle on the farm, and by the dunghills fcraped together
by cottagers. Turnip fields, when once brought into good
order, and into a regular rotation, generally get a fcantier
fupply of dung, not above 14 or 15 cart-load, or from 10
to 12 tons; the deficiency being made up, fometimes by a
fmall quantity of lime or marl, but more frequently by the
dung and urine of fheep when eating the turnips. Fine
fields are raifed often by lime or marl without dung,

Marl was firft ufed, about 40 years ago, by a gentleman
of confiderable property, and by an actual farmer. Sir
Gilbert Elliot of Minto*, then a Lord of Seffion, and afterwards Lord Juftice-Clerk, obferving the good effect of
marl on fome lands in the county of Angus, drained a morafs

* Father to the late, and grandfather to the prefent Baronet of the fame
name.

tafs on his own eftate, about the year 1755, and laid fhell marl on 200 acres, or thereabout, of inclofed land, all in tillage, but immediately laid into grafs [a]. The attempt excited the wonder of fome, and the ridicule of others. A young farmer, who took the marled inclofures at what was then thought an exorbitant rent, declares that he has never fince had fuch cheap and productive land, although the foil is a ftiff clay, to which of all others marl is leaft adapted. About a year or two before that time, Mr Dawfon, returning from England, immediately began to lay clay marl, on part of a farm at Harpertown, below Kelfo, then poffeffed by his father, at the rate of 336 coop-carts *per* acre. Inftead of dropping the attempt, as Lord Minto feems to have done, he perfevered for feveral years, till better accefs was opened up to lime, and till he found, that, owing to the trouble and expence attending marl, the number of labourers it required, and the high wages they demanded, he could manure a greater extent of ground yearly with lime at a cheaper rate. Clay marl has been little ufed ever fince. But fhell marl was fearched for and found in different parts of the county. Moraffes were drained, and pits dug at Eckford, Clarilaw, and other places. But none had accefs to them, except the tenants of the different proprietors. In the year 1772, it was firft expofed to public fale at Whitmoorhall, towards the N. W. extremity of the county, at 4 d. the fingle-horfe cart, containing about two bolls, or 16 cubic ft., wet as it comes from the pit. It is now raifed to 10 d. Purchafers generally fend a number of fervants and carts to the pit. The carts are filled alternately, and unloaded on fome adjacent fpot, fo

near

---

[a] At that time, it was not a common practice to meafure land, far lefs to allot a certain allowance of dung or marl to the acre. The fields are known to contain the number of acres fpecified above; but the quantity of marl laid on the acre can only be gueffed by thofe who faw it at 35 carts.

near that from 50 to 60 carts can be filled and emptied in a day : The marl remains there till it becomes dry, and loses about one-fifth part of its bulk and weight. About 25 carts brought wet from the pit, shrunk into 20 when carried home, are laid on an acre of light land. This is the least quantity, and thought rather a scanty allowance. Most people give 24 or 25 carts of dried marl, and some to the extent of 50. The length of carriage, as well as the nature of the soil, frequently determine both the size of cart-loads, and the number of them given to an acre. Clay lands require the largest dose, and receive the greatest benefit from marl laid on the surface of grass. In two or three years, it is completely incorporated with the sod, enriches and sweetens the pasture, and yields luxuriant crops when the fields are afterwards in tillage. On such lands it is not unusual to lay 80 or 100 bolls, and often a much greater quantity. The average prime cost of marl, to an acre of light soil, may be from 25 to 40 s., and of heavy, from 2 guineas to 50 s. The expence of carriage must depend very much on the distance and the roads. In tolerable roads, the same man and horses can go and return, 4 times every day when the distance is only 3 miles, thrice every day when the distance is 4 miles, twice when the distance is 5 or 6 miles, and thrice every two days when the distance is 7, 8, or 9 miles. Estimating the labour of a man with 2 horses and 2 carts only at 5 s. 4 d. *per* day, the carriage of every boll will be 4 d. for 3 miles, nearly 5¼ d. for 4 miles, 8 d. for 5 or 6 miles, and 10¼ d. for 7, 8, or 9 miles. Thus, an acre of light land, according to its distance from the pit, may be marled at the under-mentioned rates :

Prime cost of 30 carts of marl from the pit, at 10 d. each,   -   -   L. 1   5   0

Carried forward L. 1   5   0

Brought forward L. 1 5 o
Carriage of 24 carts of dried marl 3 miles, at
  8 d. each, - - o 16 o

Total, L. 2 1 o

Prime cost of 60 carts as formerly, at 10 d.
  each, - - L. 2 10 o
Carriage of it dried into 48 carts for 3 miles,
  at 8 d. each, - - 1 12 o

Total, L. 4 2 o

Again,

Prime cost of 30 carts from the pit, at 10 d.
  each, - - L. 1 5 o
Carriage of it dried into 24 carts 8 miles, at
  1 s. 8 d. each, - - 2 o o

Total, L. 3 5 o

Prime cost of 60 carts as formerly, L. 2 10 o
Carriage of it dried into 48 carts 8 miles, at
  1 s. 8 d. each, - - 4 o o

Total, L. 6 10 o

Hence the average expence of marling light land, at the distance of 3 miles, is L. 3 : 1 : 6 *per* acre; and, at 8 miles, is L. 4 : 17 : 6. And every reader, who may take the trouble of making similar computations, will find, that the average expence of marling heavy land, at the distance of 3 miles, is L. 3 : 7 : 6, and at 8 miles, is L. 5 : 12 : 6, allowing 90 bolls or 45 single-horse carts to each acre. But a much larger quantity is frequently given, and several extensive fields have been marled at the rate of L. 10 Sterling *per* acre.

S Besides

Besides the diſtance and expence of carriage, marl is attended with the diſadvantage of retarding corn from ripening. Though this effect is chiefly felt in cold and expoſed lands, yet it takes place in ſome degree in warm and early ſoils. In ſeveral places, the grain, ſown on one half of a field manured with lime, will be 12 or 15 days earlier ready, than the ſame grain ſown at the ſame time on the other half manured with marl. The grain, too, on the marled land, will be a tenth part lighter. But, in a favourable ſoil and climate, the difference is not ſo diſcernible. The one is generally ripe, or nearly ſo, as ſoon as the other is cut down, and the grains are almoſt of equal quality. It is alſo obſerved, that after lands, properly marled gently cropped and laid in graſs, are broken up again by the plough, they bring crops as early, if not earlier, to maturity, than if they had not been marled. In all ſoils and climates, marl, when judiciouſly applied, is found to make excellent graſs. Hence high and bleak lands, eſpecially if inclining to clay, after being marled, ſhould be kept in hay or paſture: and even in low and rich fields, when ſufficiently marled and properly managed, clover will always be a luxuriant and profitable crop. The effects of marl are ſeldom immediate, but generally laſting, except when the land manured with it has been exhauſted by over-cropping; an evil which has been felt, but is not much to be dreaded from the preſent experienced farmers in Roxburghſhire.

Lime as a manure was known and uſed as early as marl; but want of fuel prevented it from being burned in thoſe parts of the country where it abounds, and owing to bad roads little of it was brought from a diſtance. It was not till the great road to England, by Coldſtream-bridge, opened a readier acceſs to the kilns in the eaſtern parts of Northumberland, that it began to ſuperſede marl in the
lower

lower parts of Roxburghshire, and till turnpike roads were made in the county itself, that the use of it became general. Mr Brown, late of Elliestoun, * deserves to be recorded, both as a principal promoter of a road thro' the centre of the county, and also as one of the first great proprietors, who brought lime by that road, and the western road by Gala-water, from Mid-Lothian, and by cross-roads from Northumberland, each 27 or 28 miles from his estate, in such quantities as to manure completely at least 150 acres; at a time, too, when such an undertaking was apt to be considered as a certain indication, either of a disordered mind, or of an overflowing purse. Since that time, lime has recommended itself to such favour in every part of the county, as a quicker and more powerful agent than marl, and in most places obtained at an easier rate, that there is frequently a greater demand for it than can be answered.

Farmers towards the north are supplied with lime from Mid-Lothian; at the distance of from 20 to 30 miles, and bring it as return carriage, mostly in two-horse carts, containing 3 bolls each, tho' sometimes in one-horse carts, containing 2 bolls each. The boll is 4 firlots Linlithgow measure, and costs now 1 s., formerly only 10 d., at the kiln. Those towards the east get lime from the lower parts of Northumberland. The distance is less only from 12 to 24 miles; the lime is of a better quality; and the measure is larger; but the advantage of a double carriage is lost. The boll here is about $2\frac{4}{5}$ Linlithgow firlots; it costs at an average $7\frac{1}{4}$ d.; and 5 bolls load a double cart. Hence the load is only $1\frac{1}{2}$ d. higher than from Mid-Lothian, and it contains a Linlithgow firlot more. For several years, the neighbourhood of Jedburgh have been furnished with lime from the higher

* Now a Commissioner of Excise in Scotland.

higher or north-west part of Northumberland, on Reed-water. It is carried from 16 to 30 miles. Empty carts are sent for it. It costs 7 d. per boll, which is nearly equal to 2¼ Linlithgow firlots; and 5 of them is the common load of a two-horse cart. But it is of a superior quality to every other lime known in the county, and the road is excellent, though carried through a hilly country, and in one place about 1500 feet above the sea. The western district is supplied with lime burned in the county, or in the neighbouring county of Dumfries. The lime made in the county sells for 11 d. per boll of 2 Linlithgow firlots; but its inferiority confines the demand within the narrow space of 9 or 10 miles. That got in Dumfries-shire is so much better, that it is brought above 30 miles. It costs indeed only 7 d. per boll. The measures are the same, and 6 bolls load a double cart. Lime equally good is found in Liddesdale, but it has already been observed, * that for want of roads little of it is used. It is highly worthy of honourable mention, in a work of this kind, that a farmer, at an equal distance of 26 miles from the two Northumberland lime-kilns, on the east and south, in one season, carried lime from each nearly in equal quantities, for 130 acres, at the rate of 6 carts per acre or 31 Northumberland bolls; each boll, including carriage, being 2 s. 8¼ d.; each acre being nearly 4 guineas; and the whole sum laid out amounting to L. 545 : 14 : 7. I have the pleasure of adding, that this spirited exertion has been abundantly rewarded by three excellent crops, of turnips, barley, and clover with grasses.

The quantity of lime here given may be considered as the general average for an acre of light land. Heavy lands require at least 8 such carts, more frequently get 10, and

sometimes

* Chap. I. Sect 5.

sometimes 16; this last making the expence of manuring an acre at the same distance of 26 miles L. 10 : 16 : 8, and at 30 miles about L. 12. The carriage may be stated at 4½ d. *per* mile for a two-horse cart. Allowing 10 of these as the average for clay, and 6 for light soils, the expence of liming an acre of each may be easily calculated, according to its distance from the lime-kilns.

Greater pains are taken to incorporate both marl and lime with heavy than with light soils. After they are spread on heavy land, it receives always 2, and often 3 ploughings, and as many harrowings. Light land, when previously well pulverised, is generally but once ploughed, and sometimes lime is only harrowed into it : but marl must be earlier and more thoroughly mixed with the soil, that it may operate more quickly ; and after all, its beneficial effects may not be fully felt on the first, or even on the second crop. Lime is seldom, if ever, laid on the surface of grass fields.

Composts of different kinds have been used, though not so frequently as might be expected, from the distance of lime, and the toil and expence of marl. When first tried, having been unskilfully made, the roots and seeds of weeds adhered to the component parts, retained their vegetative quality, and overran the fields on which composts were laid. On this account they were for some time in disrepute, but begin to be better understood, and more skilfully managed. Lime or marl is always one principal ingredient. Lime is mixed with earth, moss, turf, straw, rubbish, the stuff dug out of ditches and drains, or scraped together from streets and roads, and the refuse of gardens. All, or part of these, are thrown together in larger or smaller quantities as they can be got. Care is taken to keep them free from weeds, and

to

to apply as much lime in regular strata as will completely reduce them to powder. Composts are also made of lime, and weeds alone freed as well as possible from earth, the proportion of lime being always sufficient to destroy their power of vegetation. In all these composts, much depends not only on the quantity of lime, but also on its being attentively embodied into the other materials, and allowed time to operate its full effect on them. Marl is only mixed with moss, straw, or rubbish. With moss it has been found to answer vastly well on lands inclinable to clay; and both with moss and the other ingredients it fertilises lighter lands. But the mixture must be carefully made, and not too soon carried to the land. Time must always be given for the materials to corrupt and to coalesce.

Composts are likewise made of lime or marl with earth. But the earth is erroneously taken from the surface, where baneful seeds may lurk unperceived. By dipping below it for fresh soil never before stirred, purer and richer composts might be made with smaller proportions of lime or marl, and at less expence. Virgin earth is itself a manure, readily unites with lime or marl, ferments soon and vigorously, and becomes a mass of complete putrefaction.

SECT. IV.—*Weeding.*

ALL that can be observed, on this particular, has been already anticipated in Chap. VII. Sections 4th and 5th, to which the reader is referred.

SECT.

Sect. V.—*Watering.*

WATERING has not hitherto been attempted; but there are so many places in the county, to which it would be advantageous, that some gentlemen and farmers propose, either to bring down a skilful operator in that line from some part of England where it is practised, or to send some person of education and intelligence thither to be instructed in the art.

CHAP.

CHAP. XIII.

LIVE STOCK.

Sect. I.—*Black Cattle.*

IF ever there was a breed of black cattle peculiar to this county, it cannot now be distinguished. For several years, a number of the Northumberland, Lancashire, Galloway, and west country kinds, a few of the Dutch and Guernsey, and many from the northern counties of Scotland, have been brought into Roxburghshire; and their offspring, from various crosses with each other, forms the principal part of its present motley stock. The milch cows are in general short-horned, deep-ribbed, and of a red and white colour; but are also found polled, and of every various horn, shape, and colour. In the more level and richer part of the county, they approach in size and quality towards the large improved breed, which has of late been carefully reared in the contiguous district of Northumberland. Their milk and butter are excellent, and they weigh when fattened from 45 to 60 stones*. Those of a lesser size somewhat

exceeding

* From 56 to 78 or 80 stone English.

exceeding half that weight, are found to thrive best in the
higher grounds. Two kinds begin to obtain a preference,
as giving from 8 to 12 Scotch pints every day during summer of rich milk, yielding butter of an admirable flavour,
and being easy feeders; one of them is the polled or Galloway kind, whose properties are well known over all the
island; and the other is a breed with small horns of a middling length, thin necks, round deep bodies, and short stout
legs. Each of these will reach, when properly fed, from
32* to 45 stones. And from 36 to 40 stones may be considered
as the average of fat cattle through the county. As some
gentlemen and farmers, of late, are at great pains in the
choice of their bulls, there is reason to hope that these two
breeds may be brought to greater perfection, or that a better than either, with all the best properties of both, may be
procured from some judicious or fortunate mixture.

But great attention will not probably be paid to this object, while the markets at Kelso and Jedburgh maintain their
character for fine veal, and while farmers draw greater profits from feeding than from their dairies. About 620
calves are killed every year by the butchers in Kelso
alone †, and 1400 more may be safely allotted to Jedburgh, Hawick, and other lesser markets in the county,
besides what are carried out of it, and fed by private families for their own use. The prodigious quantity of milk,
necessary to fatten even 2000 calves ‡, and to rear nearly as
many, is one reason why very little cheese is made, and
no more butter than is barely sufficient for the consumpt of
the inhabitants, and for salving the sheep. Liddesdale is to
be

T

* From 40 to 56¼ stones English.

† See Statistical Account of Kelso, vol. 10. p. 590.

‡ The average rate is about 7 or 8 pints per day, for 5 or 6 weeks each,
to calves when fattening, and about four or five pints to such as are reared,
for thirteen or perhaps fifteen weeks.

be excepted, where butter and cheese are fold to the amount
of L. 1000 a-year; and where the nature of the foil will probably call the attention of farmers to increase the number
and improve the breed of milch cows. In the reft of this
large county, they are objects of inferior attention to fpayed
queys and oxen intended for the ftall. Yet the number,
reared annually for this purpofe, bears an inconfiderable proportion to thofe, which are bought in autumn and the beginning of winter in Northumberland, at the northern tryfts, or
on their road paffing to England. Thefe, and many others,
bred in the neighbourhood, or collected from different corners, when of a proper age, and in tolerable condition, are
fed on turnips, and fold as foon as they are decently fat, or
kept on till the end of fpring in hopes of higher prices; but,
when very young or lean *, they get only ftraw, coarfe hay,
and the refufe of turnips, till they are turned out to grafs
about the beginning or middle of May, and, if not fit for the
butcher by the end of harveft, are then brought into the turnip ftall. They are tied to the ftake by the neck or by the
horns; and there are feveral contrivances to prevent them
from raifing their heads fo high as to fwallow, without chew-
ing it, a fmall turnip, or a piece of a large one, by which
they run the rifk of being choked. To chain them by the
horns, befides anfwering this purpofe, has the further advantage of keeping them from licking themfelves, which
both carries hairs into their ftomachs, and difcolours the
flefh of the parts expofed to the tongue. Care is taken to
rub them well with old curry-combs and brufhes, to remove
their dung,. and to give them frefh litter, at leaft twice or
thrice every day, and oftener if neceffary. The bulbs of
turnips

* It is thought that the prefent high price of butcher-meat will induce
farmers to feed even *young* and *lean* cattle as quickly as poffible, inftead of
keeping them over winter to be fattened on next fummer's grafs.

turnips are thrown before them every morning and after-
noon till they are satiated *. At night they get a little straw
and sometimes hay; and they lie down 4 or 5 hours at mid-
day, and 9 or 10 during the night. They are never loosened nor allowed to taste water, and by some they are bled as
often as occasion requires. Some farmers are of opinion that
they will fatten as fast, and that their flesh will be better, by
allowing them liberty, at times, to breathe the fresh air in
the straw-yard. There can be no doubt of this treatment
being salubrious, if there is no danger of their hurting each
other. Their increase in weight and price depends, in a
great measure, on their tendency to grow fat, on their management, and on the length of time they are fed. In 4 or.
5 months, they add, at an average, about one fourth to the
weight at which they were tied up, and yield about 36 *per
cent.* of profit on the money paid for them. When kept
over two winters, their weight is generally more than doubled, and their profit is commonly above *cent. per cent.*
Three of them will nearly fatten on two acres of good turnips, the average value of which may therefore be computed at L. 3, 15 s. or L. 4 *per* acre. There cannot be fewer
than 6000 † black cattle of all ages and sizes fed annually.
                                                    But

---

* Some farmers allege, with great plausibility, that cattle ought never to be
satiated, but to get a certain allowance regularly, and to be left with a cra-
ving appetite; and that they ought also to get a little straw or hay in the
middle of the day.

† This number may be thought wholly inadequate to the great quantity of
land stated to be in turnips, (Chap. VII. Sect. 4.), especially if 3 bullocks can
be fed on 2 acres. But it is given as an average for several years, and the
average quantity of land in turnips, during that period, was at least 6000 acres
less than it is at present. Allowing it to be 18000 acres, one-third of it must
be computed to fail altogether, or to yield little produce; the largest half of
the remainder is consumed by sheep designed for the shambles, or by the stock
on the farm, whether black cattle or sheep, to enlarge their size, and keep
                                                    them

But this number will probably decrease, in proportion as sheep are found equally profitable with less trouble.

Few oxen are employed in husbandry, nor is it probable that here they will ever come into great request. For tho' they are more easily maintained than horses, can be trained both to the plough and cart, and can be fed to great advantage after being wrought, yet they are unfit for the long carriages of grain, lime, and coals, they are less docile than horses, must be oftener renewed, and cannot stand fatigue so well, or perform any work so expeditiously; and dispatch is of vast importance to a farmer, especially in an inland county, where his profits may often depend on his getting manure brought quickly to his land, his feed, particularly turnips, quickly sown, and his grain sent quickly to market. They may be of considerable use, however, in breaking up new ground, while horses are fetching marl or lime to it. And it is not improbable that, in many places, they may be yoked in thrashing machines, to free horses from a motion which some allege is hurtful to them, and to prevent them from being taken from other labours, where speed is more requisite.

Black

them in good plight; so that scarcely more than 5000 or at most 6000 acres are left for the feeding cattle; and these, at an average, cannot be reckoned so very good as to feed more than a bullock each, or perhaps 4 of them may feed 5. On the other hand, the number of fat cattle may appear disproportionately great to the 700 annually killed at Kelso (Statistical Account, vol. 10. p. 590). But the quantity of veal sold there bears a much larger proportion to what is used in the county, than the quantity of beef does. More than three times that number of beeves are annually killed in the other markets and by private families. And nearly two-thirds of those fed in the county are carried to Northumberland and Mid-Lothian. According to both these views, the actual number of black cattle should exceed 7000, and I must be quite safe in stating it above 6000.

Black cattle, in every period of their lives, are subject
to several diseases. Calves, during the first three or four
weeks, are sometimes seized with an inflammation in the
intestines, provincially called the *liver-crook* or *strings*. It
is attended with a strangury and seldom cured ; though
bleeding gently, in an early stage, has been successful, and
it may be prevented by cutting the navel-string of the
calf, when newly dropped, till it bleeds. About the same
age, they have been attacked with a swelling in the joints
of their hind-legs, which may be cured by frequent fomen-
tations and poultices of chamomile and other herbs, and by
rubbing the parts with flannel immediately after the fo-
mentation, and on changing the poultice. There are likewise instances of their being carried off by water in the
head, called here a *sturdy* ; but none of these diseases are
frequent, though the first mentioned is the most common.

Young cattle, from one to three years old, are subject to
a disease called the *rot*, a kind of consumption, occasioned
by improper exposure to damps either from the atmosphere
or soil, and sometimes by want of wholesome food. It appears in a kind of soft watery swelling below the jaws,
which has been in one or two instances let out with success ;
but the disease for the most part, especially in warm weather and in good pasture, terminates in a violent and mor-
tal flux.

Aged cattle, especially females, are liable to be hide-
bound, a disease known here and in the neighbouring counties by the name of the *fell-ill*. The *fell* or skin, instead
of being soft and loose, becomes hard, and sticks closely to
the flesh and bones, a state in which no creature can thrive.
The cure is bleeding, and laxative and nourishing food.
Herbs, boiled in new ale or mashes of malt, with some butter and a little grated ginger, should be given lukewarm,
till

till the difeafe begins to yield, and then green food, or boiled meat well cooled. This difeafe is very often accompanied by another in the tail. One of thofe grifly members,
of which it is compofed, becomes foft, and muft be freed
from hair, flit longwife till it bleeds freely, plaftered with
garlic and foot, and covered for fome days with a rag till it
heals. By eating fome venomous plants, their tongue fometimes fwells, and puftules rife upon it. Till thefe are opened and wafhed with falt and water, cattle cannot pluck and
chew their food. When reared on open pafture, and afterwards carried to fields where there is heath or brufhwood, they are feized frequently with a ferious and alarming difeafe, called the *wood-ill*, and fometimes the *moor-
ill*, generally afcribed to their eating fome herbage growing among the heath or bufhes, to which they were
not accuftomed from their infancy. Their head fwells,
their eyes are inflamed, their urine is red, and they become
very coftive. A handful of falt mixed with a mutchkin *
or more of their own blood, as it comes warm from their
veins, poured down their throats, is a common and fuccefsful
remedy. Port-wine and bark have alfo been attended with
a good effect. An Englifh pint of falt and water, given twice
a-day for a week or more, till they are reconciled to the
pafture, and then gradually leffened, is a good preventive.
Vermin, which fometimes infeft them in fpring, are deftroyed by tar-water and falt, by black-foap made into an
ointment with gunpowder, and by tobacco-juice. The
fcab, or a kind of itch with incrufted and virulent puftules,
with which they are alfo, though rarely, vifited, is more
infectious, and difficult to be cured. They are bathed or
rubbed with preparations of fulphur and nitre; but without care to keep them warm, this remedy has proven fatal.

---

* Somewhat lefs than an Englifh pint.

tal. A strong mercurial ointment will remove both vermin and scab more speedily, and with less danger, if the animals are kept, for two or three days, on aperient food and drink gently warmed, and get a purgative when the outward application is over. In wet weather, ulcers arise in the clefts of their hoofs, which are easily cured by washing and rubbing them till they bleed, applying a little spirit of vitriol, and keeping them dry for a few days. Cows sometimes cast their calves in spring; and, as this misfortune generally happens to more than one of a herd, it is attributed to improper food, especially to coarse hay, when much spoiled and smelling disagreeably; which shews the vast importance of giving wholesome provender to cattle. When bad hay is not quite corrupted, it may be corrected, in some degree, by being exposed to a keen penetrating air, and sprinkled with salt and water immediately before it is used.

Cows, when put upon good pasture to be fattened, are apt to suffer much from bealed udders, occasioned by the milk not going entirely from them, or by its returning through the influence of the grass, after having left them while eating dry fodder. If the suppurated matter, with some assistance from a skilful hand, does not find a proper vent for itself, it becomes necessary sometimes to cut off one of the dugs to allow it a full discharge. In either case, the part is frequently anointed with a mixture of tar and butter, to keep the wound open and free from flies. The best preventives are, to milk the teats perfectly dry without leaving the least drop, and not to touch them again though milk should gather, to bleed the animal every ten or twelve days, and to give her for some days draughts of tar, alum, madder, vinegar, and other astringents mixed with or dissolved in water.

SECT.

SECT. II.—*Sheep.*

ROXBURGHSHIRE has long been famous for the number and excellence of its sheep. Those, with black faces and legs, short bodies, and coarse wool, are now wholly given up as a breeding stock. A few of them are kept for the table, because their mutton has a delicate flavour. The vast superiority of their wool has, every where, obtained a decided preference for the white-faced and long-bodied kind; and attempts are daily making to improve their carcases, without injuring the quality of their fleeces. Their chief defect is low and thin shoulders; to remedy which, three farmers, viz. Mr John Edmistoun, late of Mindrum, and Mr James Robson, then at Philhope, both in Northumberland, and Mr Charles Ker, then at Riccaltoun in this county, went to Lincolnshire about 40 years * ago, before the breed there had degenerated, and purchased 14 rams, picked out of threescore in the possession of one man. These rams were white-faced; had excellent forequarters; carried a great quantity of fine and close wool with little *waste* or coarse in it; and throve well. They improved Mr Ker's sheep very much in shape and carcase, and increased both the quantity and quality of their wool. Mr Robson sold the first wedders produced from crossing his ewes with them at a considerable advance. He brought their progeny into

Roxburghshire .

---

* This fact is mentioned in the General View of the Agriculture of Northumberland, p. 21. as having happened *thirty-three* years before 1794; but as Mr Robson came to Scotland in 1760, and had these rams four or five years before he left Northumberland, it must have been about forty years since the experiment was tried. I embrace this opportunity of acknowledging the instruction and assistance which I have received, in drawing up this work, from the sensible observations made in that publication, and in Mr Culley's Treatise on Live Stock.

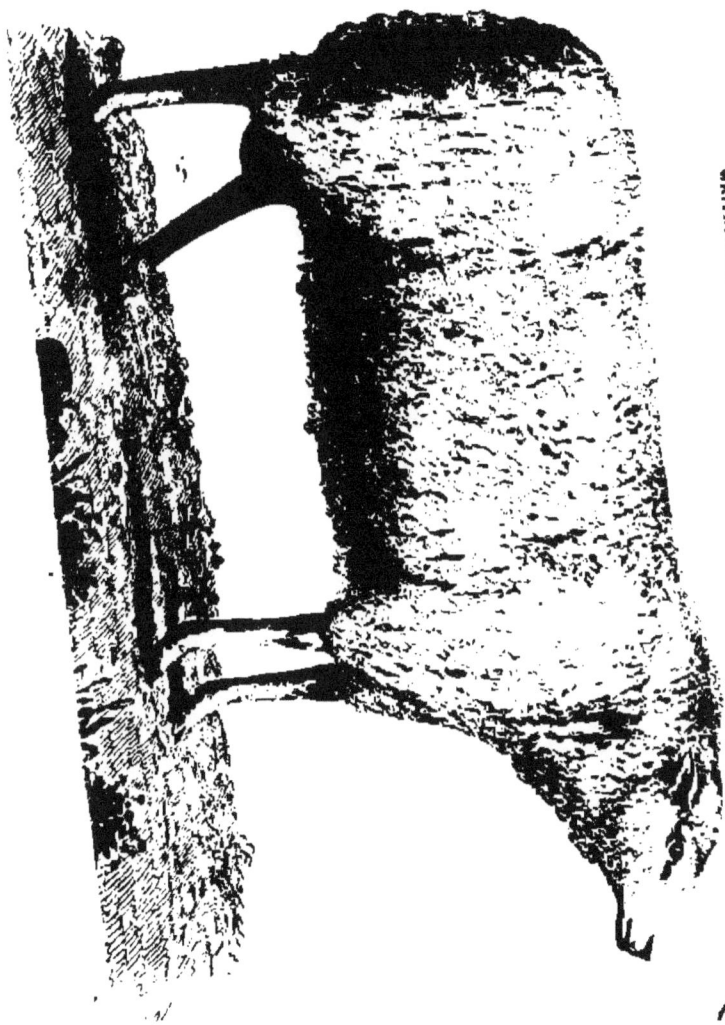

WHITE-FACED or CHEVIOT RAM, with a cross between of the DISHLEY BLOOD.

Roxburghshire in 1760, and is decidedly of opinion, that the effects of this cross, in meliorating the chine, the fore-quarter, and the wool, still remain in his flocks. Since that time, by various changes of rams, some of which have a portion of the Dishley breed, and by a judicious selection of shapely ewes for breeding, several neighbouring flocks may vie with those of Mr Robson; and there is reason to hope, that a continuance of the same spirit of inquiry and enterprise may bring them to still greater perfection.

Wethers of such improven flocks, when sold by the breeders a little fed at $3\frac{1}{2}$ years old, are at an average about 14 lib. [*] per quarter; ewes scarcely eleven. The former feed to 18 lib. [†] often higher, according to the season, the pasture, and the time they are kept at grass or turnips; the latter are sold lean, to breed from a year or two in other places, and then are fed on turnips, when they reach from 14 to 16 lib. In the northern parts of the county, where this improved breed is only slowly making its way, wethers on the hill rarely exceed $10\frac{1}{2}$ lib., and ewes $8\frac{1}{2}$ or 9 lib.; and feed, the former to 14 or $14\frac{1}{2}$ sometimes to 15 lib., the latter generally to 12 lib. or perhaps a little more.

It seems to be admitted, that an acre will nearly maintain a sheep to the south of Jedwater, but that to the north of it about $1\frac{1}{4}$ of an acre will be requisite, and that in a great part of Liddesdale a sheep will eat almost the whole produce of two acres. Intelligent farmers, in different corners, who are well acquainted with the whole county, agree that somewhat more than $1\frac{1}{2}$ of an acre, and somewhat less than $1\frac{1}{4}$ of an acre, may be allowed to each sheep. The former would make their number 206,438, the latter 193,538, and

U   the

[*] About $17\frac{1}{4}$ lib. English.

[†] Above 22 lib. English.

the exact medium is a mere trifle below 200,000, which cannot be far from the truth. Hence their real value can be easily ascertained, both at their present high prices of 20 s. or a guinea, or at their former and more common rates of 15 s. or 16 s. a-piece.

The relative proportion of wethers, ewes, and young sheep, kept on different farms, varies, according to the nature and exposure of the pasture, and sometimes according to accidental circumstances. Grounds, where young sheep are liable to diseases, are naturally stocked with those which are aged; while the weaned lambs, here called *hogs*, are sent to more healthy pastures. In some farms ewes only are kept, and in others wethers, which last are bought young, and, after two or three years, are sold to the grazier or butcher. One-half of the stock upon a breeding farm, when enumerated at the time of salving, is generally supposed to consist of ewes from which lambs are expected the following season; somewhat more than two-thirds of the other half are wethers young and old; and the remainder are ewe-hogs, to supply the place of such old ones as may be sent to market during the next year, either because of their missing a lamb, or of their growing too old for breeders.

A few years ago, salving sheep with tar was, in several places, on the decline, from the higher price given for white wool, but is again gaining ground, as the same advanced price cannot now be obtained. Of white wool about 10 fleeces are requisite to make a stone, and in 1795 it brought L. 1, 3 s. which is only 2 s. 3$\frac{3}{10}$ d. *per* fleece; whereas a stone of salved wool has scarcely 8 fleeces, and that year sold for L. 1, 1 s. or 2 s. 7$\frac{1}{2}$ d. *per* fleece. This increase, indeed, will barely defray the expence of salving

the

the sheep; but while farmers are not tempted by larger
profits, they will return to a practice, which has been found,
by experience, to keep their flocks warm and free from
vermin during winter, and to produce wool of a finer pile
as well as in greater abundance. It should also be mentioned, that 8 fleeces of salved wool weigh rather more than
a stone; for $7\frac{1}{4}$ or $7\frac{1}{2}$ fleeces are reckoned an average stone
of all the wool in the county: And considering the many
parcels, which are annually produced, of fleeces from 5 to
7 *per* stone, in comparison of the few which require 9 and
10 to the stone, that average must be pretty just. Allowing, however, 8 fleeces to every stone, the annual quantity in the county will be 25,000 stone, which in 1795 a-
mounted to as many pounds Sterling, and this year was
about one-fifth more.

At the end of autumn the operation of salving begins,
and, except in a very unfavourable season, is finished before
Martinmas. It can only be performed to advantage when
the fleece is dry. The general rule, formerly, was to use
equal quanties of tar and butter; and little regard was paid
to the quality of either. Such a load of indifferent tar both
hurt the wool, and was an unnecessary burden on the sheep.
Care is, now, taken to procure good tar; and a much greater proportion of butter is added, at least a third part, commonly more. With two gallons* of tar some mix $1\frac{1}{4}$ †
stone of butter, as a sufficient allowance for threescore of
sheep. But, for the same number, it is more common to
allot only one stone of butter to two gallons of tar ‡. To
incorporate

---

* English measure	† Equal to 36 lib. English.		
‡ 1 stone butter,	-	L. 0 13	4
2 gallons tar,	- -	0 3	0
For 60 sheep,	-	L. 0 16	4
And for each sheep about		0 0	$3\frac{1}{4}$

But

incorporate them completely, the butter is flowly melted
and poured upon the tar, and they are conftantly ftirred till
they become cool enough for ufe. The wool is diftinctly
parted into rows from the head to the tail of the animal,
and this mixture is rubbed carefully with the finger on the
fkin at the bottom of each row. A man will, at an average, falve 20 in a day. When of a proper kind, ufed in
moderation, and fkilfully applied, tar is univerfally found
to be falutary to fheep, an improvement to their wool, and
eafily feparated from it during the procefs of making it into cloth. But it ftill remains to afcertain, what is the precife
quantity which will beft anfwer thefe good purpofes, and
whether the quantity fhould not vary, according to the expofure and foil of different farms, the nature of different
fheep, or fome particularity in their circumftances.

The period of geftation with ewes is 21 weeks; and the
ram is not admitted to them till the end of November or
beginning of December, that they may lamb about the
20th of April. In fome of the lower and warmer farms,
lambs are allowed to come a few weeks earlier; in the
colder diftricts, they are made ten days or a fortnight later. Their prefervation and health being of the greateft
importance, many precautions are taken to fecure both.
Some wool is pulled from the udders * of the ewes to give
them readier accefs to the teats; farmers are naturally defirous of their being brought forth, when there is a probability

But, as both the proportion of the ingredients, and the quantity put upon each
fheep, vary in different parts of the county, fo muft alfo the expence, and
4 d. or 4½ d. is thought to be nearly the average, efpecially as the addition
of ¼ ftone of butter makes an increafe of 1¼ d. on each fheep.

* All fheep are udder-locked, as it is here called, that being thought re-
frefhing and falutary.

bility of the weather proving mild, and of the grafs being plentiful for their mothers; endeavours are conftantly ufed to keep pregnant ewes in good condition, and to put them on the beft paftures before the expected time of their lamb- ing, as well as to continue them upon it while they give fuck; and, with this view, though flocks may fometimes range promifcuoufly in winter, yet early in fpring they are fepa- rated into different parcels (provincially *hirfels*) of hogs, gimmers *, wethers, and ewes, each of which, under a dif- tinct fhepherd, is kept on a different part of the farm, left fuch, as are uncumbered with lambs, fhould eat up the moft nutritive food from the ewes and their young.

Lambs, when three or four weeks old, are attentively infpected, when a few of the moft likely males, produced from fhapely ewes by good tups, are felected for rams, and the reft cut for wethers. Mild and dry weather is al- ways preferred for performing this cruel though neceffary operation, the extremes of heat and cold bearing equally hard on the young animals. After being fuckled from nine to thirteen weeks, according to difference of fituations, fea- fons, and circumftances, they are weaned, and fubjected to a fecond infpection, that the farmer may pick out the moft promifing to fupply his flock with breeding ewes and we- thers, and fell the remainder as they become ready for the fhambles or the market. There are fome, but very few inftances of lambs being allowed to fuck longer than thir- teen weeks.

A confiderable time before the ewes are deprived of their lambs, the other fheep on the farm are plunged, as often as is neceffary, over head and ears into a deep pool, and left
to

* A *gimmer* is the name given to a young ewe after being once fhorn. When fhorn a fecond time fhe is called an *ewe*.

to swim out of it. The ewes undergo the same operation, sometimes before, but more generally after, their lambs are taken away. This is intended to free their fleeces from the mud and sand which adheres to the salve; and they are clipped or shorn as soon as they are sufficiently dry. An expert shearer will clip 50 fleeces in a day; but 42 may rather be taken as the average. Their wool is kept in distinct parcels, that of young sheep being more valuable, and fetching a higher price when rated separately, or increasing the lumped price of the whole. At sheep-shearing *, a mark is given, or renewed, for distinguishing the different properties of neighbours, and the sex and age of sheep on the same farm.

The diseases, incident to this useful animal, may be ranked, according to their prevalence and inveteracy, in the following order, adopting the names by which they are known here, viz. sickness, louping-ill, sturdy, rot, and braxy. The three first attack chiefly young sheep, and the two last old ones.

The sickness † is a kind of inflammation and stoppage in the bowels, resembling an iliac passion, for the most part incurable, and occasioning, sometimes a speedy, and at other times a lingering death. When the carcase is opened, the flesh is always discoloured, and the urine has a fetid smell. Wether hogs are much subject to it, especially towards the close of autumn, and also, though more rarely, in spring. It is supposed to arise from different causes. It is imputed to their eating too greedily certain grasses, which spring up quickly after rain, and which produce a more

violent

* The reader is referred for a poetical description of this operation to Thomson's Summer, and may be assured that it is as just as it is beautiful.

† I understand this disease is called the Braxy in many places both in England and Scotland.

violent effect on their irritable intestines, than on those of
older sheep. This conjecture is confirmed by the distemper losing both its frequency and its virulence in some
farms, where, during the dangerous seasons, the young and
old were brought into the same pasture, and the former
were prevented from devouring too much of the sweet yet
noxious food, by the equal fondness shewn for it by the latter, and their superior strength to secure the largest share
for themselves. This disease has also been engendered by
the hard and dry food, on which sheep are constrained
to subsist in the end of autumn or beginning of winter,
when little else is produced on their pasture, and especially in a severe frost, descending, in an undigested state,
into their bowels, and remaining there till an inflammation
is excited. In this case, the obstruction might be prevented or removed, by green food of an aperient nature, or even
by a little salt timeously administered. In a more advanced state, but before the disease has made too great progress,
perhaps 50 or 60 drops of laudanum, in some insinuating
and powerful purgative, like castor or even lintseed oil,
might be of service*.

                                                    The

* After having digested and compressed the information, which I received
concerning sheep, as well as I could, I was favoured by Sir John Sinclair with
the following note from another publication, with a desire to insert it. To
render my compliance with this request more extensively useful, I shewed the
note to several sheep-farmers, conversed with them on the subject, and took
down from one of them some observations, which are distinguished from the
note by wanting inverted commas.

" The distemper, called the *braxy*, which in Scotland is so fatal to the
" flocks, merits to be particularly attended to. Lambs are most subject to
" this disorder; it in common makes its first appearance with the hoar frosts
" at the latter end of the year, and is most felt by those kept in cold and
" exposed situations; when they are dead, their bladder either is burst, or is
" found quite full of urine, and that of a very strong smell. This disorder,
" most probably, proceeds from the following cause: Sheep, when left to
" follow their own natural habits, retire to rest early at night, nor do they
                                                    " rise

The louping-ill affects the whole or part of the body, like
a palfy, or apoplexy, flopping the circulation of the blood,
                                                                and

" rife to feed till day-light. At the feafon of the year above mentioned,
" the fheep, and more efpecially the lambs, not liking to feed on the grafs,
" till the fun has taken off the froft, remain longer in their layers than in
" common; during which time, fo large a quantity of urine is collected
" in the bladder, that it caufes a fuppreffion, and the fheep is not able to
" ftale. All animals breed more urine in cold frofty weather, than in mild,
" in confequence of their perfpiring lefs, and of courfe, if in health, ftale
" more frequently. The following may be found of ufe in the above dif-
" order: Nitre pounded fmall 60 grains (or a teafpoon-full), liquid laudanum
" 20 drops, to be given in a teacup-full of water, and to be put down the
" throat of the lamb with a fpoon.—Or two tablefpoon-fulls of caftor-oil
" with twenty drops of liquid laudanum.—Or fixty grains of nitre, with
" twenty drops of laudanum, in a teacup of cold water, may be found to
" anfwer; if they do not operate, and produce the defired effect in an hour,
" the dofe muft be repeated.—Or a little Hollands gin may be of fervice,
" with twenty drops of laudanum, remembering, after the medicine is given,
" the fheep ought to be drove about gently, and fuffered to ftop at times
" that it may have an opportunity to ftale; and by being drove about gen-
" tly, it will caufe the medicine to operate the fooner, as no time is to be
" loft; they are not to be made to run, as the weight of water in the blad-
" der would increafe the inflammation; this diforder might, certainly, in a
" great meafure, be prevented by bringing the lambs, at the end of the
" year, into warm inclofed grounds; and, if the owner of the lambs has not
" an inclofure, the fhepherd ought to be amongft them very early in the
" morning, with his dogs, to make them quit their layers, that they may
" ftale."

This laft practice has been frequently tried, from a fufpicion that the difeafe might proceed from the caufe here affigned, but did not always prove
effectual. And befides the fuppreffion of urine, there are other kinds of this
difeafe, or perhaps rather concomitant and inveterate fymptoms of it. One
of them is an inflammation between the *fell*, or lower fkin, and the flefh,
which foon becomes a mortification and is incurable. Another is hard, con-
creted, and indigefted food, obftinately adhering to the inteftines, which may
be obviated by an injection of fweet oil, if early given. Sometimes, too,
there is an inflammation in the gut, which has been cured by bleeding and
moderate exercife.

                                                                Thus

and cauſing a total or partial ſuſpenſion of motion. It is
moſt common in bleak and cold ſeaſons. It has the appearance,

Thus far go the note and the farmer's obſervations; and on them I take
the liberty of remarking, in hopes of making the ſubject more generally underſtood, that it is not lambs, but hogs or young ſheep from ſix to 18 or even
21 months old, which are moſt ſubject to this diſtemper; and that, from all
the facts which I have been able to collect, concerning the manner of their
being ſeized, the remedies which have been tried, and the appearance of the
carcaſes, it is doubtful, whether the ſuppreſſion of urine be a cauſe, or an
effect of the diſeaſe. For though the urine has always a ſtrong rank ſmell,
and though this may ariſe from its being ſuppreſſed, yet it ſeems leſs probable,
that the ſuppreſſion ſhould be occaſioned, by the hogs lying a few hours
longer than uſual in a froſty morning, than by ſome prediſpoſition in the habit
to irritation, either on their eating ſome particular food in ſo great quantities,
and in ſuch a ſtate, as not to be eaſily diſſolved in the ſtomach, or on their
drinking water that is noxious, or any water when they are too warm, or on
their being expoſed to ſudden tranſitions from heat to cold. There are ſome
human conſtitutions much more prone to inflammatory diſorders than others;
and why may not this likewiſe be the caſe among ſheep? The farmer's account of the diſeaſe ariſing from indigeſted food is ſubſtantially the ſame
with that given in the text; and the inflammation in the gut may be ſuppoſed
to be a natural conſequence of this obſtruction. His cures merit attention, eſpecially the injection of ſweet oil. With reſpect to the cures propoſed in the
note, I am happy to find the author concurring in my idea of the caſtor oil
and laudanum; but cannot approve of ſo large a doſe of the oil and ſo little
laudanum. A teaſpoon-full, or at leaſt 50 drops of the latter will throw the
animal into a ſtupor for ſome hours, ſtop the progreſs of the inflammation,
and afford time for the former to operate. The proper quantity of oil muſt
be aſcertained by experience; but I ſhould think, as one tableſpoon-full is a
ſufficient doſe for a ſtout man, in any ordinary caſe, it may well operate on
a young ſheep.

The note proceeds as follows: " Houſe-lambs, brought to the London mar-
" kets, with their legs tied, are ſubject to a diſorder like the braxy, their
" bladders being full of urine, as they will not ſtale with their legs tied; the
" butchers, after they have brought them home, give them a little clean
" ſweet, oat-ſtraw, which they like to pick amongſt, and with it a pail or
" two of clean water; when they find themſelves at liberty, and have the
" ſtraw under them, they moſt probably ſtale, and are well of courſe; but
" an

X

ance, in fome cafes, of being hereditary, purfuing the fame
flocks when removed to a different pafture, and, in other
cafes, of being attached to particular grounds, vifiting all
flocks which are brought upon them. Thefe circumftances
lead to a conjecture, that it might arife from ftrange fheep
catching cold, by lying down after fatigue to reft upon wet
and unhealthy ground, and communicating to their offspring
the latent feeds of debility or difeafe, which then had deeply infected their blood. But others infift, with no fmall
plaufibility, that it is nothing elfe than a numbnefs and inability brought on by the ticks * fucking their blood, till the
fheep become faint and powerlefs from the want of it, and
allege, in confirmation of this opinion, the following undoubted facts; that neither the vermin nor the difeafe were
known in this county half a century ago; that both made
their appearance at the fame period; that ticks are always
found in the fields, where the louping-ill prevails, and on
the bodies of every fheep that dies of it, except perhaps in

a

" an experienced butcher looks at them, after they have been in his cellar or
" yard an hour or two, and at night before he goes to bed; if at any of thofe
" times, he finds a lamb to be ill from the above diforder, which he knows
" by its hanging down its head, drooping its ears, grinding of the teeth,
" fetting up the back, &c. he kills it, and finds the bladder ready to burft
" with urine; and if it has been fuffered to remain long ill, the fweetbread
" will be found much fhrunk and wafted from the pain.

" In defperate cafes, the fhepherd might-cut the fkin of the belly over
" the bladder, then open a fmall orifice in the bladder, with a knife or other
" inftrument to let the water out, and afterwards few up the fkin of the
" belly, as in fpaying animals, and cover it with a pitch plafter; the blad-
" der will heal of its own accord. Whilft this operation is performing, the
" lamb is to be held up by the hind legs, till the water is difcharged, and
" laid on the back till the fkin is fewed up."

What follows in the note, I have omitted, as it relates to the *black-water*,
a difeafe altogether unknown in this county.

* See an account of them below, p. 165.

a very few inflances, where enough of blood was not left
for maintaining them.   Zink, and white vitriol, have both
been tried, and fometimes fucceeded in removing it, but oftener failed. A warm bath, and bleeding in the belly, have
likewife effected cures, and one or other of thefe is thought
to be the fafeft remedy, when applied before the difeafe has
got too firm a feat.   Its yielding to bleeding feems to over-
throw the theory of its being the confequence of wanting a
fufficiency of blood.   But upon the fuppofition of its being
occafioned by ticks, it may be prevented by anointing the
animals infefted by them with mercurial ointment, which is
known to deftroy every kind of vermin, and by fprinkling
copioufly with lime-water thofe parts of the pafture where
they abound.   It may even be worth a farmer's expence,
upon a leafe of moderate length, to lime fields overrun with
them, and to rub with fome mercurial preparation, or tie a
fmall leathern bag with a little quickfilver in it around every fufpected fheep in his flock, a few weeks before the di-
ftemper commonly becomes moft prevalent.   If all the
fheep, thus treated, efcape the louping-ill, the preventive is
obvious and eafy.   Thefe two are the moft common and
the moft fatal difeafes to young fheep.

The fturdy, too, or water in the head, is not unfrequent
among them, and is firft difcovered by their appearing ftu-
pid and giddy.   Experienced fhepherds have a needle,
which they thruft up through the nofe to open a vent for
the water.   In other cafes, when the fkull is felt to be foft,
they cut a piece of it, take out the fmall bag * which contains the water, replace the piece, and plafter it firmly over

with

---

* I have heard it alleged that, fometimes, there are feveral diftinct bags or
cells full of water; and I have been referred to very refpectable authority
for fatisfaction on this point; but I have never had an opportunity of afcertaining the truth of it.

with pitch and wool. Patients have recovered by both operations, but oftener die; and there are instances of the disorder returning the following season. Some farmers, destitute neither of ingenuity nor observation, are of opinion, that the water originates in the tail, and gradually ascends along the ridge of the back to the head. But its appearing in sheep, whose tails were cut off immediately on their being lambed, and its return in several instances after being extracted, are not in favour of this theory.

The rot is properly defined, in Johnson's Dictionary, to be " a distemper among sheep which wastes their lungs." Yet unlike the consumptions, to which the human species is subjected, it is not infectious, at least much less so than other diseases among sheep. There can be little doubt of its proceeding from the same cause with the *sickness*, as it abounds chiefly in wet growing seasons, and in farms, where there are numerous oozing springs of water, or soft rich earth thrown up by mole-hills and on the sides of drains, producing a rapid growth of sweet and tender grass; a large quantity of which, swallowed hastily by young sheep, occasions an inflammation, and, eat more slowly and constantly by old ones, brings on the rot. The preventive here is obvious, and is attended to as far as it is practicable: salt and corn, given in an early stage, effect a cure; but the disease, when far advanced, admits of none.

The braxy, or perhaps rather *breakshaw*, is the name given in this county to a severe flux, which weakens and often carries off old sheep, especially ewes, and is so much dreaded as infectious, that, on its appearance among a flock, every sheep attacked by it is confined in a small inclosure, and carefully kept from drinking any thing but lime-water. Fortunately it rages chiefly at a season when there is plenty of grass; yet such is its inveteracy, that, in spite of good feeding, and astringent medicines, it generally proves fatal to a great

proportion

proportion of thofe whom it vifits. Might not ground rice
or ftarch, with a few drops of laudanum, be tried as an injection, or the rice boiled to a jelly and a little laudanum be
poured down the throat?

Sheep, too, are much infefted by vermin of different
kinds, the moft troublefome of which are ticks, little blood-
fucking animals, which pierce and tenacioufly adhere to the
fkin, peftering their victims fo inceffantly, that they cannot
fettle at their pafture, and fometimes caufing their death.
Ticks are always found, with a very few exceptions, on the
carcafes of fheep, which have died of the *louping-ill.* But
there are alfo inftances of lambs being deftroyed by ticks,
without any fymptoms of that diforder.

Both fheep and lambs are often loft from carelefſneſs, or
by accidents. Mothers, who are unnatural or want milk,
puſh away their new-dropped lambs, and others are forcibly
deprived of them by ftronger ewes ftill heavy with young.
In fuch cafes, the lambs, if not immediately noticed, fometimes die, and commonly are reduced greatly by hunger before they are relieved. A cold night, too, carries off fome
of them, efpecially when newly cut for wethers. Sheep
are frequently hurt by tumbling into holes, or being caught
in buſhes; and, if not fpeedily extricated, are in imminent
danger of perifhing. Many of them alfo are rendered lame,
by prickles running into their feet, and, in fome feafons,
by an excoriation or forenefs in their feet, which is conta-
gious, and known by the name of *foot-rot.* Every kind of
lamenefs muft be a manifeft difadvantage to animals, whofe
daily fubfiftence depends on the range they are able to take,
and, when it rifes to a great height, muft emaciate and deftroy them. But thefe loffes are trifling, in comparifon of
thofe which are fuftained from fnow. A number of fheep,
in a ftormy night, are fmothered by huge wreaths of prodigious

gious extent and depth, formed by eddies of the wind. Some
of them have been dug out alive and well, after being en-
tombed for many days, but, in general, they are found, either dead, or so weak as to require care, time, and the choi-
cest pasture, to bring them again into good plight. When
the ground is deeply covered with snow, there is a necessity,
either of feeding sheep with hay, or of driving them from
their hills to turnip-fields, sometimes at the distance of many
miles. The hay is carried in trusses on horseback, and given at the rate of a stone each day to every score of sheep.
A greater quantity is reckoned too high feeding, and the
cause of disease and mortality, when they return to their ordinary food. A less quantity would not keep them in proper condition, either to bring up lambs, or to take on fat.
This dry food, even when given with the utmost caution, is
hurtful to sheep; and the fatal effects of it are more or less
felt, in proportion to the length of time during which it is
eat *. Farmers would gladly have recourse to turnips, if a
sufficient quantity of them could be got. But as there are few
fields to be purchased, and these sometimes at the high price
of L. 6, and even L. 7 *per* acre, a sheep-farmer reckons himself very fortunate, if he can raise, on his own possession, or
procure, even at a high price, as many as will put his breeding ewes in good order for giving milk, and is obliged to rest
contented with hay for his other sheep during a lying snow,
and such food as the fields afford when it goes off. The average expence of feeding a score of sheep, on hay, is 5 s. 3 d. *per*
week, estimating the hay only at 9 d. *per* stone, whereas it is generally much higher, and on turnips, is 7 s. 6 d. or 4¼ d. each.
The continuance of snow for 4 or 5 weeks must thus cost
                                                    him,

---

* Perhaps the noxious effects of dry food might be lessened, by sprink-
ling a little salt and water on it, or giving the sheep daily a little salt dissolved in water.

him, at leaft, a guinea for every fcore he poffeffes; befides
the lofs to which he is expofed from difeafes and deaths after
its departure.   But this is really a faving on the whole, as
he would fuffer much more by leaving the fheep, like his
fore-fathers, to glean a fcanty fubfiftence on fome dry knolls,
from which they have fcraped or the wind has blown the
fnow, or by nibbling the tops of long heath, rufhes, or bent-
grafs.

The condition of fheep has been much improven, of late,
by keeping fewer of them on the fame ground which gives
them more food, by draining which both meliorates and increafes their pafture, by falving with better materials more
fkilfully proportioned and applied, and by giving breeding
ewes and young fheep a few turnips, or the beft feeding on
the farm, during winter.   By thefe means they grow to a
larger fize; they acquire a better fhape, for though they may
not rife much higher in the fore-quarter, they become round-
er in the ribs, and broader in the back; they are ftouter,
healthier, fatter; and they carry heavier if not finer fleeces.

There are 5 or 6 fmall flocks of the Difhley breed, kept
by gentlemen in rich inclofures, and by one or two farmers
in the arable diftrict.   They are remarkable for the beauty
of their fhapes, their tendency to fatten, their thin pelts *,
and their heavy fleeces.   Their bones are fmall and neat,
their backs broad and flat, and their bodies round like a barrel.   Wethers, at 2 or 2½ years old, weigh, at an average,
                                                      about

* Though their pelts are much thinner than thofe of any other large and
long-wooled fheep, yet they are a good deal thicker than thofe of the common Cheviot, and black-faced kinds.   The pelts of thefe laft, when in good
condition, are generally thought to be thinneft and to make the beft leather.

about 20 lib. * the quarter, and fold at two guineas or 40 s. each for feveral years in the neighbourhood, and this year (1796) at 50 s. in the county. Ewes, at 3, 4, or 5 years old, weigh, according to their age, from 17 to 20 lib. * the quarter, and fell from 1¼ guinea to 2 guineas a head. Their fleeces weigh from 6 to 9 lib. Englifh; and about 3½ of them will, at an average, make a † ftone of wool. The weight of their carcafes and fleeces renders them unfit to travel far for food; but on an eafy pafture, though coarfe, it is aftonifhing how fat they will grow in a fhort time, and how little they eat. Rams of this breed, reared in the county, were hired, both by gentlemen and actual farmers, at the rate of from 8 to 15 guineas for the feafon, with a view of improving their former breeds. Ewes have been tupped in the neighbourhood at no lefs than 2 guineas each. Some of them, noted for breeders, have been brought from different quarters, at a vaft expence. There is, at prefent, an appearance of their becoming more general in the lower parts of the county, and of further experiments being tried by croffing Cheviot ewes, in hilly paftures, with rams having more or lefs of their blood.

A few Spanifh, Herefordfhire, and Southdown fheep have been introduced into different parts of the county, and thrive tolerably well. I have not heard of a direct crofs between the Spanifh and the native breed of the county; but the iffue, of a crofs between the Spanifh and Southdown, has been croffed again with a Cheviot ram, and the young fheep produced by this fecond crofs, when clipped for the firft time, had much heavier fleeces than their dams, or any of

the

* Dutch weight, the lib. = 17½ ounce Englifh.
† The ftone = 24 lib. Englifh.

the real Southdown ewes on the farm. The Herefordshire, from their apparent delicacy, and the lightness of their fleeces, will not probably become favourites, notwithstanding the fineness of their wool. The Southdown, on the contrary, whose wool is little inferior, and who are lively, active, and hardy, bid fair to answer on high grounds, and to improve the wool of Cheviot sheep, without materially lessening or hurting their shapes. Yet two actual farmers [*], who gave some Herefordshire and Southdown ewes the same rams with the other ewes upon their farms, can perceive little or no difference between the progeny of the Hereford and Southdown ewes, either in size of carcase, quality of wool, or weight of fleece. The wool of both in 1795 sold for 2 guineas per stone, while the wool of Cheviot sheep only fetched 22 s. or 23 s. And the fleeces of both were nearly equal; eight of them when salved weighing a stone, and ten of them being requisite when not salved. A ram, from this cross, promises well both as to shape and wool. A few ewes at Riddel, partly Southdown, and partly a cross between them and Spanish, gave as much wool per fleece in 1795 as the average of the Cheviot sheep through the county, and of a much finer quality, having fetched 36 s. per stone instead of 22 s. The lambs of these ewes, by a Cheviot ram, are handsomer than their dams, and carry wool nearly as fine. The following note, obligingly communicated by Sir John Buchanan Riddel, shows the comparative weight of the fleeces of different kinds of sheep and their crosses, which were clipped on his estate in 1796, and sold for 45 s. per stone.

	lb.	oz.	dr.
Southdown ewes 2 years old per fleece,	2	6	9¾
Southdown ewe hogs, -	2	5	10
			Southdown

	lb.	oz.	dr.
Southdown croffed with Spanifh, -	2	0	0
Herefordfhire ewes (very old), -	1	12	5¼¾
Hogs got by a Cheviot ram out of the two			
laft-mentioned lots, -	2	11	7

Allowing the wool of the laft to be worfe than that of the
others, yet it is fo much heavier and finer than any wool
produced by pure Cheviot fheep as to recommend a fimilar
crofs to general attention. What may be the final refult of
various mixtures already attempted, or of other mixtures between rams from fome of the prefent croffes, or rams brought
down from improved ftocks of Hereford or Southdown
fheep, and Cheviot ewes *, time muft determine.

There is a fpecies of fheep at Faldanefide, towards the
north-weft extremity of the county, different from all that
have been mentioned. In their faces, fore-quarters, and general appearance, they feem to have fome remote relation
to the Difhley breed ; but are larger both in bone and fize,
not fo broad in the back, or round in the ribs, or thin in the
pelt ; refembling, in thefe defects, a fpecies of fheep formerly
very common in Berwickfhire and the lower parts of Northumberland, but now fcarcely to be found without fome
mixture of the Difhley blood. In other points, they feem
to partake of the Cheviot fheep, being active and hardy ;
and their fleeces, both in weight and length of pile, holding
a middle place between the long and fhort wooled fheep,
weighing, at an average, about 3 lib. each †, and requiring from 5 to 5¼ of them to a ftone. Their wool, though
long, approaches nearer to the clothing than to the comb-
                                                          ing

* See Mr Culley on Live Stock, p. 137.

† Or about 72 oz. Englifh.

ing kind, but, owing to its inconvenient length, does not bring a price equal to its fineness. Several of them are black, or rather grizzled, and yet, what is rather uncommon, their wool is not coarser than the white fleeces. Wethers weigh, on the pasture, about 17 lib. *per* quarter, and may be fed to 24 lib. One of them was sold in 1791 for L. 3, 2 s. Sterling.

The existence of such a breed, not original and distinct, but an evident mixture of short and long wooled sheep, may give birth to many speculations, concerning the advantages which may be obtained by crossing the Dishley and the Cheviot sheep, and the inconveniencies and dangers attending the attempt. Increase of the fore-quarter, enlargement of carcase, and greater weight of wool, are to be laid in balance, with the deterioration of the wool, not in quality but in usefulness and consequently in real value, with the inferiority of the pelts, and with the danger of such heavy animals, both in body and fleece, finding comfortable subsistence in cold, exposed, and steep districts, which are not, like Faldanefide, fertile and sheltered by nature, and highly enriched by marl. Lambs, from Dishley rams, by following Cheviot ewes through mountainous sheep-walks, and by being afterwards constrained to take a wide range for food, may be supposed to acquire the activity and hardiness of their mothers; but whether this really will be the case, or whether the exercise, by which they attain qualities so opposite to those of their father, may not prevent their growth in the fore-quarter, as well as in size and roundness of body, must be the result of many fair and careful experiments. On this subject Mr Ure remarks *, " The general laws, respect-" ing the economy of the animal system, seem to have a " near

* p. 59. L. 12.

" near refemblance, in many refpeds, to the general laws by
" which the vegetable fyftem is directed. In many fitua-
" tions, animals, equally with oats, &c. will infallibly dege-
" nerate, unlefs they are kept up by interchanges from foils,
" climates, and breeds, which, in many refpects, differ wide-
" ly from one another. This interchange, or mixture, is
" particularly neceffary in thofe fituations which are not
" natural to the animal, or fpecies of grain, with which
" they are flocked or fown. By this neceffity of an
" intermixture in the propagation of fubjects belonging
" to the kingdoms of nature, the admirable chain of mu-
" tual dependence is, in a great meafure, kept entire. The
" time is, perhaps, at no great diftance, when mankind, by
" an accumulation of experiments, will become proficients
" in a fubject, the knowledge of which is, probably, only in
" its infancy."

This paffage has given rife to the following anonymous
annotation on the margin of one of the printed reports tranfmitted to me. " Thefe obfervations, on mixing the breeds
" of fheep, feem to be founded more on theory than prac-
" tice. Some old experienced graziers think, that many a
" good native breed of fheep has been fpoiled for a particu-
" lar foil and climate, by croffing with other forts. Soil and
" climate will produce a breed, which may be kept from
" degenerating, by a proper felection of male and female to
" fave rams from; and fuch a breed will, on the whole, be
" generally found more profitable, than any croffed or mon-
" grel breed, which nature did not defign for that particular
" foil and climate."

Without prefuming to obtrude an opinion on a queftion
fo curious and important, I may be allowed to ftate the following general facts relative to it, which come within my
own obfervation. 1ft, There are feveral farms in this county, where fubftantial and permanent improvements have

been

been introduced into the breed of sheep, without any other precaution to preserve them from degenerating, than a proper selection of ewes for breeders, and of likely rams, either reared on the farms, or borrowed from neighbours. 2d, There are other farms, where the true Cheviot breed will degenerate either in wool, shape, or weight, or in all these respects, unless constant care is taken, every year, or at least every second year, to procure proper rams from flocks less apt to degenerate. 3d, In many farms, an entire change has been effected from the black-faced to the white-faced sheep, by using Cheviot rams for a succession of years. The distinguishing peculiarities of the one gave place to those of the other, in a slow and gradual manner; and in the course of four or five generations, or eight or nine years, all traces of the black face and legs, short shapes, and coarse wool, wholly disappeared. And it is the general belief, that a similar change may be brought about in the same period, in any farm whatever.

These facts shew, that very much may be done by judicious crosses, and that a good deal also, depends on soil and climate. Whether any alterations in these, produced by drains and plantations, will prove more favourable to one breed than to others, or prevent or lessen the tendency of particular breeds to degenerate in certain situations, remains yet to be ascertained. If any defect in the soil or climate makes a race of sheep to decline, it seems reasonable to suppose, that they should thrive when that defect is removed. The benefit resulting from drains * may be felt in a very few years; but a long time must elapse before trees newly planted can grow up to give shelter, and till that time shall arrive

* All the farms, where the most valuable Cheviot sheep are bred, have been very completely drained, and have a bottom of red granite. Very few farms, on any other bottom, have hitherto been as well drained.

arrive, the queſtion, reſpecting the influence of climate on particular kinds of ſheep, cannot receive a ſatisfactory ſolution.

A conſiderable quantity of butter and cheeſe is made of ewe-milk. Little attention is, in general, paid to the manufacture of butter, as it is ſeldom eat, and chiefly intended to be mixed with tar for ſalve. All the farmers and their ſhepherds have cows, the cream of whoſe milk plentifully ſupplies their families with butter. During the ſhort ſeaſon of milking ewes, a ſmall quantity of butter may ſometimes be made from a part of their milk, mixed with that of cows, and kept for different purpoſes of cookery. But, were it not for the difficulty and expence of procuring a ſufficient quantity of this article for ſalving their numerous flocks, farmers would employ every drop of their ewe-milk in making cheeſe, which is a conſiderable article of ſale, and much eſteemed, by ſome for its peculiar reliſh, and by others as an excellent ſtomachic. From 5 s. 6 d. or 6 s. it has lately ariſen to 7 s. and ſeveral parcels to 8 s, and even to 8 s. 6 d. per ſtone *, owing, chiefly, to the practice of milking ewes being difuſed in many places from a perſuaſion that it is hurtful, though partly, alſo, to the increaſing demand for this commodity. Concerning the expediency of milking ewes, opinions have fluctuated, and ſeem not yet to be quite eſtabliſhed. In expoſed ſituations, where ewes cannot bring forth their lambs early, it is generally thought adviſable to prolong the period of ſuckling them, till the ſeaſon of milking is far advanced, and only to draw the teats a few days to eaſe the ewes. The lambs become thus fatter for the market, or ſtouter to ſupply vacancies in the flock, and the mothers are

in

* Of 16 lib. trone, each lib. being near 24 oz. Engliſh, hence the ſtone is about 24 lib. Engliſh. In 1796, ſome parcels were ſold for 9 s.

in better order, either for being fold to a grazier, or for ftanding the feverities of winter. In more fheltered and richer farms, where lambs may be allowed to come earlier, and are fooner weaned, it may neverthelefs be more profitable to abftain from milking their mothers, that both may fatten more fpeedily and bring a higher price. Much certainly depends on local fituation, and accidental circumftances. And farmers muft be left to judge for themfelves, either according to their own experience, or the more fuccefsful practice of others. It is pretty generally admitted, that ewes may be as much weakened by their lambs fucking a long while, as by being milked; and that there is a certain period when lambs fhould be weaned, without any difadvantage to themfelves, and greatly to the relief of their mothers; but that this period may be fhorter or longer, in different farms, and fhould be regulated by the ftate of the ewes, the lambs, and the pafture. It is alfo allowed, that ewes are rather eafed, than hurt, by being milked for a fhort while after the lambs are weaned, but that the length of time fhould be determined by their condition, their age, the nature of the pafture, and the degree of convenience with which they can be gathered into the folds. Young ewes, generally, are only milked for a few days; and are feldom if ever milked fo long as thofe who are older.

In thofe places, where this practice is ftill continued, feven or eight weeks are the common period of its duration. A pint * of milk, at an average, is given by a fcore of ewes, and about 36 pints will make a cheefe weighing a ftone. But fome cow-milk is generally mixed with it, the proportion varying according to the number of ewes and cows on different farms; fo that fome cheefes are made

almoft

* Somewhat lefs than a Englifh quarts wine meafure.

almost wholly of ewe-milk. and others have as large a
share of cow-milk as 22 to 40 pints. The latter not being
nearly so rich as the former, when a third, or even a fourth,
part of it enters into the composition, 40 or 42 pints will
be requisite for the stone of cheese. Hence it may be calculated, that, from a flock consisting of 50 score of ewes, whereof
about 36 score are milked every evening and morning at
the rate of 36 pints each time, with the addition of a fourth
part of cow-milk, a cheese should be made every day,
weighing somewhat more than two stone, and that, where
a larger number either of ewes or cows are kept, cheeses
may frequently exceed 3 stone, or two cheeses may be
made daily of a less size. Hence too, the cheeses made on
a moderate-sized farm, whose flock of ewes amounts nearly
to the number specified, may be reckoned at 120 stone in
eight weeks, which, at 8 s. per stone, is L. 48 Sterling. It
is not unusual for farmers to let the milking of their ewes,
formerly for a penny each per week, or 8 d. for the season
of eight weeks, and now for 1½ d. per week, or 1 s. for
the season. At this highest rate, the milking of 36 score
of ewes is precisely as many pounds. And the farmer
just loses L. 12 Sterling for the sake of being freed from
the trouble of hiring, maintaining, and managing ewe-
milkers, furnishing and keeping in order a number of u-
tensils, and conducting the whole process of making the
cheese.

This operation merits a description *. The milk is gently
heated, and coagulated with a rennet. The curds are broken,
by stirring them with the hand or a stick, and then compressed by a coarse cloth, which bears them down, but affords an easy passage for the whey to rise and float on the

top,

---

* This account is chiefly abridged from Mr Ure, with a few necessary alterations and additions.

top, whence it is skimmed off by a large flat dish made for the purpose. When no more can be obtained in this manner, the curds are put into a canvas bag very coarse and stout, and placed on a strong barrow, with three or four spokes about two inches broad and about three inches from each other. The barrow is set over a tub to receive any whey that may come from the curds. Across them is laid a heavy and long deal or plank, on each end of which a woman sits, alternately pressing it down, and being herself lifted up with it. The jolt and violence of this motion squeezes out all the remaining whey, which is generally white and thick. The curds are then tumbled out of the bag into a dry tub, broken into very small particles, and salted. They are sometimes subjected, a second time, to be squeezed as already described, to force away any drops of whey, which might have adhered to the lumpy curds, but which must easily filter through them after being carefully broken. In this case, they are again separated, and wrought by the hand, and get a little more salt if it is thought necessary. After all these operations, they are thrust into the cheese vat, and put under the press for 24 hours, during which time they acquire the form of a cheese, and it is changed as often, and receives more or less pressure, as is thought necessary. The presses are commonly moved by a screw, and are made, sometimes of wood, and sometimes of stone. They are also constructed on the principles of the lever, admitting weights to be applied at the extremity or at any intermediate distance, and the cheese-vat to be placed nearer or farther from the weight, according to the degree of pressure required. After coming from the press, the cheeses are laid on a floor, where there is a free circulation of air to dry and harden them slowly, and they are regularly turned, at first once if not twice every day, afterwards

Z once

once every second or third day, and latterly perhaps every week or ten days, till the end of September or beginning of October, when they are weighed and delivered to the purchaser.

The whey, first taken off, is given warm for consumptive complaints, and violent coughs; or, mixed with milk and oatmeal, is heated in a kettle, but not allowed to boil, and stirred till it acquires a top like a posset, which is skimmed off and eaten by servants, and the thin beneath it is carried out to swine. What is forced out by the subsequent operations, when thin, is poured into the kettle, but, when thick and rich, is kept over night, and throws up a kind of butter, very useful for combing wool, or mingling with tar for salve.

SECT. III.—*Horses.*

THERE are many different kinds of horses in this county, though none are peculiar to it. For draught, a breed, with a considerable mixture of *blood*, for which Northumberland is justly famous, was much esteemed some years ago. Their mettle, and speed are admirably adapted for post-chaises, but they want strength to bring heavy carriages from a distance through a hilly country. The Lanarkshire horses, able for any weight, cannot stand long journies. But their stallions produce excellent foals from Northumberland mares, uniting the strength of the father with the spirit of the dam. The issue of this cross are fast rising into esteem. There are also several Irish horses both strong and active, but they are mostly geldings or mares. An handsome stallion from that kingdom, covering the progeny of a cross

between

between the Lanarkſhire and Northumberland breeds, would
probably produce the very beſt kind of draught horſes for
this unequal and inland diſtrict, where compactneſs, bone,
and mettle, are equally requiſite. Ponies, from the north
of Scotland, are very common in moſt families for children,
and make uſeful drudges. A croſs between them and blood
horſes often poſſeſſes the hardineſs of the one and ſpeed
of the other. Some of them, too, are very handſome, and
well fitted to carry ladies, or gentlemen of a middling ſize.
They are indefatigable travellers, and by no means nice
with reſpect to food. A ſpecies of leſſer draught horſes,
ſtout, compact, and active, is much uſed by ſmall tenants,
cadgers, &c. and very proper for going long journies, with
moderate loads. Some of them come from Fife, others
from Galloway, and are here croſſed with other breeds.
Moſt of the gentlemen, and ſome farmers, keep horſes of
full blood for their own riding or for hunting, but none for
the turf. It is a queſtion not eaſily ſolved, whether a greater
number of horſes is bred or brought into the county. Formerly the importation from other counties was more conſiderable than it has been of late ; and, if the paſſion for
raiſing foals continues to increaſe, the county in a few years
may ſupply itſelf with horſes.

Their number, in the diſtricts of Jedburgh, Hawick and
Melroſe, in the year 1789, under the operation of the old
law reſpecting ſtatute-labour, was 2994. The number, at
that time in the Kelſo diſtrict, cannot be aſcertained from
any authentic documents ; but the twelve pariſhes, of which
it conſiſts, being moſtly ſituated in the populous and arable
part of the county, could not contain fewer than 1350 horſes, or from 110 to 112 at an average for each pariſh, making the total number in the county then 4344.

The

The surveyor has kindly furnished the following note and remarks, most distinctly shewing their exact number in 1796 :

LIST of Horses in the County of ROXBURGH.

Parishes.	Carriage & Saddle Horses.	Work ditto.	Young ditto.	Total.
1. Ashkirk, part of,	13	51	34	98
2. Ancrum,	26	163	36	225
3. Bowden,	11	137	47	195
4. Bedrule,	6	37	9	52
5. Cavers,	32	189	44	265
6. Castletown,	26	134	63	223
7. Crailing,	19	98	30	147
8. Ednam,	15	91	10	116
9. Eckford,	12	138	28	178
10. Hawick,	39	210	23	272
11. Hobkirk,	18	111	26	155
12. Hownam,	14	44	18	76
13. Galashiels, part of,	4	26	7	37
14. Country part of Jedburgh,	29	216	32	277
15. Kirktown,	10	45	16	71
16. Kelso,	55	162	13	230
17. Lilliesleaf,	20	121	29	170
18. Lessudden, or St Boswells,	8	64	9	81
19. Linton,	10	59	2	71
20. Morebattle,	15	119	13	147
21. Makerstown,	11	53	14	78
22. Minto,	9	65	20	94
23. Maxton,	6	60	13	79
24. Melrose,	27	284	31	342
25. Oxnam,	17	105	17	139
26. Roberton, part of,	11	57	14	82
27. Roxburgh,	14	115	21	150
28. Sprouston,	13	158	28	199
29. Smailholm,	11	69	17	97
Carried forward,	501	3181	662	4344

PARISHES.	Carriage & Saddle Horses.	Work ditto.	Young ditto.	Total.
Brought forward,	501	3181	662	4344
30. Stitchill, - - -	14	53	20	87
31. Southdean, - -	13	89	19	121
32. Selkirk, part of, - -	3	32	4	39
33. Wilton, - - -	19	140	19	178
34. Yetholm, - - -	9	106	2	117
Total county, -	559	3601	726	4886
Burgh of Jedburgh, -	27	83	0	110
Total county and burgh,	586	3684	726	4996 *

REMARKS.

" *The preceding List being furnished by the Surveyor of*
" *Taxes, it becomes necessary to observe,*

" *That though the number of horses may be reckoned pret-*
" *ty accurate, yet it must not be supposed that there are 586*
" *employed solely as carriage and saddle horses, as by far the*
" *greatest part of that number is made up of horses belong-*
" *ing to tenants occupying farms at L. 70, or upwards of*
" *yearly rent, which subjects them to the riding-horse tax,*
" *though they only ride one of their work-horses.—In the*
" *number of young horses are included all work-horses be-*
" *low 13 hands high, and perhaps some of the young horses*
" *may have harrowed a little in seed-time.—The number of*
" *work-horses employed in carrying on, and managing the*
" *husbandry in each parish, is very exact; but in each pa-*
" *rish*

* When from this number, are deducted the 726 young horses, it would
appear, that the late taxes have occasioned a small decrease since the year
1789.

" *rifh are alfo included the horfes belonging to* carters or
" *jobbers and cadgers.*"

SECT. IV.—*Hogs.*

THE number of fwine cannot be calculated with any degree of exactnefs, as it varies very confiderably at different
feafons. Some time ago, about 600 * were killed at Kelfo
every year; and perhaps twice as many in the reft of the
county; but of late they have rather decreafed. They are
kept chiefly by millers, brewers, and farmers, and fed
on duft, grains, whey, and the refufe of potatoes, and corn.
Servants, alfo, who have houfes of their own, villagers,
cottagers, and tradefmen, frequently have one, to glean offals from the roads, ftreets, and gardens, to lick the difhes,
to confume fuch potatoes as are too fmall for the table, and,
at laft, to be fattened by corn, or meal foaked in warm water. But they are found to do fo much damage to grafs-
fields and thorn-hedges, and to be fo expenfive in times of
fcarcity, that they are now much given up. They are generally of a middle fize, become fat at every age from fix
to fourteen months, and weigh from 8 to 20 ftone †. Few
are under or exceed this fize and weight; but feveral, formerly were, and fome ftill are, much larger. Neither pork
nor bacon is much ufed by the common people, though they
are not reftrained by any fuperftitious averfion. Hence, probably, more fwine are fattened than confumed in the county. The overplus finds ready purchafers in the merchants
of Berwick, who cure pork for the London market.

SECT. V.—*Rabbits.*

THERE are no rabbit warrens in the county; and, though
they burrow in feveral places, their numbers are not fo great

* Stat. Acct. Vol. X. p. 590.   † Each ftone equal 17½ lib. Englifh.

as to make them objects of attention, either to the proprietors in the view of profit, or to the farmers as a nuisance.
A few of them are sometimes taken and kept tame by way
of amusement, but they fetch too trifling a price to be hunt-
ed by poachers for gain.

Sect. VI.—*Poultry.*

Though very few farmers rear poultry of any kind for
sale, yet there are many of them in the county, especially hens, which in most leases make a part of the rent, under the name of *kain*, and are generally kept for conveniency or profit. A chicken in summer, and a fat hen
in winter, is always a good dish at command for an un-
expected visitor. Those, which are not needed in this way,
are sold in the neighbouring markets, chickens from 4 d. to
6 d. and hens from 9 d. to 1 s. Their eggs, also, are both
exceedingly useful for domestic purposes, and form a considerable article of gain. A hen, who lays every day, only three months in the year, and whose eggs sell only at
4 d. *per* doz. yields 2 s. 6 d. yearly. And when people, in
Hawick alone *, carry eggs, to the value of L. 50 at an average every week through the year, to Berwick, carriers
in the whole county may reasonably be supposed to draw
at least four times that sum, after every allowance for eggs
collected and brought from neighbouring counties. That
farmers, notwithstanding these profitable considerations,
should not be fond of hens, may easily be accounted for,
from the sad havock which they make in land newly sown,
and among corn, both while ripening, and after being stacked. But they are naturally great favourites with house-
wives, on account of their flesh, eggs, and feathers, and
likewise

* Stat. Acct. Vol. VIII. p. 530.

likewife with fuch villagers, and cottagers, as have no crops to be injured by them.

Ducks are not nearly fo numerous, though they lay an immenfe quantity of eggs, are eafily reared, and are reckoned agreeable food; but they cannot be ufed in fuch various ways as dunghill-fowls, and many people have a prejudice againft their eggs.

Geefe and turkeys are reared by gentlemen for their tables, and by fome farmers for fale; but not in fuch confiderable numbers, as to exceed greatly what are confumed in the county. Their average prices are, a goofe, about 2 s. 6 d. a turkey, 3 s. 6 d. a duckling, 7 d. or 8 d. and a duck, from 10 d. to 1 s. 2 d.

SECT. VII.—*Pigeons.*

THERE are many pigeon-houfes, but very few pigeons can be purchafed. The prices are from 1 s. 6 d. to 2 s. 6 d. the dozen.

SECT. VIII.—*Bees.*

IT is impoffible to afcertain, with the leaft pretenfion to accuracy, either the number of breeding hives intended to be preferved through winter, or their actual produce in the following fummer. Many are deftroyed by inclement weather; fome perifh through neglect; few or none can thrive in a bleak and cold feafon. Every thing depends on their getting favourable opportunities of collecting their winter's ftore.

ftore. Yet they have been the fource of comfortable fubfiftence to feveral, and of wealth to one or two individuals,
who, by obfervation and experience, have acquired uncommon fkill in their management. The price of honey,
at an average, may be ftated at 6 s. the Scotch pint, and of
honey-comb at 1 s. *per* lib. More is annually made than
ufed in the county.

A 2   CHAP.

CHAP. XIV.

RURAL ECONOMY.

SECT. I.—*Labour, Servants, Labourers, and Hours of Labour.*

THE nature and prices of several different kinds of labour have already been incidentally stated, under those articles, in the preceding chapters, to which they respectively belong; and, for the conveniency and satisfaction of the reader, the substance of these scattered particulars shall be here collected together, and such information added, concerning other particulars, as I have been able to obtain.

Much less work is done by the piece than might be expected from the advanced state of agriculture. It was only
introduced

introduced a few years ago, and is slowly becoming more general.

On ground that is easily wrought, ditches are dug, five feet broad by three feet deep, at 8 d. or 10 d., and three feet broad by two feet deep, for 4 d. 5 d. or 6 d., and thorns are planted, but not furnished. Drains, four feet wide at top, three feet or two and a half feet at bottom, and three and a half feet deep, cost from 8 d. to 1 s. When twenty-six or thirty inches wide at top and the same in depth, they are from 4 d. to 7 d. Those, two feet wide, and only one foot eight inches deep, are sometimes as low as 2 d., and generally about 2½ d. or 3 d. Open drains on sheep-walks, about sixteen or twenty inches broad and twelve or fourteen deep, cost about 1 d. and often not so much. But, on hard and stony land, the above prices are about one-third more: And they all refer to the rood of six English yards, the only measure by which such works are done here. The proprietors or tenants always fill up and cover drains, with their own servants, horses and carts.

Hay has been cut from 1 s. 8 d. to 3 s. 6 d. *per* acre. About 2 s. 2 d. or 2 s. 3 d. is thought to be the average. Very little corn has been cut by the piece. From 5 s. 6 d. to 6 s. 6 d. has been given for reaping an acre, binding the sheaves, and setting them up in shocks. There is an instance or two of its having been cut with a scythe at 2 s. 6 d. *per* acre, and the expence of gathering, tying it, &c. is computed at 2 s. 6 d. or 3 s. more. It was commonly thrashed, in the lower parts of the county where there is a good deal of wheat, for the twenty-fifth part of the produce, and, in the higher parts where there is little wheat, for the twenty-first part. Thrashers frequently get 4 d. or

5 d.

5 d. *per* boll and their meat, and from 8 d. to 1 s. without meat, according to the price of provisions, the quality of the grain, and local situation.

There is no regulation for the carriage of goods, either by measurement, or weight. Much also depends on their nature, and the distance they are carried. Timber is charged at the rate nearly of 1 d. the cubic-foot for every seven miles. A cart-load of coal, lime, and marl generally costs about 4¼ d. *per* mile, when drawn by two horses, and about 3 d. when drawn by one; but a specific bargain being for the most part made for a certain number of cart-loads, at a stipulated price, which often includes the prime cost, the rate of carriage *per* mile may of course vary. Merchant-goods are carried at the rate of 1 d. *per* stone English for every nine miles; but more is demanded for brittle wares, and parcels that are easily damaged. Wool being a bulky commodity, about six packs are laid upon a two-horse cart, and about 6 d. *per* mile is generally paid for carrying them.

It was formerly the practice for smiths to work the iron of others wholly by the piece, receiving a stated allowance yearly in corn, meal, and fuel, according to the number of horses, carts and ploughs, belonging to the different farmers who employed them, and money for all extra jobs. But of late it is becoming more common for their employers, still furnishing iron, to pay them 1½ d. or 2 d. for making and 1 d. or 1¼ d. for removing a horse-shoe, from 2 d. to 3 d. *per* lib. for making the iron-work of a plough, from 4 d. to 8 d. for repairing and 2 d. for sharpening a coulter and sock, from 5 s. to 10 s. for putting an iron-ring around the wheels of a cart, according to its weight, and 2¼ d. or 3 d. *per* lib. English for all the necessary appendages.

When

When ſtones are laid down, maſons build ſtone-walls, without cement, four and a half feet high, for 1 s. 6 d. and lately for 1 s. 10 d. the rood of ſix yards; and, when cement is furniſhed and prepared, they get from 30 s. to 36 s. for the rood of 36 by 1 yards, according to the height of the wall or houſe. For the ſame rood, ſlaters receive from 16 s. to 20 s. when ſlates are brought to the ſpot. No other kind of work is done by the piece.

The wages of maſons are from 1 s. 8 d. to 2 s.; of wrights *, from 1 s. 4 d. to 1 s. 8 d.; with a deduction, formerly of 4 d. or 5 d. and lately of 6 d. or 7 d., when they get meat. Labourers, from the 12th November to the 12th February, receive 8 d. or 9 d. and their maintenance, and from 1 s. to 1 s. 2 d. without it. Through the reſt of the year, they get 10 d. and ſome of them 1 s. and their meat, and 1 s. 2 d. or 1 s. 4 d. without it. In hay and corn harveſt, their wages are ſtill higher.

Men-ſervants, when maintained in the houſe, receive from L. 8 to L. 10 yearly of wages. About L. 9 or 9 guineas is thought to be the average. Women receive about L. 4. Their maintenance is eſtimated at 6 d. per day in theſe dear times. When farm-ſervants have families and houſes of their own, their various emoluments amount to L. 18 or L. 20. The following is the moſt ſimple ſtatement of their annual income:

Wage,	-	-	L. 9 0 0
A cow, maintained ſummer and winter,			3 10 0
		Carried forward,	L. 12 10 0

---

* *Wright* in Scotland is the general name of all thoſe who work in timber. The particular branch, which they purſue, is often prefixed to this name, as *mill-wright*, *ſhip-wright*, *wheel-wright*, *houſe-wright*, *cart-wright*, *plough-wright*, &c. Even coachmakers are ſometimes called *coach-wrights*. Nothing is prefixed to it when it ſignifies a joiner.

Brought forward,	L.	12	10	0
Weekly allowance for meat, 1 s. 6 d.,	-	3	18	0
House-rent, - -		1	0	0
Two carts of coals,		1	4	0

	L.	18	12	0

Though this is the fum that goes out of the mafter's pocket, yet the profit of the cow will bring more into that of the fervant. Nothing is reckoned on his meat during harveft, which the mafter furnifhes, nor on a crop of potatoes or lint on a fpot manured with his dung, (though from thefe his family derives confiderable advantage), becaufe he generally provides a reaper either for thefe privileges or for his houfe. Many married fervants receive meal, and other perquifites, but their weekly allowance is withdrawn, and their wages are proportionally lefs.

The wages of fhepherds are ftill higher, owing to their being allowed to keep a few fheep along with thofe of their mafter. This practice is more profitable to them, and interefts them more in the fafety and welfare of the flock. Their earnings, thus arifing from a complication of fources, cannot be eafily calculated, but were generally fuppofed fome years ago to be L. 18, and cannot this year (1796) be below L. 20.

There is a general complaint, through the whole county, of labourers being fcarce. Thrafhers, efpecially, cannot be found, though fewer of them are now needed fince the introduction of machines. When a fervant faves a few pounds, he is ambitious of poffeffing a horfe and a fmall tenement, that he may turn cadger, and will undertake no work except where his horfe is employed. Hence labourers are not numerous, and confift chiefly of thofe, who have failed in other employments, or have thrown them up for want of

health ;

health; which accounts, in part, for their unwillingness to work by the piece, and their preference of days wages. There are, however, a few clever fellows, who handle a pick and a shovel with great dexterity; and strangers, sometimes, sojourn for a while, and perform piece-work. Better accommodation in point of houses and fuel may induce good labourers to settle here. There is no fear of their getting plenty of employment.

The hours of labour are, from six o'clock in the morning till six in the evening, while there is day-light, and, in winter, from the dawn of morning till the twilight, with an allowance of an hour to rest at breakfast, and another at dinner. Servants rise earlier and work later when occasion requires, but, in general, do not work, at an average through the year, above 10 or 11 hours a-day.

The houses, both of cottagers * and shepherds, have been already described. They live chiefly on bread, oatmeal, potatoes, milk, cheese, eggs, herrings and salted meat. Their bread is made of barley and peas ground into meal, kneaded into bannocks, and toasted on a thin plate of iron, suspended over a moderate fire. They also use oat-cakes made much in the same manner, but thinner. Wheaten bread, ale, and whisky are accounted dainties, and only presented on great occasions; such as baptisms and marriages. House-servants fare better. Their breakfast is a mess of oatmeal-*porridge* (or hasty pudding) and milk. Their dinner is, broth and boiled meat warm, twice every week, and, the other days in the week, either broth heated again or milk, with cold meat, eggs, cheese, or butter, and as much bread of mixed barley and peas-meal as they choose. Their supper is, either the same as their breakfast, or, often during winter, boiled potatoes mashed with a little butter and milk. The time of their meals varies according to

the

* Chapter III. Sect. 3.

the feafon, and their work. In winter, they breakfaft before day, that they may be ready to begin their work as foon as there is light, and do not dine till the twilight; but they get a luncheon, and their horfes a little corn, about mid-day. During the reft of the year, they work four and a half or five hours before breakfaft, reft or do any job in the middle of the day, dine about one o'clock, and work again four and a half or five hours in the evening.

Sect. II.—*Provifions.*

Butcher meat of every kind may be purchafed weekly, at a moderate rate, in the markets of Kelfo, Jedburgh, and Hawick. The firft holds a juft pre-eminence over all the markets in the fouth of Scotland, and north of England alfo, Morpeth alone excepted. It is famed for beef and veal; and for pork it is unrivalled. The mutton and veal of Jedburgh are fully equal in excellence, but not in quantity, and its beef is not much inferior. Hawick, too, is well fupplied with good beef and mutton, but here, and through the reft of the county, there is little veal or pork. Lamb every where abounds, in its feafon, of an admirable quality. There are regular butcher-markets, alfo, in Melrofe, Yetholm, and Newcaftletoun in Liddefdale; and feveral families on the confines of the county get meat from the neighbouring markets of Lauder, Selkirk, and Langholm; but Kelfo and Jedburgh fend more to Berwickfhire, Northumberland, and even to Mid-Lothian, than is brought into the county. A great number of falmon and of falt-water fifh is fold, in the proper feafon, in different markets, efpecially at Kelfo. Their prices vary, but are feldom exorbitant. There are breweries at Kelfo, Ednam, Jedburgh,

burgh, Hawick, and Melrofe, which fupply the county and neighbourhood with excellent fmall and ftrong beer. Scotch porter is made at Kelfo and Ednam, a ftout, cheap, and wholefome beverage, though very unlike what comes from London. There are bakers in all thefe places, and likewife in many villages. And, befides what they make, a good deal of bread comes weekly from other counties. Before the late high prices, the average rate of butcher-meat and poultry through the year might be nearly as follows:

* Beef,	-	3¼ d. or 4 d.	Turkeys, each,	3 s. 6 d.
Mutton,	-	3 d. or 3¼ d.	Geefe, -	2 s. 6 d.
Pork,	-	3 d. or 4 d.	Ducks, -	1 s. 0 d.
Veal,	-	3¼ d. or 4 d.	Hens, -	0 s. 9 d.
Lamb,	-	3 d. or 3¼ d.	Chickens, -	0 s. 4¼ d.
		all per lib.	Pigeons, per doz.	
			from 1 s. 6 d. to 2 s. 0 d.	

The average prices were, of butter when frefh, 9 d. and when falted, 10 d. per lib †, of ewe-cheefe, 7 s. or 7 s. 6 d. and of cow, 4 s. 6 d. or 5 s. per ftone †. All thefe articles are higher at prefent; and milk is fold, in all the villages, at the low rate of 1 d. the Scotch pint as it comes from the cow, and for the half of that price when the cream is taken from it. Few pot-herbs are fold, as moft families have gardens. Potatoes, fome time ago, were at an average about 9 d. or 10 d. the firlot, except at feed-time when they rofe to 1 s. 4 d. or 1 s. 6 d.

A very large quantity of grain is exported from this county, as it comes from the winnowing machine. Much,

B b   too,

* Butcher-meat is fold by the Dutch pound, which is feventeen and a half Englifh ounces.

† The pound of butter and cheefe is equal to 24 Englifh ounces, and the ftone is equal to 24 Englifh pounds.

too, is fold to be manufactured in the neighbourhood, and fome brought from the neighbouring counties to be manufactured here, and carried, in meal or pot-barley, to the hilly parts of Northumberland, Dumfries, and Selkirkfhire, to Peebles, and to Mid-Lothian. There is no way, therefore, of calculating the quantity actually confumed in the county, except by allowing ¼ ftone *per* week to every foul in the population, and fuppofing the adults to make up the deficiencies of infants. On this principle, the population being 32,103,—the weekly confumpt will be 16,051¼ ftone, and the annual 834,678 ftone, including grain of every kind. By a moderate computation, every working horfe will require twelve bolls of oats yearly. Allotting only one half of that quantity to all other horfes, including young horfes, carriage and faddle horfes, and ponies, but not foals, the number of working-horfes being 3684,—they will confume 44,208 bolls yearly, and that of other horfes being 1312,—they will confume 7872 bolls yearly, in all 52,080 bolls.

The following is a Table of the Fiars *, and of the monthly returns fent to Government of the average prices of grains :

A.

* The *fiars* are the county average prices of the different grains, fixed twice every year, a few weeks after Candlemas and Lammas, and properly refer to the fix months immediately preceding thefe terms ; fo that the fiars for Candlemas 1792 nearly correfpond to the monthly returns for the end of 1791 ; thofe for Lammas 1792 to the returns for the firft fix months of that year, and fo on. But in the fubjoined table, the Candlemas fiars are placed oppofite to the monthly returns of the firft fix months, and thofe for Lammas to the laft fix months of every year.

A TABLE, of the average Prices of Grain returned monthly to Government since September 1791, and of the County Fiars since Lammas 1791. Opposite to the Returns for the last 4 Months of the 1791, are the Fiars for Lammas 1791. Opposite to the Returns for the first 6 Months of every succeeding year are the Fiars fixed at Candlemas that year; and opposite to those for the last 6 Months are the Fiars fixed at Lammas.

	MONTHLY RETURNS.					FIARS.				
	Wheat.	Peas.	Barley.	Oats.	Oatmeal.	Wheat.	Peas.	Barley.	Oats.	Oatmeal.
1791, last 4 ms.										
1792, 1st 6 ms.										
—— 2d 6 m.										
1793, 1st 6 ms.										
—— 2d 6 ms.										
1794, 1st 6 ms.										
—— 2d 6 ms.										
1795, 1st 6 ms.										
—— 2d 6 ms.										
1796, 1st 6 m.										
—— 2d 6 ms.										

N. B. These prices all refer to the county bolls: That for wheat and peas containing 5 firlots of 2274,888 cubic-inches each, and = 5 bushels 1 peck 2 pints and a fraction English standard measure; and that for oats and barley, containing also 5 firlots of 33 pints or 3412,332 cubic-inches each, and = 7 bushels 3 pecks 11 pints 16,3 cubic-inches English standard measure.
The boll of oatmeal is 16 Dutch or Scotch troy stones.

Sect. III.—*Fuel.*

COALS, peats, turf, and wood are all used for fuel. Coals are brought from the north-east of Northumberland to the lower parts of this county, in two-horse carts, containing from twelve to fourteen bolls each, the boll being about a firlot barley measure, and costing at the pit 2d or 2¼ d. To the neighbourhood of Jedburgh, small coals, the same which abound around Newcastle, are carried both in carts and on horseback from the north-west of Northumberland. A cart drawn by two horses, containing six loads or twelve bolls, costs at the pit 4¼ d. or 5 d. *per* load; and three narrow bags, measuring 2¼ firlots at the pit, form the horse-load, and sell at Jedburgh for 2 s. 2 d. after being brought by the border coal-drivers about twenty miles. The southern extremity of Liddesdale has coal of the same kind within itself, which is sold at 3 d. *per* bushel, or 6 d. the load. The bushel there is equal to 3 Winchester ones. Similar coals, sold by the same measure in Dumfries-shire, are carried to the neighbourhood of Hawick, generally in two-horse carts, which hold six bushels * each. Coals also come as far as that village from Mid-Lothian, at the vast distance of thirty-six miles; and all the north-west parts of the county are supplied from the same quarter. They are there sold by weight, and cost at present 3½ d. *per* cwt. Peats are chiefly dug towards the centre and north-west parts of the county; but the labour and risk of making and bringing them home render them as dear as coals: And, in proportion as good access is opened to the latter, the former will be less used. Turfs, too, are found to impoverish the ground so much, that they, likewise, are fast giving place to coals. And wood is wholly local, although in 20 or 30 years hence,

when

---

* They are of late sold chiefly by the waggon-load for 1 s. 6 d. at the pit. The waggon is 16 cubic-feet, and one and a half waggons fill one of the largest double carts.

when the numerous plantations, now going forward, shall stand in need of being weeded and pruned, fires of this fuel will become more general. At present coals are the moft prevalent, and, on the whole, the cheapeft fuel; though they cannot be purchafed any where in the county below 9 d. the cwt., and in feveral places coft 1 s. 3 d., nor can 1 s. or 1 s. 1 d. be reckoned an improper average.

CHAP.

CHAP. XV.

POLITICAL ECONOMY, AS CONNECTED WITH, OR AFFECTING AGRICULTURE.

Sect. I.—*Roads.*

BEFORE the 1764, this county was in a miserable situation with respect to roads and bridges. There were few places, where wheel-carriages could safely pass, without skilful drivers and close attention; and there were only two bridges over Tweed * and other two over Teviot † of any real utility, all the rest being either aukwardly placed, or incommodiously constructed. In that year, an act of Parliament was obtained, for making part of the great road from Edinburgh to Carlisle, by Selkirk, Hawick and Langholm, which runs through the west of Roxburghshire.

It

* At Kelso and Melrose.

† At Hawick and near Ancrum.

It was succeeded, in 1766, by another act, for making a road, from the confines of the county towards Lauder, by Kelso, to the Marchburn, which divides it from Northumberland *. A third act passed, in 1768, for a road, from the same confines near Lauder, by Jedburgh, to the Redswire †, or summit of the Carter, on the north-west border of Northumberland, and for another, from Maxwellheugh near Kelso, to Hawick. Each of these acts has been renewed; and a fourth one was procured in 1793; in virtue of all which, the following branches, or additional roads, have since been made, viz. one from Kelso to St Boswell's Green ‡, where it falls in with the road from Jedburgh to Lauder; one from Kelso, north of Tweed, to the confines of the county towards Coldstream by Highridgehall, where it is joined by a cross-road made from Newton-mill; one from Kelso, south of Tweed, towards Cornhill, to Carham-burn; one from Kelso, towards Eccles and Dunse, by Ednam; one from Hawick, to join the road from Jedburgh to Redswire near the Carter toll-bar; one from Jedburgh towards Abbotrule and different places on Rule-water; one from Jedburgh to join the road from Kelso to Hawick at Spittal; and another to join it at Jedfoot-bridge; one striking off, near Newton toll-bar, from the road between Jedburgh and Lauder, through Melrose, to the bridge over the

* This road joins, near Wooler, the one by Greenlaw and Coldstream-bridge.

† From this point, a road is now made to Newcastle by Elsdon and Cambo, and another to West Auckland by Corbridge near Hexham. From West Auckland, there is a good road, by Pearce-bridge and Catterick through Leaminglane to Boroughbridge.

‡ In a direct line from Kelso towards Selkirk, to which latter place it should be carried forward.

the Gala clofe by Galafhiels; and a fmall part of the road from Kelfo to Peebles, north of Tweed, from the bridge over Leeder-water to the end of Melrofe-bridge, where it joins the road laft mentioned. Thefe various roads contain 153 miles. Befides leffer bridges, thrown acrofs rivulets, and hollows which are only occafionally filled with water, no fewer than twenty-four * ftone ones have been built, fince the 1764, over the more confiderable ftreams and rivers, including a beautiful one over Teviot, near its junction with Tweed, recently finifhed, and that very fubftantial and elegant one over Tweed at Drygrange, whofe middle arch has à fpan of 105 feet. Two of the former ones have alfo been rebuilt. Exclufive of the contributions of individuals, which on different occafions have been very liberal, the expence of making thefe roads and bridges, and of erecting toll-houfes and bars, amounts to L. 46,813 Sterling. The average annual expence of reparation and management is L. 1709 Sterling, including the reparation of the bridge over Tweed at Kelfo, though built prior to the turnpikeacts, but not including the reparation of the branch to Carham-burn, which is fcarcely completed. The real produce of the newly-erected toll-bars, except thofe on this laft mentioned branch, and the average produce, for the laft ten years, of thofe erected fome time ago, being, in whole, 26 bars and 2 pontages, amount only to L. 1793 Sterling; fo that the gentlemen concerned draw only the fmall furplus of L. 84 Sterling yearly for all the money they have funk. Yet moft of them are amply repaid, in another refpect, by the great increafe of their rents; and, without any pretenfions to a prophetic fpirit, it may be predicted that thefe

will

* Among thefe is not reckoned one built over the Ale by Sir John Buchanan Riddel at his own expence.

will rife flill higher, in proportion as eafier communications are opened up to fuel, manure, and markets *.

Crofs-roads were formerly made and kept in order, by what is called *ftatute labour*, under the authority of an old act of the Scotch Parliament, which obliged the inhabitants to work at them in perfon, or fend their fervants and horfes, or pay a fmall converfion in money. This law was found to be very inefficacious. They, who came, wrought carelefly and without fkill; and the converfion was often not demanded, or tardily paid. A fuccefsful application was made, in 1789, for a new act, empowering certain truflees to exact annually, from the occupiers of land in the different parifhes, fuch a fum as the roads in each parifh might require, to the extent of 1c s. Sterling on every L. 100 Scotch, according to the valued rent of their poffeffions, and alfo a fmall proportionate rate from houfeholders, carriers, cadgers, &c. This meafure was oppofed, not without fome colour of juftice, by feveral farmers, on the ground of its making a material alteration in the terms of their leafes, by fubjecting them to a heavy, fixed, and unavoidable affeffment on land highly valued, inftead of an affeffment on their horfes and fervants, which they had the option of leffening. But the quick and confpicuous effects, arifing from its vigorous operation, in accommodating the community at large, and feveral individuals in remote fituations, with excellent roads, have filenced all murmurs. Under the former act, the annual exaction might fluctuate extremely, but could not, in any year, greatly exceed L. 1000 through the whole county, and feldom was the half of that fum received: Whereas, by the prefent act, the annual

C c   affeffments

---

* The value of Lidftefdale, efpecially, muft be vaftly increafed, when the roads, prefently in contemplation, fhall be completed, one to Hawick, and another to Jedburgh.

affeffments may amount to L. 1573 Sterling, and have, in general, ever fince its commencement, been drawn in moft parifhes nearly to their full amount.

In making both turnpike and crofs roads, too little attention was at firft paid to avoid acclivities, and conduct them in the moft level and neareft direction. The Gentlemen were inexperienced, unwilling to break into inclofures, or to injure the property of any individual, defirous of ftudying each other's conveniency, and, above all, anxious to obferve œconomy. Hence the line of former roads was followed as much as poffible, to prevent both caufe of offence, and unneceffary expence. A road, already partly done, could be completed at an eafier rate, than a road wholly new. And proprietors had lefs caufe to complain when an old road was widened, than when a new one was carried through their fields. There was alfo fome faving in taking the advantage of bridges already built, inftead of erecting others. On the fame principle, the making of roads was committed to thofe, who gave the loweft eftimate, and who were both fparing of their materials, and unfkilful in laying them on. In a few years, there was a neceffity, in fome inftances to alter the direction, and in others to renew the roads. Thefe errors, however, have long ago been perceived and corrected. The later roads are made with an evident regard to eafe, conveniency, and beauty; and are pleafing indications of the judgment and good tafte of thofe by whom they were planned. Yet not only here, but in the greateft part of Scotland, the art of road-making is imperfectly underftood; and perhaps the following hints, on this fubject, may not be unacceptable to the public.

The firft care fhould be to get a firm foundation. All the foil, and any foft fubftance that may be under it, muft be thrown afide, till gravel, rock, or hard till is found. In cafes, where this would be difficult or expenfive, let the

bottom

bottom of the road, after paring off the furface, be laid with brushwood, bramble, the branches of trees, especially those which have numerous twigs, or such weeds and roots as are tough and cohesive. These form a kind of thick net, to prevent the stones from sinking, and the mud from rising. The stones should all be hard, broken very small, and none of them smooth or round. The rough sides and sharp edges and angles of those pieces made by the hammer, adhere together, detain the particles of sand and gravel which are forced down among them, and become a compact and firm body. Whereas large stones, and even small ones when smooth or round, invariably work their way to the surface by the jolting of heavy carriages. The greatest depth of stones should always be on the middle of the road, and there should be a very gentle slope towards each side, not above an inch or thereabouts to every three feet. When the slope is less, water will not descend readily; and, when it is much greater, all carriages will shun the declivity on the sides, and go along the highest part, crush it down, form ruts, and destroy the road. A slope of five or six inches in fifteen feet is too trifling to be felt as an inconveniency by any carriage, and affords reason to expect an equal pressure on every part of the road, than which nothing is more essential to its durability. It is also of vast importance to spread the gravel thickly, and equally, so that the teeth of a common garden rake may pass along, and draw aside the largest of those smooth and round stones with which it abounds, without reaching the broken stones laid below. These round and smooth stones, however small, should be subjected to the hammer, and mixed with the other ones which are still uncovered. If the road, after being thus gravelled, was carefully beat down with a rammer, or if a heavy roller was drawn along the summit and each side, all inequalities and hollows would sooner ap-

pear,

pear, and could easily be filled up with coarse gravel. A smooth equal surface, by not occasioning jolts, removes one manifest cause of injury to roads. And a little care for a season or two to fill up and consolidate the ruts, will present a road, which of all others bids fairest to last long and need little reparation. It is, indeed, attended with extraordinary trouble and expence at first; but will prove a saving in the end. By attending to these principles, Trustees on turnpike-roads may be assured, that they shall be no losers in the course of 30 years.

All the acts, hitherto procured, are limited to 21 years. It would save much expence, and be in other respects of advantage, could their duration be prolonged, if not to a perpetuity, at least to three times that period. And it is not easy to see any danger that would arise, from thence, to the British constitution, or any harm to individuals. At any rate, the Trustees of the roads in this county would do well to consider, in future applications to the Legislature, whether it would not be greatly for the general interest, to have all the four acts consolidated into one, and to dispose the toll-bars on the different roads and their branches in such a manner as to be less oppressive to individuals, and more productive on the whole. Several instances might be produced, wherein, by abolishing some toll-bars, and altering the position of others, the revenue would be increased; but the present mode being more lucrative to the Trustees of particular districts, no such alteration can be expected to take place, while the different districts have separate interests.

SECT.

Sect. II.—*Canals.*

THERE are no canals in this county, and very little probability of any being made. About feven or eight years
ago, a gentleman in the neighbourhood of Kelfo fuggefted
the plan of cutting one from Berwick, or at leaft from
Cornhill *, to Kelfo; and there was afterwards a propofal
of carrying it ten miles further along the Teviot to An-
crum-bridge, near the centre of the county. A fubfcrip-
tion was opened; a furvey of the propofed track was taken
by Mr Whitworth; and Inquiries were made concerning
the probable amount of the imports and exports; the refult of which was a full conviction, that, though a canal
was practicable, at an expence which could not be thought
immoderate, yet, if made, it could not fupport itfelf. After finking above L, 30,000 Sterling †, all the dues and
fares, which could reafonably be expected, would not keep
the canal in proper order, repair its banks, locks, bafons, and
boats from time to time, furnifh and maintain horfes, and
afford ordinary wages to the hands neceffarily employed. The
fcheme of courfe was dropped. Every perfon, acquainted
with the county, muft perceive, that, towards no point the
influence of a canal could extend above ten miles, and towards the fouth fcarcely fo far. Beyond that diftance, the
                                                    inhabitants

---

* The former 23, the latter 10 miles, as meafured by the common
road.

† Mr Whitworth's eftimate of a canal from Cornhill to Kelfo was
L, 15,000. Other L, 14,000 would be neceffary to carry it to Ancrum-
bridge. And a greater fum to continue it from Cornhill to Berwick. Befides, the real expence of all fuch undertakings, generally exceeds the eftimate.

inhabitants could bring coals and lime, thofe great articles
of water-carriage, at a cheaper rate from other quarters,
and find a more profitable market for their grain *. The
neceffary addition, of land-carriage from the pit or kiln to
the quay, and of freight, to the prime-coft of coal and lime
brought into the county, would raife their price too high
to find a market, except in the near neighbourhood of the
canal. And to lower the rate of water-carriage fo much
as to tempt purchafers to come from a diftance, might indeed increafe the imports, but would nearly annihilate
the fmall revenue, which the canal might be expected to
yield †.

Sect. III.—*Fairs.*

Few counties have a greater number of large fairs, efpecially for black-cattle, horfes, and fheep. In Kelfo there
are three weekly markets in the beginning of March for
horfes, at each of which there is commonly a good fhew.
Here

* While, however, Berwick continues, as it certainly is at prefent, to
be the principal market for grain, a canal to that port would be of vaft
importance to corn-farmers, and grain would form one chief fource of its
fupport. But fhould the great demand for grain come from other quarters, the canal would be neglected. And very little wool would be exported by it; as the greateft part of what is carried out of the county
grows at a diftance from its propofed track.

† The following note was furnifhed by Sir John Sinclair: " It may be
" proper here to mention, that, though a canal on a great fcale might
" be too expenfive, yet one for fmall boats, with inclined planes inftead
" of locks, as propofed by Mr Fulton, is well entitled to the confideration
" of thofe who are interefted in the profperity of this county. And, for
" the particulars of Mr Fulton's plan, the reader is referred to his work
" on the fubject in one vol. 4to."

Here likewife are two fairs, on 10th July for cattle of different kinds, and on 2d November for hiring fervants, and for cattle to be fed on turnips or kept on ftraw during winter. St James's fair (Auguft 5.) is held on a beautiful green oppofite to it between the confluence of the Tweed and Teviot, and prefents a large fhew of horfes and of cattle for aftergrafs and turnips. A good deal both of linen and woollen cloth, alfo, is fold wholefale. Jedburgh has a confiderable fair, in the beginning of June, for milch-cows, lean cattle to be laid on grafs, and young cattle; another on 25th September for cattle defigned to be put firft on aftergrafs and then on turnips; and a third about Martinmas like the November fair at Kelfo. At all thefe fairs, there is a confiderable number of horfes. There is, at Hawick, a tryft for Highland cattle between Falkirk and Newcaftle fairs, a large fair on 8th November for fat and lean cattle, and another on 17th May for hiring fervants, particularly ewe-milkers and fhepherds. Melrofe has three fairs, one on the firft Wednefday of June for milch-cows and other cattle, one in Auguft for cattle to pafture on the fecond growth of clover, and a more confiderable one than either of thefe on 22d November for cattle, feveral of them fit for the fhambles, others in proper order for being fed on turnips, and not a few to be kept on ftraw. In June, there is a fair at Town Yetholm for lambs, and another at Kirk Yetholm for young and old fheep who have not loft their fleeces. At Rink, near the Carter, there is one for lambs on 12th July. And, at both thefe laft mentioned places, there is a fair in October for *draught* or *caft* ewes. The greateft fair in the fouth of Scotland is held on St Bofwell's Green on 18th July for lambs, fheep, black-cattle of every kind, horfes of all defcriptions, linen and woollen-cloth, and an incredible variety of leffer articles. Yet it is much on the decline; the cuſtoms, which ſome years ago brought at an average about 40 guineas, yielding this year (1796) only L. 33. At this fair, and at the ſummer fairs at Yetholm and Rink, wool is chiefly ſold; or rather the price of it is fixed. There are ſeveral leſſer fairs for particular purpoſes: And a conſiderable number of farmers and cattle-dealers in this county frequent the neighbouring fairs; particularly one at Earlſtoun on 29th June for milch-cows, black-cattle for grazing and fattening during ſummer, and horſes; one at Selkirk on 21ſt Auguſt for cattle half-fed fit for the ſecond growth of clover; one at Whitſonbank near Wooler on Whitſun-Tueſday for black-cattle, ſheep, and horſes; one at Stagſhawbank near Hexham in the beginning of July for cattle of all kinds, ſheep, lambs, and horſes, eſpecially young ones; and one at Rothbury in the beginning of November for lean cattle. A few of them go annually, to Falkirk and Crieff tryſts for black cattle, to Skirling and fairs in the county of Lanark for horſes, to fairs in Dumfrieſſhire for polled cattle, and to Newcaſtle for horſes chiefly though partly alſo for cattle. Some ſeldom ſtir abroad either to markets or fairs, but diſpoſe of their ſheep, lambs, wool, cattle, and grain to purchaſers, who come to their houſes; and, when in want of any of theſe articles, endeavour to procure them by a private bargain.

SECT. IV.—*Weekly Markets.*

THERE is a weekly market at Jedburgh on Tueſday, at Yetholm on Wedneſday, at Hawick on Thurſday, at Kelſo on Friday, and at Melroſe on Saturday; at each of which there is a regular ſupply of every kind of butcher-meat in its ſeaſon. The market at Kelſo is in every reſpect

spect best furnished and attended. Much cattle and grain are sold every week, besides a variety of lesser articles. It is frequented, by cattle and corn dealers from the northern part of the county, and from the contiguous parts of Berwickshire and Northumberland, and by victuallers from Berwick. Farmers, from the south part of the county, and from the north-west of Northumberland, who raise little or no corn, and all the shepherds, labourers, and artisans, who inhabit these hilly regions, are generally supplied with that necessary commodity, as well as with butcher-meat, &c. and sell their fed sheep and calves to the butchers, in the weekly markets at Jedburgh. People of this description, towards the S. W. W. and N. W. extremities of the county, and in the skirts of Selkirkshire, are in like manner furnished with these common articles at Hawick, and have an opportunity of selling their sheep and lambs. The markets at Jedburgh and Hawick are always attended by farmers from the arable part of the county, to purchase their weekly provisions, and to dispose of their grain to mealmongers, who manufacture it into flour, meal, and pot-barley: And these are carried, sometimes by the sellers, and sometimes by the buyers, into those districts where little corn grows. A good deal of grain is likewise sold at Melrose, but, in other respects, the markets there and at Yetholm are rather insignificant.

Sect. V.—*Commerce.*

If an inland county can, with propriety, be said to have any commerce, that of Roxburghshire consists, in importing some common necessaries and a few luxuries, and in exporting sheep, lambs, wool, cattle, and grain. It is impossible to ascertain the actual amount and value of these with any degree of certainty. According to the facts sta-

ted

ted in different parts of this survey, they may be compated as under:

Sheep, 56000, † at L. 1 each,	L. 56000,	† at 16s. each,	L. 44800
Lambs, 14000, † at 6s.	4208,	at 5s.	3500
Wool, 25000 ſt. at L. 1, 4s.	30000, † at L. 1,		25000
Turnip-cattle, 6000, † at L. 3,			
12 s. -	21600,	-	21600
Graſs-fed do. 6000, † at L. 2, 2s.	12600,	-	12600
Oats, 41008 acres, at L. 4,			
10 s. per acre, -	184536, † at L. 3, 10s.		143528
Barley, 16404 do. at † L. 4, 4s.	68896,	at L. 3, 10s.	57414
Wheat, 9842 do. at † L. 6,	59052,	at L. 5,	49210
Peas, 6562 do. at L. 4, 10s.	29529, † at L. 3, 10s.		22947

Total price of the county, L. 466393   L. 380599

Taking the medium between theſe two computations, - - - -   L. 423496 0 0

From it there muſt be deduſted,

1. The rent of the county, as in Chap. II. Seſt. 1. - L. 171941 12 0
2. The grain conſumed by the inhabitants and by horſes, as in Ch. XIV. Seſt. 2. viz.

832364 ſtone meal, at 2 s. per ſtone, - L. 83236 8 0
52080 bolls oats, at 16 s.   31664 0 0
                              —————— 114900 0 0

Carried forward,   L. 288642 0 0 L. 423496 0 0

† ‡, &c. Theſe marks were prefixed, by an intelligent friend, to thoſe articles, in the different calculations, which, in his opinion, are neareſt to the truth. According to him, the whole produce of this county amounts to L. 413,823 Sterling annually, which is only L. 9673 Sterling leſs than the medium taken in the text.

Brought forward, L. 286842 0 oL.423496 0 0

3. About one-fifth of the sheep,
   lambs and cattle sold, u-
   fed for home consump-
   tion,   —   —   L. 17690 0 0

   ————————   304532 0 0

Remains of gain to the county, after paying rents, and feeding people and cattle,   —   —   —   —   * L. 118964 0 0

* The reader will perceive, that all these calculations are founded on the information contained in the preceding pages; and particularly, that the number of sheep and lambs correspond exactly with the sales of a sheep-farm given by an actual farmer in Chap. IV. Sect. 6 *On Expence and Profit*. A gentleman, however, well acquainted with Roxburghshire, and the management of sheep, is of opinion, that fewer old sheep are sold annually, and many more lambs. Supposing the county to be wholly stocked with ewes, the annual sales would consist of, one-sixth of them, and about five-sevenths of the lambs produced by two-thirds of them. After making the usual allowance for mortality, one-sixth of 100,000 ewes would not exceed 30,000, and five-sevenths of 133,331 lambs would be reduced to 93000. These he reckons

The former or 30,000 old sheep, at 16 s.   —   —   L. 24000 0 0
The latter or 93,000 lambs, at 7 s.   —   —   —   32550 0 0

Thus making the annual produce,   —   —   —   L. 56550 0 0

which is a mere trifle above the value of sheep alone, according to the highest calculation in the text, but considerably above the value of both sheep and lambs, according to the lowest. But the difference will be less if either of the prices in the text are adhered to in both calculations.——
Thus,

30,000 ewes, at 20 s.   L. 30000 0 0   at 16 s.   L. 24000 0 0
93,000 lambs, at 6 s.   27900 0 0   at 5 s.   23250 0 0

   L. 57900 0 0   L. 47100 0 0
Amount, as stated in the text, L. 60000 0 0   L. 48300 0 0

Perhaps, however, the safest way is to take a medium both between the numbers of sheep and lambs, and their prices. The medium between
56,000

Sect. VI.—*Manufactures.*

The manufactures in this fine county are very inconsiderable. From the large quantity and good quality of the wool produced, and from the excellent situations which every where abound for water-machinery, there is every reason to expect that the woollen branches might prosper. But the few clothiers, scattered through the different towns and villages, are chiefly employed in what is called *country-work*, that is making small parcels of wool and yarn, sent to them by different families, into cloth, flannels, or worsted-stuffs, according to the instructions they receive. Hence it is not easy to ascertain the precise quantity of wool manufactured by them on their own account, especially as those, who do most in this way, live in the very suburbs of Galashiels in the county of Selkirk, from whence they moved only a few years ago, have a great part of their machinery, and nearly all their principal hands, in that village, and are in every respect so connected with the clothiers there, that an account of their manufactures falls properly to be included in the Agricultural View of Selkirkshire. Setting aside the wool used by them and by private

---

56,000 and 30,000 is 41,000 sheep; the medium between 93,000 and 14,000 is 53,500 lambs; and the medium prices are, for sheep, 18 s. and lambs, 6 s.

41,000 sheep, at 18 s. - - - -	L. 38,500 0 0
53,500 lambs, at 6 s. - - -	16050 0 0

L. 54,550 0 0

How very near is this to the exact medium between the two calculations of these articles in the text, which is L. 54250!

vate families, the whole quantity wrought by actual manufacturers may be estimated as under:

Carpets at Hawick,	–	–	–	–	St. *2700
Woollen-cloth there and through the county,				–	1300
Flannels and blankets,	–	–	–	–	900
Stockings and worsted-pieces,	–	–	–	–	300

St. 5200

The carpets are allowed to be admirably fabricated, and
are found to wear well. The proprietors, instead of selling those parts of the wool, which are picked out as too
fine, or not of a proper nature for carpets, have, of late,
made them into carpet and table-covers, rugs, saddle-cloths,
&c. ǂ At Hawick, the woollen manufacture is still in its
infancy, but makes such rapid progress, that more wool is
used there than in all the rest of the county. It is there,
too, that stockings are chiefly made, though weavers of
them are to be found, venturing on a small scale at their
own risk, in many corners of the county. The greatest
quantity of flannel and blankets‡ is made at Kelso and Jedburgh.

* The Stat. Acct. Vol. VIII p. 529. makes the quantity 220 packs
of twelve stone each, or 2640 stone. Since the 1792 or 1793, when the
Stat. Acct. was written, the quantity used has rather increased.

† Stat. Acct. of Hawick, p. 528,—9.

‡ Carpets cost 3 s. 8 d. and 3 s. 10 d. per yard. Coarse and narrow
woollen-cloth is made from 2 s. 8 d. to 4 s. per yard. Flannels, 7-8ths
wide, from 2 s. to 2 s. Blankets, 3-4ths and 7-8ths wide, from 10½ d.
to 1 s. 4 d.; and yard wide, from 1 s. 4 d. to 2 s. 2 d. Stockings, made
of wool, at L. 1, and from that to L. 3 per doz. and of cotton, from
24 s. to 50 s. per doz.

burgh. Premiums have been gained, by the manufacturers of these articles in both places, from the Honourable Board of Truſtees.

Though much lint was never raiſed here, yet formerly a great deal more of linen-cloth was made than at preſent. Foreign flax was chiefly uſed; and the ſpinning of it conſtituted the principal work, during winter, of maid-ſervants in every family, and of the wives and daughters of cottagers and mechanics. The populous neighbourhood of Melroſe was particularly famous for the number of its ſpinners and weavers, and the quantity of excellent webs produced there. But now foreign flax has riſen too high to yield a reaſonable profit. There is not enough raiſed in the neighbourhood to give employment to ſo many hands. Women earn more by ſpinning wool or working in the fields, and weavers by working cottons for manufacturers in Glaſgow. Yet a bleachfield *, ſet on foot there about forty years ago when the weaving of linen was in its zenith, continues to thrive. This is to be aſcribed to its being now the only one in the county, to the attention and good management of the bleacher, and to the number of pieces made, by private families for their own uſe, or by the wives and daughters of cottagers, labourers, artizans, and farm-ſervants, from the ſmall lots of lint they frequently obtain permiſſion to raiſe for the dung which they furniſh, though, indeed, ſuch people commonly bleach their webs themſelves, when they have the conveniency of a green ſpot and a clear ſtream near their dwelling-houſes, and ſell what is finer than their homely wearing, for a little money to anſwer any emergent occaſion. More lint is raiſed, ſpun, and wrought, in the lower parts of the county, where the woollen manufacture has not found its way, and

where

---

* Stat. Acct. of Melroſe, Vol. IX. p. 81,—2,—3.

where a lady * from Fife had the merit, of introducing the
two-handed wheel about sixteen years ago, and of teaching
her neighbours to use it, by which they nearly double the
quantity of yarn they formerly spun in a day. But there
is no manufacture carried on, except one in Kelso for co-
loured thread †, which employs above an hundred spinners,
and one at Hawick of inkle †, which consumes annually
ten tons of linen-yarn. Both are conducted with skill and
enterprize, and are in a flourishing condition. There are
two mills in the county for switching lint, and both are
kept pretty constantly at work.

Both tanned and white leather is manufactured at Hawick
and Jedburgh. A good deal, also, is tawed at Kelso and
in the neighbourhood of Galashiels, belonging to this county. The tanning branch, though succeeding very well,
and yielding a higher duty to Government than the other,
is not carried on to such extent. The vast number of sheep
and lambs, which are slaughtered, or die in severe or unhealthy seasons, is a strong inducement to attempt the manufacture of their skins. There are twenty tawers, here
called *skinners*, in Kelso, and about twelve more in the rest
of the county ‡. In Kelso, about 120,000 skins of all kinds are
manufactured annually. If the half of that number be allowed for the other places in the county, nearly as many
skins will be annually dressed as there are sheep in it, and
more than double the number of those which are sold or
die

* Mrs Morison, wife to the Seceding Clergyman at Morebattle, Stat.
Acct. Vol. XVL p. 510.——Mr Ure, p. 71.

† Mr Ure, p. 71.——† Stat. Acct. of Hawick, p. 519.

‡ This includes apprentices and journeymen as well as masters. There are
only fourteen who pay duty to Government, Stat. Acct. of Kelso. Vol. X.
p. 586 and p. 590.

die annually. The tawers muſt therefore be ſupplied from other places.

Jedburgh was once deſervedly celebrated for its candles. They are ſtill made there, and at Kelſo, Hawick, and Melroſe, but not in ſufficient quantities to ſerve all the families in the county. Many make their own candles, or get them from other places, eſpecially from Edinburgh, Leith, and Dalkeith.

But the chief article of manufacture is grain into meal, flower, pot-barley, malt, beer, and porter. The mills, beſides the conſumpt of the county, grind annually not leſs than 40,000 bolls of all grains. There are brewers and maltſters at Kelſo, Jedburgh, Hawick, Melroſe, Ednam, Yetholm and Smaillholm.

The exciſe paid to Government, from the 6th July 1794 to 6th July 1795, on all theſe articles, was as follows:

TABLE.

T A B L E.

	Malt Liquon.			Malt.			Tanned Lea-ther.			Tawed ditto.			Candles.			Total paid by each Place.		
	L.	s.	d.	L.	s.	d.	L.	s.	d.	L.	s.	d.	L.	s.	d.	L.	s.	d.
Kelfo, —	350	0	6	146	10	11	—	—	—	120	7	3½	186	8	0	803	6	8½
Jedburgh,	111	0	3	54	3	0	100	4	0	8	7	4½	58	0	2	331	14	8½
Hawick,	333	9	1	127	6	3	170	17	3	4	2	9½	32	13	9	568	9	1½
Melrofe,	150	19	8	89	12	11	—	—	—	*44	4	9½	12	16	1	297	12	5½
Ednam, —	637	9	9	158	5	4	—	—	—	—	—	—	—	—	—	795	6	1
Yetholm,	0	18	0	2	9	4	—	—	—	—	—	—	—	—	—	3	7	4
Smailholm,	2	3	4	22	5	5	—	—	—	—	—	—	—	—	—	24	8	9
	1485	11	7	600	13	2	271	1	3	177	2	3	289	17	11	2824	5	2

* This duty is paid for the white leather tawed in the suburbs of Galashiels which are in Melrose parish.

E

SECT. VII.—*Poor.*

THE principal facts relative to the poor will be found
under the article *Poor-rates*, Chap. IV. Sect. 4. and in
the annexed table. It may not be improper to add here,
that the county is often infested with gangs of tinkers and
horners from the neighbourhood of Berwick, and sometimes from the shires of Ayr, Renfrew, and Lanark. They
travel with their wives and children on asses, mules, or
ponies, loaded with their wares and tools; and, though
they disdain the name of beggars, are a sore burden on the
farmers for lodging and provisions to themselves and cattle.
At the time of sheep-shearing, too, sturdy women, chiefly
from Edinburgh and Dalkeith, provincially called *Randies*,
traverse the pasture district, under pretence of gathering or
asking locks of wool, and are suspected of taking more
than is given them. Some of both classes are so mischievous, as to assault those who are weaker or more timid
than themselves, to break the windows, and in other respects to demolish the property of such as refuse their demands. Quacks, jugglers, and strolling players not unfrequently pick the pockets of the industrious. And old sol-
diers and sailors glean some contributions which they commonly leave at the next alehouse. Nobody, who resides
in the county, ever begs, except perhaps a blind fidler, or
such as labour under mental imbecility. Gleaners in harvest became so great a nuisance, that farmers, in the lower
and arable parts of the county, allow none to enter their fields
till the corn is removed; and, in general, only the infirm or the
young, who can do nothing else, are permitted any where

to

to follow the reapers. By this mode of charity, children have sometimes picked up as much grain, as, with frugal management, maintained the family of a cottager for six or eight weeks. A few, who have been unfortunate in better stations, find a welcome reception at the tables, and are supplied with decent apparel at the joint expence, of their friends and former companions. To the honour of all concerned, let it be mentioned, that no where is more liberal provision made for the poor in times of real charity. In every parish, during the winter 1795–6, the assessment was increased, or a voluntary contribution was raised. The high prices of provisions bore harder on families in the middle ranks of society, than on the parochial poor.

Sect. VIII.—*Population.*

It is a pleasing consideration, that, after all the complaints made of depopulating the country, by the union of farms, by the demolition of villages, and by emigrations to avoid oppressive laws, there is, on the whole, a small increase in the number of inhabitants in this county since the year 1755. There may, indeed, be reason to suspect that the numbers were not then accurately returned, but might be stated, from conjecture, in some parishes above, and in others below the truth. But there can be no doubt, from the testimony of many attentive observers still alive, that several villages, farm-houses, and cottages have disappeared within these forty years, and that several districts have been almost wholly deserted. On the other hand, it is equally certain, that during that period many farm-hou-

ses

fes have been built in new fituations, that fome villages have been created, and others enlarged, that the manufac- tures in Hawick have confiderably increafed the popula- tion there and in the neighbouring parifhes of Wilton and Cavers, that the manufactures at Kelfo * and Ednam have had the fame effect on the population of thefe parifhes, that the fkirts of Melrofe parifh have received an addition of inhabitants from their contiguity to the flourifhing manu- factures at Galafhiels, and that the defire of independence has drawn numbers to villages for the fake of purchafing houfes and fmall fpots of land fufficient to maintain a cow, a horfe, or both. Thefe ways, however, of increafing the population are by no means favourable to agriculture, as neceffary and ufeful hands are removed to a diftance from farms, where there is the greateft occafion for them, and be- fides acquire a diflike to every kind of work which does not employ their horfes as well as themfelves. Proprietors and tenants will find it their mutual intereft, to have villages on every confiderable eftate, and cottages on every farm, and, that labourers may be induced to fettle among them, to make the houfes comfortable, and to let them at low rents. For in a county, diftant from fuel and from fome of the moft neceffary articles of confumpt, where fuch evi- dent and great profit arifes from bringing thefe, and per- forming

* The Statiftical Account of Kelfo, Vol. X. page 587. afcribes the great increafe of population in that place to widows and fingle women li- ving more conveniently, and getting *employment* more readily there than in the country, and to the deftruction of villages fending the occupiers thither for habitation and *employment*. But ftill *employment* in one line or another is allowed to be the caufe of their flocking thither; and in all places as large as Kelfo, the different branches of manufacture, either in a direct or indirect manner, afford the chief employment to the inhabi- tants.

forming various other works with horses, to counterba-
lance this obvious advantage, every encouragement should
be held out to that useful class, which is most likely to engage them in the different branches of manual labour, that
the operations of husbandry may be carried on in a speedy
and effectual manner.

A

A TABLE of the Population, Poor, Expence of maintaining them, number of Acres in Natural and Planted Wood, and Valued Rent of the different Parishes in ROXBURGHSHIRE.

Parishes.	Population in 1755.— 1790s	Poor. No.	Exp.	Woods. Plant. Natur.	Valued Rent.
			L. L.		L. s. d.
Jedburgh,	5816— 260	92 300 & int. of 442	460 } 150	23367 6 4
Southdean,	480— 71	22 56 *	60 }	6415 4 0
Hobkirk,	538— 700	25 76	260 90	9354 15 6
Cattletown,	1307— 1411	79 224	236 100	15860 0 0
Kirkton,	330— 34	13 30	350 }	4526 13 4
Cavers,	943— 1300	49 135	} 93	18877 6 8
Hawick,	2713— 2928	110 370	78 }	11591 11 0
Wilton,	936— 1211	35 200	80 —	7545 6 8
Minto,	395— 51	16 48 & int. of 50	420 —	5163 4 0
Bedrule,	297— 254	11 32 & int. of 56	8 8	3475 13 4
Ancrum,	1066— 1147	24 110	400 6	12332 2 0
Crailing,	387— 671	14 27 *	220 —	8733 0 0
Oxnam,	762— 691	24 76	140 —	14101 10 8
Hownam,	632— 365	9 32	50 —	10070 17 2
Eckford,	1083— 952	24 66	200 7	11180 13 4
Morebattle,	789— 784	16 int. of 1600	30 —	16781 14 8
Yetholm,	699— 1050	32 134	27 —	7049 13 4
Linton,	413— 384	14 46	30 —	5514 6 8
Sprouston,	1080— 1089	18 50 *	24 —	13263 6 8
Ednam,	387— 600	12 48	50 —	6880 0 0
Kelso,	2781— 4324	92 256	200 —	15257 9 0
Roxburgh,	784— 900	23 69	110 5	9934 6 8
Makerstoun,	165— 255	none. none.	70 —	5617 6 8
Smailholm,	551— 421	11 43	41 —	3339 16 8
Maxton,	397— 326	8 27	40 —	5495 6 8
St Boswells,	309— 500	3 14	120 —	4521 17 10
Melrose,	2312— 2446	148 87 *	300 6	19985 4 6
Bowden,	672— 860	20 65	50 3	8030 11 0
Lilliesleaf,	521— 630	5 23	350 —	8265 8 4
Roberton, ⅔.	465— 449	21 85	84 5	7413 12 4
Ashkirk, ⅓.	450— 383	7 24	80 —	5181 18 4
Selkirk, 1/11	50— 50	none. none.	26 —	1153 16 8
Galashiels, ⅓.	148— 134	2 5	8 —	2334 6 8
Stitchill, ⅓.	479— 500	none. none.	80 —	3062 9 0
Abbotrule †,	189— —	—		
	31593—32103 3159	979—2776	4682—603	

Increase since 1755. 510

* There is a considerable collection weekly in the parishes thus marked.

† Now suppressed and annexed to Southdean and Hobkirk.

GENERAL VIEW

of the

AGRICULTURE

in the county of

SELKIRK.

SING! my bonny harmless sheep,
That feed upon the mountains steep,
Bleating sweetly, as ye go
Through the winter's frost and snow ;
Hart, and hind, and fallow deer,
Not by half so useful are ;
Frae kings, to him that heads the plough,
All are obliged to TARRY WOO.

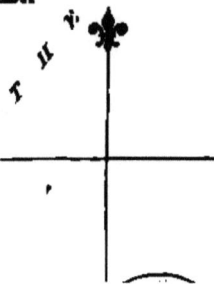

AGRICULTURAL SURVEY

OF

SELKIRKSHIRE.

CHAP. I.

GEOGRAPHICAL STATE AND CIRCUMSTANCES;

SECT. I.—*Situation and Extent.*

THE ſhire of Selkirk is not of great extent, and of a very irregular form. Nor do its boundaries, in general, run along the ſummits of mountains, or the courſe of ſtreams, which, however crooked, would afford evident marks for deſcription. A line, nearly ideal, and often whimſical in the extreme, divides it in very many places from the ſurrounding counties. Part of it ſtretches towards Mid-Lothian on the north, between the counties of Roxburgh and Peebles, having, on the eaſt, that track of the

former

former which lies north of Tweed between the waters of Gala and Leeder[*], and on the north-west and west, skirting the latter, from the northern extremity of Windlestrae-law, across Tweed, to the confines of Dumfries-shire towards the source of Yarrow-water, a distance of about twenty miles, though measured in a straight line, and much more than double that length, following the excentric line of the marches, which, jutting out into sharp angles, and shapeless promontaries, in some places nearly inclose larger or lesser portions of Tweeddale. The boundary with Dumfries-shire on the south-west and south is more regular, keeping mostly the very ridge of the mountains, from whence springs issue and rain-water descends in different directions towards the western or eastern coast, and extending upwards of fifteen miles. Upon meeting again with Roxburghshire, towards the south-east, the boundary resumes its irregularity, cutting the parishes of Roberton, Ashkirk, and Selkirk, into very unequal parts, and taking many unaccountable turns, till it falls upon the river Ettrick, about a mile above its junction with Tweed, and the same distance below the county town, and follows the course of these two rivers till they receive the Gala. It is impossible to calculate, with any pretensions to exactness, the measurement of these various curvatures, but a straight line makes the boundary with Roxburghshire about twenty-four miles. That county also completely surrounds a small circular space, nearly two miles in diameter, belonging to Selkirkshire, towards the eastern extremity of Ashkirk parish.

The whole county, thus bounded, lies between 55°. 22. and 55°. 43. N. latitude, and between 2°. c. and 3°. 20. W. longitude from Greenwich. Its greatest length, from

the

[*] See p. 1. and 3.

the fource of Ettrick water to the junction of Gala and
Tweed, is 27 miles; and its greateſt breadth, at right angles with the above, is, from Borthwick-brae to Glenſax-
burn, rather more than ſeventeen miles. Taking at a medium twenty miles for its length and twelve for its breadth,
it will contain 240 ſquare miles or 153,600 acres. But a
gentleman of accuracy, who took the trouble of meaſuring
the map *, makes its contents 257 ſquare miles or 164,480
acres. Both theſe computations are by ſome thought too
high; and, indeed, it is very difficult to aſcertain the exact area of a county ſo ankward in its ſhape, and unequal
in its ſurface. The loweſt part of it is about 300 feet above
the level of the ſea; many houſes are 600 and ſome more
than 1000 feet. With the exception of a few vallies, the
whole of it is mountainous; and moſt of the mountains
are of conſiderable height. Blackhouſe heights are 2370
feet; Windleſtrae-law, 2295 feet; Minchmoor, 2280 feet.
Ettrick-pen, 2200 feet; Lawkneis, 1990 feet; Wardlaw,
1986; Hanging-ſhaw-law, 1980 feet; Three Brethren,
1978; Black Andrew, 1968 feet; and Peat-law, 1964
feet †; beſides a great number from 1800 to 1000 feet,
all above the ſame level. It includes only two complete
pariſhes, thoſe of Ettrick and Yarrow, and three other pa-
riſh-churches, Selkirk, Galaſhiels, and Roberton, about
7⅓ of Selkirk, ⅜ of Galaſhiels, ¼ of Roberton and Aſhkirk pariſhes, ſcarcely ſo much of Stow, a pariſh in Mid-
Lothian, about ¼ of Innerleithen and a ſmall corner of
Peebles pariſhes, both in Tweeddale.

SECT.

* By Ainſlie in 1772.　　　† All taken from Ainſlie's map.

Sect. II.—*Divisions.*

From the elevated and exposed situation of the county, it is not well adapted for tillage, and is scarcely susceptible of any division in an agricultural view. The arable part of it, at present, may amount to about 8800 acres. And a regular course of crops could not be raised on double that quantity, to the advantage of the farmer, and without injuring the sheep-walks. Considered as a pasture district, it may be divided according as it is stocked with black or with white faced sheep. The former are preferred on the higher grounds towards the sources of Yarrow and Ettrick waters, from Ladhope above Yarrow church on the one, and from Deloraine and Hindhope on the other. Through the rest of the county, they are rarely to be seen, and of late a few of the latter are introduced into these upper regions.

Sect. III.—*Climate.*

In the lower part of the county, there is not so much humidity as might be expected, from its elevation, and the numerous mountains with which it is surrounded. Less rain falls at Selkirk than at Wool * about five miles nearly due

* See pages 4, 5. I regret that I cannot subjoin an extract, from a register of the weather kept at Selkirk, to contrast it with the one given from Wool, but, for the reader's satisfaction, I copy a note from the Stat. Acct. of that parish, Vol. II. p. 438. " By a regular attention to the " pluviameter

due fouth of it ; and only about ¼ inch more than at Hawkhill * near Leith. Branxholm † or Wool † may be taken as
a pretty juſt ſtandard of the climate, about ſix or eight
miles above Selkirk, on the waters of Ettrick and Yarrow. And there are very few places, even in the higheſt
parts of the county, ſo very moiſt as Langholm † ; though,
in proportion as it riſes, there is a greater quantity of rain,
the air becomes more cold and penetrating, froſts are more
early and ſeverely felt, and ſnow lies deeper and longer.
On ſome vallies 600 feet above the ocean, the rays of the
ſun; reflected by the ſurrounding mountains, throw a degree of heat that brings the crop very quickly to maturity. The number of ſprings, which are obſtructed in their
courſe, form marſhes ‡ more or leſs ſhallow and extenſive.

There

---

* pluviameter, barometer, and Fahrenheit's thermometer, for ten years,
" the mean quantity of rain yearly was found to be 31¼ inches; the me-
" dium height of the barometer, 19 ⁸⁄₁₀ ; the medium of heat 43 degrees,
" Nor did the medium of heat differ one degree during theſe ten years."

● Stat. Acct. of Selkirk, Vol. II. p. 431. Hawkhill probably is, in
every reſpect of climate, not unlike Dalkeith, p. 4, 5.

† See the Tables, page 4. 5.

‡ By a marſh I mean a ſurface kept perpetually wet, and generally
overgrown with ruſhes, by the obſtruction of ſprings and the detention of
rain-water. Marſhes are always ſhallow, and are now moſtly drained. A
moraſs is flat, of conſiderable depth, apt to be overflowed in winter, but
in ſummer ſo dry as to be paſtured, or to produce coarſe hay, though ſome
of them, or rather ſome ſpots of them, never acquire as much ſolidity as
to bear the weight of a man. A moraſs, from whence peats are dug, is
called a moſs, (ſee p. 7.). The ſurface of many places, on the ſides, ſummits, and hollows of hills, is covered with this ſubſtance, which is always more or leſs retentive of moiſture.—This is meant by moſſy land.

There are many moraffes, fome of them of an unknown depth; a good deal of moffy land; and feveral lakes. The moifture, exhaled from the vaft quantity of water collected in thefe, cannot fail to increafe the dampnefs of the atmofphere, and to produce frequent mifts and fhowers. Nor can this inconvenience be effentially leffened by thofe numerous drains, which are daily making, though thefe muft doubtlefs contribute, in fome degree, to meliorate the climate. The general courfe of the weather and feafons is much the fame as in Roxburghfhire.

Sect. IV.—*Surface and Soil.*

The general appearance of this county is a continued fucceffion of mountains, gradually rifing one above another in loftinefs, very different in fhape and magnitude, moftly green and bare, though feveral are heathy, and a few are covered with trees. Their naked and bleak afpect, when feen at a diftance in cloudy weather, is loft, upon riding among them, and beholding the rich fward with which they are covered, the clear ftreams which iffue from their fides, the fleecy flocks broufing on their green paftures, and their lambs frifking around. The animation of the fcene is heightened, by patches of brufhwood and fmall clumps of trees with which in a few places the hills are adorned, the fertility of the vales by which they are feparated from each other, and the romantic banks of the waters which wafh their bafes. The windings of Tweed and of Yarrow form a fcenery, which is finely variegated, and which may. vie in beauty with the celebrated * vale of Langollen.

The

---

* Rendered famous by the pen of Mifs Seward, and by the refidence of two young ladies of quality from Ireland.

The soil of the sheep-walks, with some exceptions, is found and dry, generally from its lying on a bottom of gravel, granite, or whinstone, and even a good deal of it, either inclining towards clay, or incumbent on clay or till, is prevented from retaining a hurtful quantity of water, by its steepness, and the firm consistence of its surface. There is very little pure clay in the whole county; and most of the land, where a mixture of it appears, or where it forms part of the substratum, lies on the sides of hills, nearly at an equal distance from their summits and the vallies below. There are some, though very few marshy spots, near the sides of rivers, and on the tops of high mountains. There is, indeed, an extensive flat, in an elevated situation between the waters of Ettrick and Borthwick, of a soft and spongy nature, and full of morasses, which may be considered as the only exception to the general assertion that deserves to be noticed. Heath grows vigorously on dry soil, but becomes rare and stunted, according to the wetness of the land, and in very wet land disappears altogether. Detached portions of it are found in every corner. It is only on the higher grounds towards the sources of the waters, that the mossy soil prevails; sometimes appearing in its native dark and sterile hue, but more frequently presenting a thin sward of beautiful and tender grass, through which the feet of cattle sink more or less, according to the depth of the mossy substance, and the quantity of rain it has imbibed. It is in such places, chiefly, that the plant abounds, which hence is called *mofs*, of whose leaves and roots sheep are so fond early in spring, when other food is scarce.

The soil of the small part in tillage, is light, dry, and easily managed. Even the few places, which lie on till, have so much declivity, that a little care, in laying out and ploughing the ridges, carries off both the springs and

the

the surface-water. Very little of it is sufficiently deep and
strong for producing wheat. But nearly the whole of it is
admirably adapted for turnips, clover, barley, and oats.
Peas, too, succeed very well. The white grains, though
not large, have thin husks, are plump, and of an admirable
quality. Turnips seldom fail, and a very great weight of
clover has been raised upon an acre. I mention these facts,
as conveying to every intelligent reader the best idea of a
sharp, warm, and kindly soil, which is rather, on the whole,
deficient in depth. White clover appears, in every field
that is surrendered to pasture, without having been sown,
and indeed is found throughout the whole county, where-
ever the soil is dry.

SECT. V.—*Minerals.*

THERE are no metals, coals, lime, or freestone in any
part of this county. But there is abundance of whinstone,
and a good deal of granite. Mosses, formed of decayed wood
and other vegetables, are made into peats for fuel. Some
of them are of considerable extent and depth. And those
towards the south-east, in the parishes of Selkirk, Roberton,
and a corner of Yarrow and Ashkirk, cover large beds of excellent shell marl. In the rills, by which some of them are
fed, many small stones are found; some of them overspread
with a gleety or glutinous substance; others incrusted with
matter, very similar to that of which the shells are composed; others again with shells in every progressive state
of formation; and a few with the animals alive, in shells
completely formed, but of different degrees of consistence
and hardness. These shells, when perfected, either quit the
                                                    stones,

ſtones, or are waſhed from them by the ſtream; and though
a few of them are ſometimes left upon the graſs which it
occaſionally overflows, yet they are in general carried down
by the ſwelling torrent, and lodged in the moſs, into which
it empties itſelf, and through which with difficulty it fil-
ters its way. There they accumulate in heaps; the animals periſh; and their bodies, with the roots and fibres of
the vegetables which grow up among'them, are converted,
in a long courſe of years, into an unctuous ſlime or mud,
which, as well as the ſhells, crumbles down into a fine powder by the action of the air. In a lake of conſiderable extent and depth, called *Oakermoor-loch*, there is a vaſt quantity of marl. It is ſituated on very elevated ground,
and ſurrounded by low and ſloping banks, except in one
point, where it ſends out a ſmall ſtream. Water oozes
from the ſides of the banks towards the lake; but the oppoſite ſides of all the banks are dry above the level of its
ſurface; below that level, numerous ſprings iſſue, and, within a few yards of their ſources, are ſeen thoſe various appearances which have been deſcribed. This has led to a
conjecture, that the water of the lake may have found ſub-
terraneous paſſages, and carried, along with it, ſome ſhells
entire, others diſſolved into particles which afterwards accumulate upon and incruſtate ſtones, and a part of the viſ-
cous matter, always ſurrounding ſhells in the pit, which
by its nature tenaciouſly adheres to ſtones, and aſſumes various fantaſtic forms eaſily miſtaken, by ſuperficial obſer-
vers, for ſhells in different ſtages of perfection. But, beſides the improbability of the ſame water finding a courſe
nearly level under ground in ſo many different directions,
this theory is contradicted by two aſcertained facts; one
of which is the animal being frequently ſeen alive in ſhells
while yet ſoft and ductile; and the other is no incruſtations
or imperfect ſhells being perceived in thoſe moſſes, pits, or

G g   hollow

hollow places, where the shells are deposited and whence marl is dug. Similar incrustations, and even small balls composed entirely of the same matter, are sometimes found in the beds of brooks which do not pass through marl, and, being evidently calcareous, are supposed to be formed by springs impregnated with lime. Yet that no rocks of lime have ever been discovered in the county or within many miles of it, that there is abundance of marl in the near neighbourhood of the brooks where such incrusted stones and balls of calcareous earth lie, and that shells, especially when calcined or reduced in any way to powder, have all the common qualities of lime, are circumstances rather unfavourable to this supposition.

These particulars, while they prove beyond a doubt that marl is the production of fresh-water animals, present difficulties to be solved by naturalists, and open to them some curious sources of speculation and inquiry. To account for the incrustation of stones with calcareous earth in a county where no lime is known to exist, and to determine whether it comes, from some rock as yet unexplored, from loose fragments or particles scattered among other substances, and washed away by streams, or from pulverised shells, or from any other matter found in the neighbourhood, requires a scientific knowledge of these subjects, as well as an accurate examination of the surrounding mountains, and the different strata of which they are formed. On the supposition of the incrustation proceeding from a rock or detached pieces of lime, it may become a question, how far this substance is necessary or useful to the animals in rearing their shells, and, on the other supposition of its being occasioned by pulverised shells, it is of equal importance to ascertain the materials from which these shells are constructed.

SECT.

Sect. VI.—*Waters.*

Like all mountainous diſtricts, this county abounds in ſprings; and, as it contains no minerals, its waters are all pure, ſalutary, and agreeable to the taſte. From its ſmall extent, none of the numerous ſtreams, which riſe in it, can be expected to arrive at a conſiderable ſize, and they all loſe their names in the Tweed or the Teviot. Gala, which has its ſource in Mid-Lothian, and during its courſe in that county, flows moſtly amidſt green and naked hills, on becoming the boundary between the ſhires of Selkirk and Roxburgh, is adorned with woody banks, winds around fertile fields, and after furniſhing the fulling-mills and other machinery at Galaſhiels with a plentiful ſupply of water, empties itſelf into Tweed about half-a-mile below that village. Cadon alſo, deſcending rapidly from high mountains, pours its paſtoral ſtream into Tweed on the north. That beautiful river, during the ſhort ſpace of nine miles that it interſects this county, holds a placid and ſteady courſe, in a deep bed hemmed in by green banks moſtly covered with lofty trees, except in a few places where it is interrupted by rocks or huge ſtones. The varying aſpects of the ſurrounding hills, the venerable and vigorous woods, the cultivated or graſſy plains, and the ſmooth or rapid ſtream, preſent a new and pictureſque ſcene at every ſtep the traveller advances. Nor is the ſcenery on Yarrow leſs romantic and delightful. Riſing on the confines of this county towards thoſe of Dumfries and Peebles-ſhires, it paſſes through two freſh-water lakes; one of which, eſpecially, in extent and natural beauty, far ſurpaſſes any thing of the kind in the ſouth of Scotland. They are ſeparated by a narrow neck of level ground,

not

not above 100 yards in length, through which the water runs. The fartheſt, named the *Loch of the Lows*, is only about three quarters of a mile long, and little more than a quarter of a mile broad. The neareſt, called *St Mary's Loch*, has a bend towards its ſouth-weſt end, which will make its length about three miles. In a ſtraight line it will ſcarcely meaſure ſo much, and its medium breadth will ſcarcely be half-a-mile. Their banks, in ſeveral places, are fringed with copſe wood. The mountains, which encompaſs them, and the brooks, by which they are fed, have a ſequeſtered and wild, but not a bleak or rugged appearance. Yarrow, after leaving them, flows through dry and healthy ſheep-walks, where little wood is to be ſeen, and few ſpots admit of cultivation, for eight or nine miles, when its channel becomes rocky and hollow, its windings more violent, and its current more precipitous. The hills, at the ſame time, aſcend with a bolder elevation; their ſteep ſides, to a conſiderable height, are ornamented with wood; ſtately trees hang over the lower banks, and grow luxuriantly on the plains; while a variety of buſhes and wild flowers diverſify and embelliſh the proſpect. Ettrick takes a direction nearly parallel to that of Yarrow, but drains a country, of greater extent, more ſubject to rain, and more retentive of moiſture. It conſequently contains more water; and preſerves its name after receiving the other. It can boaſt of few trees during the firſt twenty miles of its courſe; but its vallies are wider and fitter for cultivation than thoſe of Yarrow. A little way above their junction, its ſides are ſkirted with natural wood; its plains become more extenſive and fertile, and are ſheltered by plantations on the adjoining hills. After their junction, the united ſtreams roll, often with deſtructive violence, through vallies equally rich, and adorned with ſimilar plantations of thriving wood, about four miles into Tweed, waſhing in their courſe

the

the bottom of a high bank on which the county town
ſtands, and becoming for a mile the boundary of this county with Roxburghſhire. Meggot and Douglas are the chief
tributaries of Yarrow ; the former is wholly in the ſhire
of Peebles, and falls into St Mary's loch. Ettrick is augmented by Tima, Rankleburn, and ſeveral ſmaller brooks.
Ale and Borthwick have their ſources in this county. The
former iſſues from a beautiful circular lake, about a quarter
of a mile in diameter, called *Alemoor Loch ;* and, from a ſmall
eſtate on its banks, the late Lord Alemoor, of moſt reſpectable memory, took his title. The latter riſes on the ſouthern extremity of this county towards Dumfries-ſhire ; and
its original nakedneſs is in a fair way of being ſoon removed by numerous plantations lately made both here and in
the contiguous county of Roxburgh, which the Borthwick
alternately bounds and interſects, and into which both theſe
waters run.

CHAP.

CHAP. II.

STATE OF PROPERTY.

SECT. 1.—*Estates, and their Management.*

THE greatest part of this county was once a royal forest, and a number of places are named from the
trees or shrubs which grew around them, the animals by
which they were frequented, or the sports which were practised in their neighbourhood. All appearances of a forest
are now nearly effaced. There are not more than 2000
acres of wood in the whole county. And no beasts or birds
of prey are to be seen, except sometimes a fox, or an erne
from Loch Skene, a lake in the high parts of Dumfries-
shire, towards the source of Yarrow water. Herons, hawks,
and kites are not uncommon; and hares, partridges, and
growse abound. The mountains and vallies, which formerly were covered with trees, are now mostly employed more
profitably

profitably in feeding sheep, and producing corn; though there are considerable portions of both, which might be planted, much to the advantage of proprietors, and very little to the detriment of their tenants.

Taking a kind of medium between the two computations which have been given of its contents, this county may be supposed to contain 250 square miles or 160,000 acres; and allowing 12,000 of these to be in tillage, and occupied by woods, gardens, pleasure-grounds, and the sites of houses, there will remain 148,000 acres of pasture-land; which does not yield so much rent *per* acre as the pasture district in Roxburghshire, because a greater proportion of it is coarse and poor, and the sheep, though equally numerous according to the extent of ground, are smaller and less profitable. From the best information which I could obtain, it may be rated at 2 s. 9 d. *per* acre, the 8800 acres in tillage at 10 s., the 2000 acres in wood at 25 s., and gardens and pleasure-grounds at 20 s. *, making the whole rent of the county as under:

148000 acres in sheep-pasture, at 2 s. 9 d.	—	L. 20350
8800 acres in tillage, at 10 s.	— —	4400
2000 acres in wood, at 25 s.	— —	2500
1200 acres in gardens, pleasure-grounds, and the sites of houses, &c. at 20 s.	— —	1200

160000	Total rent,	L. 28450

The

---

* I have made very little alteration of Mr Johnston's valuation of the lands in pasture and tillage. For though some farms in the lower parts of the county are let above 4 s. *per* acre, a considerable proportion of them is fit for tillage, while large tracks, in the higher parts, where nearly three acres are requisite to maintain a sheep, cannot be estimated above 1 s. 4 d. *per* acre, from which 2 s. 9 d. appears to be a pretty just medium.

The

The valued rent of the county is L. 80,307 : 15 : 6 Scots,
which, though greatly lefs than that of Roxburghfhire in
proportion to the extent of ground in each, is much higher
in proportion to the actual rent. Of this valuation, L. 36,545,
11 s. 4 d. belongs to five Peers; one of whom, however,
has no land, but draws a fmall revenue yearly in teinds,
formerly drawn by the church. The remainder belongs to
37 commoners and the burgh of Selkirk. There are fixteen of thefe commoners, who have, each of them, property exceeding L. 1000 of valued rent, and only one of thefe
is

The actual number of acres in tillage is computed, from the concurring
opinions of gentlemen and farmers in different corners of the county; and
the average rent *per* acre is gueffed on the following grounds. Including
one farm, which lets at 18 s. 6 d. *per* acre, there are about 2000 acres,
which, at an average, let for 14 s. *per* acre, =   .   L. 1400
Suppofing the remaining 6800 to be only 6 s. *per* acre, = . .   2040

The amount is   .   L. 4440

which is the mereft trifle above 10 s. *per* acre; and even the late great increafe in the rent of a few farms will not raife this average to 10 s. 6 d.
nor the average of the pafture diftrict above 1 d. or at moft 1½ d. *per*
acre.

The land in wood is valued at the low rate of L. 15 *per* acre, and the
intereft of that fum is ftated as rent, which is 3 s. 8 d. lefs *per* acre than
the average rent of fimilar land in Roxburghfhire: and it muft be obferved, that though a great deal more of valuable wood is to be found there
than here, yet more alfo has failed and become of no value.

It is difficult to afcertain either the quantity or the value of the land in
gardens, pleafure-grounds, &c. The houfes, gardens, and ftack-yards in
Selkirk and Galafhiels occupy about 450 or at leaft above 400 acres. Exclufive of gentlemens feats, there are other 200 places of refidence, to
which about 300 acres may be allowed for thefe purpofes. And an equal
allowance may be made for the fites of houfes and offices, the lawns, pleafure-grounds, gardens, and orchards of proprietors. If in this article there
be an error, it cannot make a difference of L. 200 in the whole rent of
the county.

is incapable of being a freeholder. The valuation of their whole property amounts to L. 34,380 : 11 : 10; that of the burgh is valued at L. 1053 : 3 : 4 : so that, including a mere trifle rated for a *feu*-duty, L. 8328, 9 s. is divided among twenty-one proprietors, of whom six are precluded from being inrolled as freeholders, either by the smallness of their properties, or the nature of their tenures. Of the proprietors, ten reside mostly in the county, and nine in its immediate neighbourhood; four have dwelling-houses where they may reside occasionally, and the rest are constant absentees. Many of those who do not reside, and some of those who do, employ factors to let their lands, receive and discharge their rents, examine and pay their accounts, and transact their country affairs. Particular days and places are fixed for receiving the rents of most estates, generally about three or four months after they become due. Greater indulgence is shewn to a few tenants with respect to time, but they are required to repair, with their rents, to the residence of their landlord or his factor. The resident gentlemen have all a greater or less quantity of ground under their own management, direct themselves the disposal of their pleasure-grounds and planting, and commit the cultivation of their fields and their marketings to bailiffs, here called overseers or *grieves*. Some of them farm the whole of their estates, and have leases of other lands. There cannot be less than 4000 acres occupied by proprietors, exclusive of the farms they thus possess. During the last 25 years, only seven estates have been disposed of; the largest of which was purchased by the heir of the family, by whom it had been sold a few years before. The valued rent of all these, added together, amounts only to L. 4340, 9 s. 9 d. Scots. Before that period, however, three pretty considerable estates were in the market, and, though they

H h   fetched

fetched what was then thought high prices, there can be no
doubt of their being now worth much more.

SECT. II.—*Tenures.*

THIS whole county, with very few exceptions, belonged either to the Crown, or to the Abbey of Melrofs. That
part of it, which was appropriated to the Sovereign, or re-
cognifed as his patrimony, was occupied by his vaffals at a
moderate rent, until an act of Parliament in 1594 allowed
him to alienate his lands; in confequence of which, thefe
vaffals obtained charters from him to their eftates, on paying the former rents, with fome fmall addition annually to
the Crown *. All the lands, acquired from the church, are
now poffeffed by Royal charters: And a very little part of
the whole county is held by that kind of tenure, which re-
fembles

* The following places pay *Crown-rents*, in confequence of their forming once a part of the Royal demefnes. Haining, Hartwoodburn, Brownmuir, Middleftead, Hartwoodmyres, Aikwood, Hutlarburn, Whitchaugh-
brae, Outer and Inner Huntlies, Laghope, Howford, Shaws, Helmburn,
Baillielee, Dodhead, Reidfordgreen, Hyndhope, Deloraine, Cackrawbank,
Anlethope, Oamefcleogh, Derphope, Tufhelaw, Derrybufh, Corflee, New-
burgh or Winterburgh, Gilmanfcleugh, Singlee, Eafter and Wefter Kirk-
hopes. Eafter and Wefter Fauldhopes, Carterhaugh, South and North Bow-
hill. Auldwark, Newark, Mill of Newark, Tafthrugh, Fafter and Wefter
Kerfhopes, Ladhope, Sandhope, Eldinghope, Eltrieve, Bowerhope, Corfe-
cleugh, St Mary Loch of the Lowes, Kirkftead, Dryhope, Douglaverig,
Blackhoufe, Mountberger Catflack know, Cuffackburn, Glengaber and
Shootinglees, Whitehope, Denchar, Tynnes, Lewinthope, Hangingfhaw,
Broadmeadows, Foulfhiels, Harehead, Yair, Peel, Athieftecl, William-
hope, Elibank, Flora, Glenfax, Olewpot or Fawnbunhead, Priefthope,
Sithope, Garthope, Hollylee, Thornilee, Triolieknows, Cedonlee, Fairni-
lee, Galathiels, Mofilee, Blindlee, Torwoodlee, Corklee, Redhead, White-
bank, Newhall, Knows, Blackhaugh, Windiedoon, Cadonhead.

fembles a copyhold in England. There are, at prefent, thirty-two on the roll of freeholders, of whom eight have no landed property, though three or four of them have either retained or purchafed *fuperiorities,* which give them an undoubted legal title to vote for a member of Parliament; and this roll can only receive an addition of fix actual proprietors, as matters now ftand.

CHAP.

CHAP. III.

BUILDINGS.

Sect. I.—*Houses of Proprietors.*

ONE of the Peers has a pleasant hunting-seat, where he sometimes resides for a few days in the sporting-season. Four proprietors have built excellent modern houses. Several old houses have been made snug and commodious by judicious additions and alterations, and others are easily susceptible of the same improvement. The numerous remains of strong towers, while they are monuments of the rude and fierce spirit of our ancestors, should fill us with thankfulness for the happy change which has taken place in the tempers and manners of the present age, from the secure protection of every right that is dear to men. In the whole county, there is but one ruin of a house possessed by a family in later times.

The offices, in general, are substantial, convenient, and capacious, all built with lime, and slated. In both the

houses

houfes and offices lately built, elegance is united with utility.

Sect. II.—*Farm-Houfes, Offices, and Repairs.*

The farmers are, by no means, fo well accommodated
either with dwelling-houfes, or offices; both being, in general, paultry and ill-built. Moft of the dwelling-houfes
are of one ftory, low in the roof, badly lighted, and covered with thatch. The walls, however, are of ftone and
lime; and of late a few of thefe low houfes have been flated. The offices are ftill more pitiful, meanly and rudely
conftructed, and awkwardly placed. Some ftables and cow-
houfes are fo low, as fcarcely to admit horfes and cattle of
an ordinary fize.

In the higher parts of the county, it is frequently neceffary to give all the houfes a new covering of rufhes or
fprots every year, to repair the wafte occafioned by the
tempeftuous and rainy weather. The weight, thus annually accumulated, prefling upon the roof, forces it or the walls
to give way, and often expofes both people and cattle to
great danger. A happy change, however, is taking place
in all thefe refpects. There are a few houfes of two, and
feveral of one ftory, fubftantially built with good ftones and
lime, foreign timber, excellent flates, and fizeable windows
and doors. The offices, too, are every way fuitable, and
commodioufly difpofed.

There is no occafion for any difference in the fize of
dwelling-houfes in different parts of the county, as the tenants, every where, may have families equally numerous,
and the fame calls to fhew hofpitality. Yet, in thofe diftricts which are at the greateft diftance from good inns,
the houfes are fmalleft, from a defire of rendering them
warm and comfortable, and from a fear, that, by enlarging

their

their dimensions and raising their walls, they would be more
exposed to the violent and piercing blasts so frequent in
these bleak and mountainous regions. But, though houses
were made larger and higher, this disadvantage might be
avoided, by choosing a dry and sheltered situation, by placing the gable directly towards that quarter from whence
comes the severest storms, and by joining to that gable some
necessary building of the same height with the dwelling-
house. In farms, where little or no corn is raised, a barn
might still be useful, to hold wool and cheese in their seasons, and to serve various other purposes ; and it might
stand very conveniently above an open shed or out-house,
where the ewe-milkers, farm-servants, and artificers, might
carry on their respective works till the end of autumn, and
where all the implements and utensils used in the farm, and
even some of the fuel, might be deposited during winter.
These two houses would make an admirable defence to a
dwelling-house of two stories, if placed at the end most exposed to the wind and tempest : And stables, cow-houses,
&c. might stand, either at the other end, or in some other
more eligible spot.

In the lower parts of the county, where the farms are
wholly or mostly arable, or where a considerable portion
of land in tillage is attached to the sheep-walks, many
farm-houses and offices are constructed on the same plan,
and are much of the same size as those in Roxburgh-shire.
Most of these were built at the sole expence of the proprietors. But, in some instances, in different corners of the
county, nothing was furnished, but timber, lime, and slates;
the tenants carried these from the sea-port or kiln, and paid
all the workmanship, though they had only short leases, or
rather no leases at all *. Some landlords allow a stipulated
sum,

* This was done only by the tenants of one great proprietor. They
placed

fum, others the prime coft of the materials, leaving the
tenants to make the moft of thefe meagre conditions, during the currency of their leafes. Unlefs the leafes are
long and profitable, it cannot be thought that tenants will
put themfelves to any expence or trouble, except what is
abfolutely neceffary to keep the houfes habitable till the
time of their removal. Proprietors miftake their own intereft, in not giving their tenants commodious and fubftantial houfes and offices. Thefe are powerful attractions to
all men of found fenfe ; and little can be expected, in the
way of enterprife or judicious improvement, from thofe,
who feel no defire of having themfelves and their cattle
conveniently and comfortably lodged.

Sect. III.—*Cottages.*

THE cottages, attached to farms for the refidence of
fhepherds and married fervants, are wretched habitations,
dark, fmoky, and infufficient defences againft wind and
rain. Other cottages, let by proprietors on longer or
fhorter leafes to labourers and mechanics, are not entitled
to much commendation. Being built, for the moft part,
by the firft inhabitant, on a fhort leafe at a trifling rent,
without any expence to the landlord except the prime coft
of the materials, which are by no means of the deareft and
beft kinds, the work is executed in a very fuperficial manner ;

placed an implicit truft, not without reafon, in his juftice and generofity,
and thofe of the gentlemen who manage his affairs. But the perfonal character of a proprietor or his men of bufinefs, whatever encouragement and
fecurity it may afford to tenants in particular cafes, muft only be confidered as an exception to the general and well founded rule, that landlords
fhould bear the whole expence of rearing good houfes and offices to their
tenants, and receive an addition of rent equivalent to the expence in-
curred.

ner; and without frequent reparations they would soon become ruinous. Cottages, or rather small houses of a better order, are built on long leases or *feus* *, granted for a certain premium as the value of the ground, and a small annual rent or feud 1 acknowledgment. The houses in Galashiels, the only village in the county, are mostly of the two last descriptions: and the striking superiority, both in outward appearance and in workmanship, of those built on long leases, is a strong recommendation to all gentlemen, who wish to see flourishing villages on their estates, to adopt that method, or to give *feus*.

In all inland counties, it should be a greater object, than it seems to be, with all proprietors and tenants, to provide decent and comfortable dwellings for married servants, labourers, and mechanics. Convenient and pleasant houses, besides being favourable to health, may induce many, who now rove from place to place, and change their masters and their habitations at every term, to settle, to marry, and to exert themselves for the support of their families, and may encourage both husbands and wives to be cleanly and neat in their persons, their tables, and their furniture, and to keep their children, their doors, and their gardens in good order. In all these respects, what can be expected, but discontent and disease, reluctant, careless, and slovenly exertions, from those who dwell amidst smoke and dirt?

* A *feu* is a perpetual right to the ground or tenement, for the payment of a stipulated price, and of an annual acknowledgment.

CHAP.

CHAP. IV.

MODE OF OCCUPATION.

SECT. I.—*Size of Farms.—Character of the Farmers.*

THERE are only three or four farms in the county wholly arable, or capable of being made so. None of these contains 500 acres, and only one of them exceeds L. 400 of rent. There may be about 24 or perhaps 26 other farms, whose stock and produce are divided more or less equally between corn and sheep. One-half of the remaining farms have nearly as much land in tillage as, in a favourable season, may yield a sufficient quantity of oats for the consumpt of their servants and horses. In the other half, comprehending almost a third part of the whole county, very little or no corn is raised.

The size of farms varies from 50 to 6000 acres. From 1500 to 2500 is thought to be a moderate size for a farm which is only fit for pasture, and a large size for one where there is a considerable proportion of arable land. One farm,

wholly

wholly arable, and put into excellent order at a vast expence, is subset at the rate of 18 s. 6 d. *per* acre. But all land is let by the lump; none by the acre, except small pieces around Selkirk and Galashiels. The inhabitants of these two places possess from 1200 to 1500 acres at different rents, mostly from one to two guineas *per* acre. More may be given for a few small and select spots. The lesser farms, below 300 acres, which are not numerous, and most of which keep a few sheep, bring from L. 30 to L. 100 of rent. From that sum to L. 300 is the most common rent for larger farms, whether devoted wholly to sheep, or partly employed in producing corn.

The character of the farmers admits of much diversity. A few, from being shepherds, have risen with a fair character to rent farms of considerable extent, and retain the simple and homely manners, dress, and fare of their primeval occupation. But by far the most numerous class are sons of farmers, either in this or neighbouring counties; among whom, according to the difference of their natural talents and tempers, of their opportunities to mix with good company and receive information, and of their early habits, there appears much characteristic variety in point of behaviour, living, and managing their farms. Some of them are wonderfully tenacious of ancient practices; but their number is now much reduced. Others venture on innovations with slow and timid steps, but grow bolder by the experience of their own or their near neighbour's success. And severals carry on improvements with a degree of spirit and skill, which is not easily surpassed, and which has abundantly repaid their trouble and risk; though there is much less scope here for ingenuity and enterprise than in Roxburghshire. In general, they all deserve the praise of being frank, communicative, and hospitable. Their tables are much better provided, than the appearance of their houses houfes affords any reafon to expect; and there are, in their looks and manner, a cordial welcome, and an urgency to partake of their meat and drink, which ftrongly indicate a kind heart. A few of them live in elegance and plenty, have a plain dinner well dreffed and ferved every day, and a bottle of wine or a cheerful glafs of punch for a friend. But none of them keeps a chaife, or a man-fervant for any houfehold purpofe. Being all trained up from their infancy to ride, they themfelves, their wives, and their children can manage a horfe with fome dexterity; and can climb fteep mountains, either on horfeback, or on foot, without much inconveniency. They are very fociable; and even the moft recluse are loth to part, efpecially when they meet together at markets and fairs; but, of late, there have been few or no inftances of their neglecting necef-fary bufinefs for the fake of their bottle, or companions, or indeed for any other enjoyment. Attempts to deceive and over-reach purchafers, though not wholly unknown among fome of them, are held in utter contempt by the better fort; and, upon the whole, they are very punctual in fulfilling bargains, and making payments. Their chief defect is a degree of indifference for that kind of knowledge, which can only be acquired from books, or from more fre-quent and enlarged intercourfe with mankind. Very few of them have hitherto become members of a public libra-ry at Selkirk, although they may be admitted on mode-rate terms: And very many of them difcover no defire of mixing in any other fociety, than that of their near neighbours, or of thofe with whom they have bufinefs to tranfact. Could they be perfuaded to read ufeful books, efpecially in the line of their profeffion, and to come more abroad into the company of thofe from whofe converfation profitable inftruction might be learned, they would ftore their minds with much va-

luable

luable knowledge, and find, in this acquisition, ample compensation for the trifling expence attending it.

Sect. II.—Rent.

THE farms in this county are taken, not by measurement, but according to the computations, made by the different offerers, of the number of sheep they will maintain, and the quantity of grain which may be sown on them with a reasonable prospect of an adequate return. Farmers have also respect to the nature of the soil, and prefer what is dry, sound, and healthy for sheep, and what brings corn of a good quality early to maturity. They also esteem lands, though producing coarse grasses, where sheep have an ample undisturbed range. For though it is reckoned much in favour of these useful animals, to settle and feed on little space, yet it is equally an advantage to them, especially where their food however abundant is not of the most nutritive nature, to have an extensive walk, where they are not liable to be frequently turned, by an awkwardly placed wall or by the shepherd's dog, from trespassing on the possessions of others. When forcibly restrained within narrow and irregular bounds, sheep are prevented from thriving so well, and becoming so soon in good condition, as they otherwise might. Hence a farm of this description, however excellent its pasture, will not bring the same rent in proportion to the number of sheep upon it, as another, of an inferior soil, which is more sizeable and compact. Regard is also paid to the situation of arable land; and it is of much greater value when lying all together, than when scattered in detached and straggling fields through sheep-

walks.

walks. Thefe circumftances render it impoffible to fix any general rate, at which land is rented. The grafs eat by a fheep through the year is reckoned worth from 3 s. 6 d. to 4 s. whether it grows on five acres, or on lefs than one. But the quantity of land, on which a boll of grain is fown, varies, according to climate, foil, and local fituation, from 5 s. to L. 3. A few fpots around Selkirk, occupied as gardens or nurferies, are let about that fum *per* acre; but it has been already mentioned, that the more common rate of all the lands let by the acre is from one to two guineas, and the average will fcarcely reach 30 s.

All rents are paid in money twice every year. Though Whitfunday and Martinmas are the terms fpecified in all leafes, yet it is ufual to delay exacting payment until the time of the two great fairs at Selkirk in April and in Auguft. With this indulgence, it can be no great hardfhip on the tenants to pay what is here called *fore-rent*, that is, a full year's rent before they reap a crop. Their profits arifing almoft wholly from fheep, they fell their wool, their lambs, their cheefe, their young wedders, and their caft ewes, before they make the firft half-yearly payment of their rent, and they fell fome of thefe articles the following feafon, before they make the fecond. The abfurd exactions of *carriages* *, *kain*, *dargs*, and other remnants of feudal manners, are ftill retained in fome leafes; but, in moft cafes money is accepted in lieu of them. I am forry to add, that adftriction to particular mills, is, in very many cafes, an unpleafant addition to the rent.

SECT.

* *Carriages* mean the carriage of fuel, corn, hay, &c. by tenants without payment for the proprietor. *Kain* is a certain number of tame-fowls. A *darg* is a day's work, either of man or woman, as fpecified in leafes. In fome leafes, a certain quantity of lint or tow is required to be fpun.

SECT. III.—*Tithes*

ARE quite unknown.

SECT. IV.—*Poor-rates*

ARE univerfally eftablifhed, though the weekly collections in fome parifhes are very confiderable. The fum annually levied by affeffments amounted in 1791 * to L. 343 Sterling; and, as the number of poor was then about 140, many of them muft have been able to earn fomething by working, and muft have received occafional aid, from the collections made on Sundays, and from charitable neighbours. In this account, are not included the affeffments levied from thofe parts of Stow and Innerleithen parifhes, which lie in this county, nor yet the poor who may refide there. It may not be improper to take notice, that, in general, the poor-rates do not materially leffen the voluntary contributions, becaufe thefe are fuffered to remain under the management of the kirk-feffions.

SECT. V.—*Leafes.*

THIS county being moftly paftoral, the leafes are fhort. A few have been granted, for nineteen or twenty-one years, of farms containing a good deal of arable land fufceptible of improvement. But, even for fuch farms, thirteen or fifteen

* See Stat. Acct. of Galafhiels and Selkirk, Vol. II.; of Afhkirk and Etttrick, Vol. III.; of Yarrow, Vol. VII.; and of Roberton, Vol. XL.

teen years are more common terms, and nine for the county at large. The period of some is still shorter ; and, on
the estate of one great proprietor, there are very few or no
leafes at all. Yet such is the reliance on his justice and
moderation, that tenants are rather desirous of occupying
his lands, and scruple not to lay out money in improving
their farms, and accommodating themselves with comfortable houses. I must, however, be permitted to regret, that
the respectable character of an individual should give a kind
of sanction to a practice, which, on every sound principle,
must be confidered, as the bane of agriculture, and a real
loss both to the public, and to every proprietor who adopts
it. It is a singular infelicity to any country, when the ami-
able manners of its sovereign, and the ease, plenty, and
security, which subjects enjoy under his government, engage them to make an unconditional surrender of their
rights, and entwist around their own necks the fetters of
despotism. It is impossible to calculate, how soon and how
deeply the evil, thus improvidently and tamely submitted
to, may affect themselves or their posterity. And may not
the possession of farms without leases be productive, according to circumstances, of consequences equally disagreeable
to tenants or landlords ? When a tenant dies, what security
has he, that his farm shall descend to his family ? And can
it be expected, that he will risk any expence in improving
it on such an uncertainty ? Supposing him to live, does
not his continuance in the farm from year to year depend
on the will of his master ? May not his master die, and be
succeeded (especially on an entailed estate) by an heir, who
shall construe every substantial melioration into an argument
for an advance of rent ? Or, allowing both proprietor and
tenant to live, how soon may the carelessness of a servant
in allowing cattle to destroy a hedge, or the levity of a son
in cutting a stick or shooting a partridge, or the refusal of a
friend

friend to give a political vote, or the tenant's own indiscretion in speaking rudely to some favourite minion or pointer, procure his dismissal? It is, therefore, as clearly his interest, to have a lease, that he may be independent of such capricious treatment, as it is that of British subjects to be governed by King, Lords, and Commons, a known code of laws, and regular courts of justice. Nor are leases less advantageous to landholders; of which a stronger proof cannot be given, than the certainty, in the case to which I allude, of the proprietor, notwithstanding the merited prepossession in his favour, obtaining a considerable increase of rent, and giving greater satisfaction to his tenants, by granting them leases of a competent length, and freeing them from all extraordinary expence, with respect to their houses and farms. Should the *competent length* of a lease be asked, the answer is plain. It must bear a proportion to the advance of rent. For example, to every L. 100 of rent presently paid, let L. 2 be added for every year of the lease; making an addition of L. 42 on every L. 100 for a lease of twenty one years, of L. 30 on every L. 100 for a lease of fifteen years, and of L. 18 on every L. 100 for a lease of nine years*; devolving on the landlord all expence of building, excepting the mere carriage of stones and lime; leaving, to the tenant to determine the size of the houses, and inclosures, and the length of the lease; but binding him to a general system of management, whereby the land might increase in value, and the houses and inclosures might be preserved in excellent order. It would be an improvement on this plan, if the rise in the rent was not

to

* These examples are given merely as illustrations of the principle. The additional rent may be greater or less than is here mentioned, according to the nature and local situation of farms, their susceptibility of improvement, their ready access to manure, and a variety of other circumstances.

to take place for a few years; a claufe, which, I am happy
to underftand, has found its way into fome leafes in this
county, and which deferves commendation, as it keeps money in the tenant's pocket at the commencement of his
agricultural operations, when he ftands moft in need of it.
Whitfunday is the ufual term at which leafes commence.
Tenants then enter into poffeffion of the houfes and the
land in grafs, but not of the land under corn, till the crop
is removed from the ground.

Sect. VI.—*Expence and Profit.*

THERE is fo great diverfity in the nature and fize of
farms and in the mode of management, that an account of
expence and profit can fcarcely be given, which will apply
to more than two or three farms in the county. In the few
that are moftly or wholly arable, a fmall number of fheep
are either kept or bought annually to be fattened; and young
cattle are either reared, or old ones are purchafed to confume the turnips. The portions of land in tillage, belonging to fheep-farms, are of fuch unequal fertility and extent,
and fubjected to fuch different treatment, with a view of
accommodating either the family or the flock of the tenant, that it would be extremely difficult to make any general calculation of their real produce, and of the profits
arifing from a complication of caufes and practices, from
which the reader could derive entertainment or information. The pafture diftrict is almoft wholly flocked with
ewes, either of the white-faced and long-bodied kind, or of
the black-faced and fhort-bodied. This difference, in the
manner of flocking farms, as well as in the kinds of fheep,
occafions a difference in the fales and prices both of fheep

and wool from the flatement given in the Agricultural Survey of Roxburghfhire. To enfure a plentiful ftore of food for the mothers and their lambs, it is ufual, in feveral farms, to fell a certain proportion of ewes while great with young, from whence they are called *great-ewes*. In other farms, where provifion is more abundant in the early than in the late part of the feafon, no ewes are fold till they bring up their lambs, after which thofe are picked out, who are moft unfit for breeders, and in beft condition for the markets. Thefe are called *draught* or *caft-ewes*. In one or other of thefe ways, about one-fixth part of all the ewes on the farm is annually difpofed of, the proportion of *great* and *draught*-ewes varying in different farms. It is expected that at leaft two-thirds of the ewes fhall bring lambs yearly; and fomewhat more than two-fevenths and lefs than one-third of all the lambs produced, are kept to fupply vacancies in the flock by death or fales. On thefe principles, the expence and profit, on a farm capable of wintering 2000 fheep of the white-faced kind, will be nearly as under :

The rent, at 3 s. 6 d. *per* fheep,   –   L. 350   0   0

To 1200 old ewes, at 14 s. –	L. 800		
To 380 do. two years old, at 11 s.	209		
To 400 do. one year old, at 7 s.	140		
To 20 tups, at L. 1, 10 s. –	30		
2000	L. 1179		

Intereft on this fum at 5 *per cent.*   –   55   4   0

Salving, at 4½ d. each,   –   –   37   10   0

Three herds, at L. 20 each,   –   –   60   0   0

Drains, &c.   –   –   –   15   0   0

Grofs yearly expenditure,   L. 517   14   0

The

The produce or sales will be, after every allowance for mortality,

120 great ewes, at 14 s. 6 d. — —	L. 87	0 0
200 draught-ewes, at 11 s. — —	110	0 0
800 lambs, at 5 s. — — — —	200	0 0
1800 fleeces, at 2 s. — — — —	180	0 0
Cheese, tups, *udder-locks* *, and *morts* *, —	50	0 0
Total produce,	L. 627	0 0

From which the farmer's profit appears to be, L. 109 6 0

but it may be greater, when the prices of wool and sheep are higher, when the mortality is less, and when the season is favourable to the feeding of sheep and of lambs. He cannot, in any season, sell more than a score of ewes above the calculation; but, when it is remarkably good, he may sell 80 more fleeces, and 100 or 120 more lambs.

Where no great-ewes are sold, the profit is rather larger.

Expenditure, as before, — —	L. 517 14 0	

The number of ewes will be the same as before, and their prices only 11 s. viz. 320

ewes, at 11 s. — — —	L. 176	0 0

But the number of lambs must be greater, as those of the great-ewes are to be included;

hence 920 lambs, at 5 s. — —	230	0 0

There must also be more fleeces, at least 1900,

at 2 s. — — —	190	0 0
Cheese, &c. as formerly, — —	50	0 0
Total produce,	L. 646	0 0
	which	

---

* *Udder-locks* are the wool plucked from the udders, and *morts* are the skins of sheep and lambs who die. See p. 47. and 156.

which is L. 19 more than by the former statement, and
shows the superior profit of not selling great-ewes, when
the farm has sufficient food for them. The last article may
likewise admit of a small increase, as more cheese will be
made, and there will be more udder-locks : though this is
rather problematical, as there will also be fewer skins of
sheep who die.

The comparative expence and profit of the same number of black-faced sheep, will appear from the following
statement :

Rent, as formerly,   —   —   —   L. 350   0   0
But the value of the flock must be less, at least
   1 s. 6 d. each on 1600 sheep, making L. 120,
   the interest of which must be deducted, and
   reduces the interest on the sum-total to   —   49   4   0
By using more tar, which is comparatively
   cheap, and less butter, which is comparatively dear, there will be a saving of L. 7,
   10 s.   —   —   —   —   30   0   0
The sums allowed for herds and drains, as
   formerly,   —   —   —   —   75   0   0
                                        ————————
                      Total expenditure,   L. 504   4   0

            The sales will consist of,

110 great-ewes, which, on account of the inferiority of
   their fleeces, will only sell for 13 s. 4 d.   L. 80   0   0
But the draught-ewes, by wanting their flee-
   ces, will reach the same price with white-
   faced ones ; hence 200 of them, at 11 s.
   is as formerly,   —   —   —   110   0   0
                                        ————————
                  Carried forward,   L. 190   0   0

Brought forward,   L. 190   0   0

The lambs, by being longer fuckled, will
fetch 1 s. 6 d. each more than the other
lambs; hence 800 of them, at 6 s. 6 d.   260   0   0

But the fleeces of the flock cannot be eſtimated above 11 d. each *; hence 1800 fleeces,
at 11 d.   .—   —   —   —   82   10   0

And leſs cheeſe will be made, which will require a deduction of L. 12 or thereabouts
from the laſt lumped article, reducing it to   38   0   0

Total produce,   L. 570   10   0

which leaves only L. 66, 6 s. of profit to the farmer, being L. 43 leſs than is gained on a ſimilar flock of white-faced ſheep. The reader will perceive that the greater profit is to be wholly aſcribed to the wool. And there are
no ways of increaſing the profit in the one caſe, which are
not equally open in the other.

* At the average of 6½ fleeces to a ſtone, this makes the price of the
ſtone about 6 s. 2½ d.

CHAP.

CHAP. V.

IMPLEMENTS.

ALL the implements of husbandry, which have already been described in the Agricultural Survey of Roxburghshire, are used in this county, except the snow-plough, the drain-plough, the cart with three wheels, the improved harrows, and the instrument for hoeing drilled crops. A thrashing-machine was brought into it, about the year 1792, but it was either never set agoing or soon given up. In 1796, a millwright in Galashiels made the first one that was actually employed, and it is found to answer extremely well. Three or four have been since erected; but their number cannot be expected to increase in a county where so little corn is raised.

There are no implements peculiar to it: The sledges, used for bringing home peats, and the *creels* or baskets, in which they and other articles are carried on horseback, being common in all hilly countries, where there are no roads for carts. Both here and in Roxburghshire, a kind of hoe is sometimes fixed to the small plough, instead of a coulter, for cleaning drilled crops, but it cannot answer in stony-land.

CHAP.

C H A P. VI.

INCLOSING, FENCES, GATES.

THE reader muſt be referred to what is mentioned in the Account of Roxburghſhire with reſpect to theſe particulars, eſpecially concerning the nature of different fences, and the manner and expence of executing incloſures. Great progreſs has been made, of late, in ſeparating the arable from the paſture lands in the ſame farms, and in ſubdividing into equal fields what is ſubjected to the plough. Subſtantial ſtone-walls, without cement, about five feet high, and moſtly with Galloway tops, are common in the higher parts of the county, not becauſe thorns will not grow, but becauſe it is difficult to preſerve them while young from being gnawed, and often eat over by ſheep during winter. They are found, in great luxuriancy and excellent order, around Selkirk and Galaſhiels, and on ſeveral farms where there is much tillage; and have been

reared

reared to become good fences, without the aid of pales. Walls of turf or fod are annually raifed in many places a-round thofe folds, in which fheep are confined during night, till the grain is cut and removed from the fields; the walls are then thrown down, and the fpace inclofed, enriched by the dung and urine of the fheep, is ploughed to bear a crop the enfuing feafon. Hurdles or nets are fometimes ufed, inftead of walls, and removed to another portion of the field when one is thought fufficiently faturated, which may be thought to fave expence, and get a larger quantity of ground thus manured: but when the prime coft of thefe, and the trouble of flitting them, are taken into the account; and when, at the fame time, it is confidered, that the more furface is gone over in this manner, the lefs dung it re-ceives, and that the fods, by being expofed in thin walls to the drought of fummer, are eafily fpread along the field, and converted into a fine and rich mould, fuch walls, on fpots judicioufly felected, may be pronounced, in many cafes, an ufeful improvement. Walls of this kind, raifed to protect young trees, are backed with earth like a mound, with fhort flicks, ftuck in the top, in the form of a pa-lifade.

Fences, when boundaries of property, are made at the joint expence of proprietors; when feparating pafture from arable land, are fometimes done folely by the landlord, fometimes folely by the tenant, and fometimes mutually by both; and, when fubdividing fields, are often but not al-ways reared by the tenant alone.

Nothing particular deferves to be mentioned about gates, except a fimple contrivance of three or four feparate bars, made round, with a fwivel and a ring or link at each end to go upon a hook in the posts, instead of sliding into holes, which weaken the posts, and are apt to make them rot and fail. A little time is requisite for opening and shutting them; but while hanging, they are a strong fence, and they can be laid aside out of the reach of injury from cattle and loaded carts, and consequently, by a little attention, bid fair to outlast any gate.

L l CHAP.

CHAP. VII.

ARABLE LAND.

Sect. I.—*Tillage.*

IN proportion to the quantity of land in different farms that is kept in tillage, is the attention bestowed on ploughing. It is natural to expect, that a few spots in exposed situations, which can only yield poor returns, will not be managed and defended with the same care, as large fields, on the proper cultivation of which, the farmer's profit in some measure depends. In the one case, generally, the implements are coarse, the servants are unskilful, and their work is slovenly. In the other case, all the implements are constructed in the most approved and substantial manner, expert ploughmen are procured, the horses are carefully trained, and both masters and servants pique themselves on having their fields thoroughly tilled and neatly ridged.

Two

Two horses, yoked abreast in the plough, are easily managed by one man. Three or even four, or perhaps two horses and two oxen, are used to break up new land, especially when its surface is rugged or covers large stones. Some steep places, where no strength of draught can make a furrow against the bank, are ploughed wholly downwards, the horses finding greater difficulty in dragging the plough up the hill without a furrow, than in bringing it down with a very deep one. It is evident that land of this description can never be subjected to a regular system of cropping, and that it is only broken up by good farmers, to receive manure and to be put in better order for pasture.

The size of furrows, the formation, breadth, and position of ridges, the season and the manner of ploughing for different crops, are all the same in this county as in the light lands of Roxburghshire.

Sect. II.—*Fallowing.*

Is never practised, except on land torn up from a state of nature, or in such a wretched condition at the commencement of a lease as to be unfit for turnips. In the one case, a complete season and much labour are necessary to bring it into form; and, in the other case, there is too little time, after the entry at Whitsunday, to procure manure, and to clean and dress fields for turnips with any prospect of a profitable return.

In fallowing new land, the first object is to turn over the sward so completely as to ensure its rotting, and to dig up such stones as lie in the way. After remaining in this state through winter, it is cross-ploughed in spring, and all stones, which obstruct the plough,

are

are carefully loosened and removed. Two or more ploughings are given during the summer; such stones, as formerly
escaped notice, are taken away; and the field is repeatedly
harrowed, and formed into ridges. If it is very manageable,
and not extensive, all this may be done, and manure applied in time to sow turnips broadcast. But more frequently
it requires so many ploughings, so much other work, and
such a quantity of lime or marl, that farmers, with difficulty, prepare even a few acres properly, by the beginning
of the second winter, for a crop of oats the following
spring.

Sect. III.—*Rotation of Crops.*

In the higher parts of the county, there are very few
turnips, and no peas. It is impossible to observe a regular
rotation, where oats occupy at least $\frac{6}{10}$ if not $\frac{7}{10}$ of all the
arable land, where the small remainder is divided pretty
equally between turnips and barley, and where red clover
is rarely if ever raised. There is, however, every appearance of turnips becoming more general; and farmers may
be tempted to sow red clover, although they cannot protect
it from sheep during winter, and can only reap advantage
from it for a season, not probably as a hay-crop, but at least
as enriching the pasture, till the white clover becomes
more abundant. They are all sensible that turnips and clover are desirable both for their flocks and their fields; and
this conviction seems to be gradually overcoming their fears
of attempting to cultivate these crops, and strengthening
their desires of having more of their arable ground substantially inclosed.

In other sheep-farms, which raise more corn, the most
judicious

judicious and profitable rotation, that has been adopted, is turnip, barley, clover, and oats, in equal proportions. And enough of dung, with the help of a little lime or marl, can be furnished annually for carrying it on, while the whole land in tillage does not exceed 60 acres. Where it is more extensive, the clover is allowed to remain two seasons, or a crop of peas and a second of oats, are added to the rotation.

Farms, mostly or wholly arable, are managed much on the same plan, but on a larger scale. Tenants, for want of dung, find it their interest, after enriching a field with manure, to leave it in pasture, till it can be tilled with a reasonable prospect of being dunged again in the course of a gentle rotation. Fields are thus thrown into pasture, not in any regular succession, but merely according to convenience, local situation, and the sufficiency of their fences. Other fields are subjected to the rotation already mentioned of turnips, barley, clover, and oats, with this difference, that generally a greater or less proportion of peas is substituted for a part of the black crops, and that some of the land, which should be in barley, is sown with oats. Other rotations are also followed equally agreeable to the rules of good husbandry, which are understood to consist, in an alternate succession of white and black crops, in introducing a drill crop as often as is necessary to keep the land free from weeds, and in giving it such a competent quantity of manure, during the course of every rotation, as will enable it to produce good crops of the several grains, without being much impoverished. I mean not, however, to insinuate, that these rules are observed by all the farmers in this county, in the cultivation of their fields. Some of them seem to think, that there is no occasion for resorting to a black crop while their lands can bear a white one, and that it is impossible to exhaust a kindly soil after it is well marled.

led. Others, who are sufficiently enlightened to perceive the absurdity of such maxims, have not been able to emancipate themselves altogether from former prejudices, and cannot resist the propensity, which they were early taught to foster, of taking two white crops successively from land in excellent order. But these practices are gradually giving place to a more rational and profitable system.

Sect. IV.—*Crops commonly cultivated.*

The crops most commonly cultivated are, oats, barley, peas, turnips, and potatoes.

The different kinds of oats, according to their prevalence, may be thus ranked, viz. The *red*, the *white*, the *Angus*, and the *Dutch*, all of which have already been described. In high and exposed situations, the *red*, beyond all controversy, deserve the preference; and there are few fields in the whole county, where they may not contend for it. The *white* are chiefly sown where there is some shelter, and a degree of mildness and warmth in the climate. Besides these advantages, the *Angus* require a good soil. The *Dutch* are now mostly confined to a few sheltered spots, where the *white* and *Angus* might be too late of ripening, and will probably soon be disused altogether. *Church's* oats, and the *black* oats have not been much tried. There are not many fields fit for producing the former; but the latter might be sown to advantage on several parts of different farms, where the exposure is cold, and the ground more or less retentive of moisture.

Big,

Big, a native of the county, is the only species of bar-ley, that will arrive at full maturity, and yield a tolerable increase in a very large portion of the arable land. It ad-mits of being sown late in the season, and therefore is less apt to suffer from those annual weeds, which in spite of every precaution spring up in a thin and light soil. Yet it ripens early and equally; and is a surer and weightier crop, where there is a deficiency of climate, than the other kinds cultivated in the lower and warmer farms. There the *long-eared* barley is most common and most productive; al-though it may be doubted, whether *big*, growing more quickly and being sooner ready, might not make a better nurse for clover, and whether its greater quantity, the equa-lity of its grains, and its having little refuse, might not compensate for its inferiority of weight, and of produce in pot-barley or meal. But there may be reason, on the other hand, to doubt, whether it retains all these qualities unim-paired, when sown on land highly enriched with dung and marl or lime, and whether it does not then acquire a lux-uriance unfriendly to the earliness and equality of its ripen-ing.

Battledore, or *sprat*-barley, was brought from Yorkshire in the year 1790, by George Currie, Esq; when he had the farm of Carterhaugh, about 3 miles above Selkirk. It is midle sized, rather small, plump, and remarkably thin in the skin, which makes it very heavy and productive in proportion to the measure, both in meal and in pot-barley; and, being also very equal, it will probably malt well. It has the peculiar advantage of sending forth a greater num-ber of branches or stalks from one grain than any other kind of barley, on which account about 2¼ firlots of seed are enough for an acre, or even two firlots if the land be in excellent order. But it must be sown at least three weeks

earlier

earlier than even the long-eared barley; and after all, it may be later of coming to maturity. The grains, too, are extremely apt to drop from the ear, and the heavy ears to snap from the brittle straw, in a high wind, or when the sheaves are tossed to or from the cart.

Though less peas are sown now than formerly, yet a greater quantity is annually raised. In the higher grounds, where the lateness of the climate, and the variableness of the weather made them precarious and unproductive, they are mostly given up. But, in the lower fields, where there is more genial heat, and where the soil is kindly and enriched by lime or marl, they grow luxuriantly, are extremely prolific, unless perhaps they run too much to straw, and become ready for the sickle, while the days are somewhat long and the air dry to forward their preparation for being safely stacked. In these cases, they are a lucrative and meliorating crop; they fetch a good price; their straw makes excellent fodder; their rapid growth, their tendency to cling together, and their weight bear down and crush all weeds; and the stalks of these weeds and the stubble of the peas, reduced to a state of corruption, form excellent manure for the ground.

The average quantity of these three grains, sown upon an English acre, is nearly as follows: Oats, $\frac{1}{10}$; Barley, $\frac{1}{8}$ or $\frac{11}{17}$; and, Peas, $\frac{1}{7}$ of their respective bolls. Their average produce, on the same acre, will be, Oats, $3\frac{1}{4}$ bolls; Barley, $4\frac{1}{4}$ bolls; and, Peas, 4 bolls. The times of sowing and of reaping depend much on seasons and the state of different fields. The dryness and warmth of the soil make the blade to spring and the corns to ripen so quickly, that farmers, in most cases, are rather anxious for a favourable than for an early seed-time.

It

It is unnecessary to repeat much of what has been already observed concerning the culture of turnips and potatoes, as every thing, relating to both of them, is managed in the same way as in Roxburghshire. Twenty years ago, there were scarcely ten acres of turnips in the whole county. Those, raised in some corners of corn-fields in different farms, were generally destroyed by the sheep; and the few ridges, annually sown around Selkirk and Galashiels, were greedily devoured by children and curious people, as soon as the bulb was formed. In spite of these obstacles, the culture of them has become gradually more general, and is still rapidly on the increase. Attention, care, and good fences protect them from sheep; and the depredations of idle boys are less now, that their curiosity is fully gratified, or at least are not so. perceptible in numerous and large fields, as they were in small detached spots. Turnips are here rather a more certain crop than in the sister county, and nearly as weighty. More of them are applied to rear and improve the condition of cattle and sheep, than to fatten either for the shambles.

Potatoes found their way into this county some years before turnips; though I cannot learn that they were planted, except with the spade, till the year 1772 or 1773, or that any kind was known, except the *red* and a few *kidneys*. About that time, some of the common *white* kind made their appearance, and in a few years entirely supplanted the others. About that time, too, they began to be dropped in every furrow made by the plough, which practice was tenaciously retained, till the larger returns procured by planting them in every third furrow, or in ridges at the distance of twenty-seven or even thirty-six inches, and the obvious advantage of getting the land cleared and pulverised by the plough, gradually obtained, for these two last

methods,

methods, a decided preference. They became quite common, through the whole county, about the 1778 or 1780. By that time, a change of seed was brought from Langholm; *red-nebs* were introduced; potatoes conſtituted a chief article of food for a great part of the year; and ever ſince, enough of them has been raiſed to ſupply the conſumpt of the inhabitants, and to furniſh a conſiderable quantity of seed to the contiguous parts of Mid-Lothian and Tweeddale.

It is ſtill the general practice to put dung only into that furrow on which the potato-ſet is to be planted, and to make the plough cover both the dung and the ſet with freſh earth. But though this bids fair to produce the moſt luxuriant and largeſt crop, it is liable to ſeveral objections. The potatoes, by growing immediately above the dung, are apt to bliſter and become ſcabrous by its heat: the dung, confined during a ſeaſon to one furrow and that occupying ſcarcely a third part of the whole field, cannot be brought to mix and incorporate eaſily with the other two parts, without croſs-ploughing and harrowing the land: and, by being applied only in ſpring, it favours the growth of weeds, among the potatoes, which cannot be deſtroyed without much trouble and labour. All theſe inconveniencies are avoided by laying the dung equally over the whole field during winter, and ploughing it inſtantly down. The force of its heat is allayed, by its being ſpread over a wide extent, and by its lying ſo long and ſo equally among cold earth: A great many weeds, ſpringing early up through its influence, are checked and killed before the potatoes are planted: The ſoil is mellowed, more eaſily wrought, and dreſſed at leſs expence: And the crop, if not ſo prolific, is of a better quality. The greateſt produce of an acre, which has fallen within my knowledge, was about 35 returns of the ſeed. About 9¼ firlots planted, yielded 330,

or

or 82¼ Linlithgow bolls. But 20 returns of 10 firlots planted is a good, and 18 returns an average crop.

The curl only made its appearance here about two or three years ago, and has not hitherto made any alarming progress. An ingenious neighbour has suggested, that it may be in some measure prevented, and potatoes brought earlier to maturity, by planting only one set, cut from the top* of each potato. From thence always issues the first and strongest sprout made by a potato in spring, which led him to infer, that it would grow more quickly and vigorously in the ground than any other part of the potato. And he shewed me in his garden a bed, all planted the same day, the one half with top-sets carefully kept apart, and the other with sets from the root and sides. Both were luxuriant and free from curl, but the top-sets were farthest advanced and promised to be ready, at least three weeks, before the other.

The relative proportions of these different grains may be nearly thus. Oats occupy rather more than one half of all the land in tillage or about 4800 acres. The remainder may be divided into four equal parts; three of which may be allotted to turnips, (including potatoes), barley, and clover, and the fourth to peas, and those crops which are not so commonly cultivated.

* The *top* is the part farthest from the root or tendril, by which a potato is connected with the rest of the cluster.

SECT.

SECT. V.—*Crops not commonly cultivated.*

A FEW acres are fometimes devoted to wheat. It is managed in the fame manner as in Roxburghfhire, and yields good returns; but is, in feveral refpects, hurtful to the ground.

Aftonifhing crops have been raifed of rye; but there is little demand for this grain, and it is nearly as fore upon land as wheat. The ftraw of both fells at a high price.

Beans are fometimes, though very feldom fown among peas. A fews rows are alfo to be feen, in fome fields, both of them, and of cabbages. But there is very little foil in the whole county of a fufficient depth for raifing either of thefe, or carrots, though all of them have been produced of an excellent quality on particular fpots.

The foil is much better adapted to the cultivation of yams. They have been tried in feveral places, and promife to fucceed extremely well. From their large fize, a greater number of them than of potatoes is requifite to plant an acre; but their produce, in fome inftances of which I have heard, has been twenty-four or twenty-five returns of the feed. Their culture is the fame with that of potatoes, but their growth is rather flower, and they fhould be put fooner into the ground.

There can be no doubt that Swedifh Turnips would thrive well in the whole arable diftrict. Some of them have weighed a Dutch ftone. But, without a confederacy of neighbouring farmers to raife fields of them every year, they cannot force their way into general ufe; and it is not

clear

clear that they merit so much attention. They are eat, with prodigious avidity, by every paſſenger, eſpecially in ſpring: and though cattle are equally fond of them, they are by no means ſo meliorating a crop to the ground, as common turnips.

Since the improvement of land by lime and marl, tares grow luxuriantly, and are ſown on many farms to be given green to horſes during ſummer. This laudable practice is daily gaining ground. And it ſeems highly probably that, in a very few years, every farm in the county will have ſome portion of its arable land, in tares for ſummer proviſion to the horſes, and in yams for winter proviſion to the milk-cows.

No fields of lint are raiſed, but a ſmall quantity of it is annually ſown on moſt farms by houſewives and cottagers.

It is not eaſy to form a conjecture concerning the number of acres occupied by theſe various crops. But they are ſo few, that when added to the fields annually in peas, their joint amount will not exceed what is allotted to them at the cloſe of the preceding ſection.

CHAP.

CHAP. VIII.

GRASS.

Sect. I.—*Natural Meadows and Pastures.*

Sect. II.—*Artificial Grasses.*

Sect. III.—*Hay-Harvest.*

Sect. IV.—*Feeding.*

CONCERNING the first three articles, very little remains to be added to what is already stated in the Account of Roxburghshire. In proportion to the extent of the two counties, the nature, the quantity, and the manner of making meadow-hay, are very much the same; and it consists of the same common grasses. Nor is there any material difference in the kinds of artificial grasses, the proportions of each sown upon an acre, the quantity produced, the management of hay, or the form and thatching of hay-stacks. Perhaps it should be mentioned, that yellow clover is rarely if ever sown.

From

From the small quantity of land in turnips and clover, and from the proportion of these which is given to sheep, it must be obvious that few cattle can be fed. Yet some of the older milk-cows on different farms, and even such young ones as run more to beef than to milk, and several oxen either reared in the county or purchased in the neighbourhood, are annually fattened, and are supposed to yield an ample profit on their value when put upon clover or turnips. There are several grassy fields on the banks of Ettrick and Borthwick waters, much fitter for black-cattle than sheep. These, however, are employed more in rearing than in feeding cattle; and it may be safely affirmed, that the number reared yearly greatly exceeds those which are fattened. If some profit did not arise from bringing up both young cattle and horses, many farmers would have a very scanty subsistence, whose flock consists wholly of black-faced sheep, or who pay a dearer rent than 3 s. 6 d. for the grass eat by every sheep.

Some time ago, cattle were grazed during summer, when a year old for 12 s. or 15 s., when two years old for 18 s. or 21 s., and when three or more years old for 25 s. or 30 s. All these prices are now advanced, year old cattle to 18 s. and even to 20 s., two years old to 25 s. some to 28 s., and all older cattle from 35 s. to 40 s. and even to 42 s. The summer's grass of a horse, too, has risen from 40 s. to 50 s. Taking these rates for an average, and allowing 15 s. as an advance of price for the winter's maintenance of a heifer or bullock, and two guineas for wintering a young horse, a farmer, who can bring up a dozen of the former, will add L. 27 yearly to his profits, and four of the latter will add about L. 18 more to them, besides what he may gain by his own judicious management, in selecting good breeds, improving their size and shape, and disposing of them at an advantageous time.

A

A few turnips have been carefully faved till fpring to fatten early lambs. Sheep, too, are not unfrequently put upon them in the beginning of winter, and fold to the butcher, in a regular fucceffion, as they become fit for the fhambles. But the chief ufe of turnips, and indeed of clover-fields alfo efpecially in the higher parts of the county, undoubtedly is, to prevent or remove difeafes, to make up lean fheep, to preferve others from falling away, and to keep the whole flock in a thriving condition.

CHAP.

CHAP. IX.

GARDENS AND ORCHARDS,

IT cannot be expected, that, in a county fo fmall and fo devoid of towns and villages, there fhould be gardens and orchards, producing pot-herbs and fruits for fale. But all the common and feveral rare vegetables for the kitchen, and thofe fruits for the table, which are found in fimilar climates, are raifed, of an admirable quality, in the gardens of the refident gentlemen. Thefe, in general, are kept in excellent order, and fome of them are laid out with good tafte. The adjoining fhrubberies, likewife, are pleafantly difpofed, and exhibit greater variety of plants than could be expected from their elevated fituation. The beauty of fome pleafure-grounds is heightened and animated by Tweed flowing along in a gentle current, or rolling in awful majefty. While thofe around Haining, embellifhed by a natural lake of confiderable extent, and by clumps, detached trees, and fhrubs fcattered up and down and diverfified with wonderful felicity, deferve to be particularly

mentioned,

mentioned, as attracting the notice and admiration of travellers. All the farmers have gardens; but in some places, the soil and climate will bring nothing to maturity,
except a few hardy vegetables; in most places, gardens do
not merit much attention, and do not receive even the little
that they merit; yet there are instances, though by no
means numerous, of their being managed with skill and
care. Much more can be said for the gardens belonging to
tradesmen, cottagers, and the inhabitants of Selkirk and Galashiels. Many of them are neatly dressed, yield a profu-
sion of useful vegetables, and are ornamented with shrubs,
flowers, and bushes, bearing the smaller fruits.

There are few orchards, most of the fruit at gentlemen's
tables being raised on walls, or on espaliers and standards
in their gardens. Many of them have small nurseries for
supplying themselves with young trees; and there is one at
Selkirk, where a few plants of various kinds are reared
for sale.

CHAP,

CHAP. X.

WOODS AND PLANTATIONS.

IN ſtating the number of acres in wood at 2000, I have followed Mr Johnſton. The beſt information, which I could collect from the converſation of gentlemen and farmers in different corners, made it rather leſs. But the difficulty of aſcertaining the real extent of the many ſmall and irregular clumps, corners, banks, and even narrow belts, ſufficiently accounts for the trifling difference; and I thought it ſafer to truſt to the computations of a man, whoſe profeſſional knowledge is entitled to reſpect, than to the more vague conjectures of numerous individuals.

The greateſt part of the wood conſiſts of Scotch firs, the largeſt half of which was planted above 25 years ago. Several trees, felled from time to time, were ſawed into planks from fifteen to nine inches broad, and from twelve to twenty feet long; and many others, equally large, are now

ready

ready for the axe. Thofe, which are cut down to allow
fpace for the reft to grow uncumbered, here not improperly called *thinnings* or *weedings*, while young are fit only
for the fire; but, at twelve years old, efpecially on kindly
foil, are ufed for pales and fimilar purpofes.

Several hundred acres are occupied by other trees more
valuable though of flower growth, particularly oaks, afhes,
elms, and planes, many of which have only been lately
planted, though not a few are of a great age and large fize.
Oaks have frequently been ufed, whofe trunks meafured
from 7 to 8 feet in circumference, and contained, according to their length, from 18 to 40 feet of timber, befides
nearly as much in the other parts of the trees. Inftances
might be given of a few much larger. I meafured one,
whofe circumference 3 feet above the ground was about
9¼ feet; another only three or four inches lefs, and a third
7¼ feet. The two firft are at Fairnilee, and one of them
clofe by the ground is about 13 feet 9 inches. The trunk,
being 7 feet high, contains only about 38 feet of wood,
but proceeding to a confiderable height, after fending forth
its loweft branches, with little diminution of circumference,
and having feveral large arms, there muft be at leaft 80 feet
of excellent timber in the whole tree. Afhes very commonly are five or fix feet round, and have from 20 to
30 feet of wood. One, at Yair, meafures 12 feet 9 inches
at the bottom, but is divided into two clefts about a foot
above the furface of the ground. Another, there, is 8 feet
2 inches at the height of 5 feet, and has an upright
ftem of 12 feet, which confequently contains no lefs than
48 feet of timber; and the whole tree, having confiderable fhoots and branches, cannot be eftimated below
80 feet. I have meafured feveral others from 7 to 8¼ feet,
and one at Sunderland-hall above 12 feet, but none that
has nearly as much wood. Elms are fully equal in fize to
afhes.

aſhes: Two of them, at Yair, meaſure each above 13 feet round, at the ſurface of the ground; one of them at 6 feet above it, is 11 feet 9 inches, and has a ſtraight trunk of 12 feet; the trunk of the other is 9 feet in length, and its average girth is 10 feet 4 inches: and both together muſt contain from 260 to 300 feet. There are ſeveral leſſer elms both there and in other parts of the county, which run from 5 to 8 feet in circumference, but vary very much in length of body and quantity and quality of timber. No trees are ſo luxuriant and ſhapely as planes. They grow tall, ſtraight, and large, their branches ſpread thickly and equally, and they have a full and rich foilage: At Tor-woodlee there is one, which meaſures, where it appears above the ground, 13 feet 7 inches in circumference, and, at the height of 20 or 24 inches, ſeparates into two clefts, one of which is 9 feet 4 inches, and the other 9 feet 1 inch round. Both taper ſo gently for 12 or 15 feet, that the timber in them muſt be about 120 or 130 feet, and there may be about 50 or 60 feet more in the reſt of the tree. Several other planes in the county are remarkable for height, ſize, and beauty.

Interſperſed among theſe are, in different places, many beeches, larches, mountain-aſhes, birches, different kinds of willows, limes, and ſome beautiful hawthorns. A fine beech, near Galaſhiels houſe, deſerves to be noticed, not ſo much for its ſize, being little more than 6 feet in circum-ference, as for the cleanlineſs and length of its ſtem, which cannot be leſs than 26 feet, and for the number and rich-neſs of its hanging branches. Near it is a larix, 9½ feet round at the baſe, 5 feet 8 inches at the height of 6 feet above the ground, and 5 feet 1 inch at the height of 12 feet, which conſequently will ſtand an average of 5 feet for 24 feet high, and muſt contain 37½ feet of wood. It is ſurpaſſed in tallneſs, ſtraightneſs, and quantity of wood by one at Haining, which is 11 feet 5 inches at the bottom, and 6¼ feet at the height of 6 feet, but seems to taper so quickly that it cannot be allowed a larger average for 24 feet in height than 5 feet or at most 5 feet 4 inches round; though the top of it, above that height, is of considerable size and value; and the tree, upon the whole, stands unrivalled in this part of Scotland. The other trees, especially the red sallow, thrive well and arrive at great perfection And every tree, mentioned in the Account of Roxburghshire, is also found here. The prices of different kinds of timber are likewise substantially the same.

CHAP.

CHAP. XI.

WASTES.

THERE are no commons in this county; and no part of it, either from neglect or mifmanagement, can juftly be called *wafte*, except perhaps a fpace of nearly 300 acres, which is appropriated for pafture to the horfes and cows belonging to the burgeffes of Selkirk, and for thin fods to cover the roofs of their houfes below the thatch. It is eafy to conceive, that a foil, thus employed for a long courfe of years, muft have made a confiderable progrefs towards fterility, and that the intereft of the burgh, to whom it belongs, as well as of the public at large, ftrongly dictates the immediate abolition of this pernicious practice, and the cultivation and improvement of the land by inclofure, tillage, and manure. The prejudices, clamours, and even hardfhips of individuals, fhould not be allowed to obftruct the folid and permanent melioration of a country.

CHAP.

CHAP. XII.

IMPROVEMENTS.

Sect. I.—*Draining.*

ALTHOUGH the arable land, in general, is naturally fo dry, or flopes fo equally, as not to require drains, yet there are feveral fpots on cold impenetrable till, which the greateft care and attention, and the moft fkilful and coftly drains, can fcarcely reduce to a manageable flate. In fuch cafes, the drains, being made through hard till, or fhelving rocks, or huge fhapelefs ftones, muft coft, according to the difference of their width and depth, as much as the deareft drains in Roxburghfhire. Let it be mentioned, for the honour both of proprietors and tenants, that many of them have carried and ftill are carrying forward expenfive drains with great fpirit and fuccefs, by which a new and rich appearance is given, not only to marfhy places, but alfo to

valuable

valuable fields below, which were injured and defaced by
the water in rainy feafons, when denied a natural and
free vent, either overflowing or fpringing up in them,
and deftroying the crops. This affords a happy prefage
that the little, which remains to be done, will be fpeedily
effected.

Open drains, like thofe in Roxburgbfhire, have of late
become very common in fheep-walks, and are rapidly increafing. Qne farmer fome years ago made upwards of
8000 * roods of them, at his own expence. An incredible
number of them have fince been made in different parts,
which fhews the general fenfe entertained of their utility.
At the fame time, it has been objected to them, " that the
" ground, as it becomes drier, is more infefted with moles,
" and that the new earth, thrown up in mole-hills, and af-
" terwards fpread either by accident or intention, produces
" grafs very hurtful to fheep." This obfervation I found
on the margin of a report tranfmitted to me, and I tranf-
cribe it, becaufe it is confirmed by fome farmers, who allege that even the grafs, fpringing up quickly from the
frefh earth caft out of the drains, is the caufe of difeafes,
efpecially where there is a mixture of mofs with the foil.
The dreaded mifchief, however, I fhould apprehend, may
be prevented by ufing a few timely precautions : Let landlords and tenants make a general agreement to deftroy all
moles : let mole-hills be fpread immediately over as wide
an extent as the fhovel can reach,—and above all, let the
ftuff dug out of the drains, inftead of being laid in a kind
of mound on its lower lip, be thrown to a greater diftance
and afterwards fcattered over the field, and the fods carried
to fill up holes or cover fpots bare of foil. The influence of

.O o   the

---

* Mr Johnfton, p. 10. A rood is fix yards, and cofts about 3-4ths of
a penny, or four of them cofts threepence.

the fresh earth, being thus diffused over a larger surface,
cannot any where be so strong as to produce noxious effects: The sides of drains will be less apt to give way, when
relieved from the pressure of sods and earth, and of sheep
attracted by their sweet grasses: And drains will not be
so readily choked, by the accumulation of particles, stones,
and clods, forced down from the mound, in changeable
weather, by the action of the air or the feet of sheep. The
extirpation of moles is an important improvement in sheep-
farming: and, as it does not fall under any part of the
plan prescribed by the Board of Agriculture, I shall here
take the liberty of recommending it to public notice. One
great proprietor in this county has contracted with a company of mole-catchers, to free his estate from that destructive animal for a number of years, at a certain rate according to the measurement of the lands. But this laudable
attempt must be rendered, in a great degree, abortive, unless it is adopted by contiguous proprietors, as the moles
from their estates will soon overrun the fields which have
been cleared. A general combination, therefore, among
all landlords and tenants in Great Britain, is necessary to
exterminate this subterraneous enemy: and surely the mis-
chief, which it occasions in grass and arable lands and still
more in gardens, should unite all, who are liable to suffer
from it, in some common measure for their mutual defence.
There is, indeed, something ludicrous in proposing a national league against moles; and perhaps the scheme, on
such a large scale, may be both absurd and impracticable.
But the same purpose may be answered, though not so
completely, by a number of similar combinations among
neighbouring proprietors and farmers. If they were entered into and attended with success in one district, they
would gradually become general; and they would at least

                                                lessen

leffen though they might not entirely prevent the depredations of moles *.

Sect. II.—*Paring and Burning.*

Few places in this county have a fufficient depth of foil
for being pared and burnt, and moft of thefe places want
climate to bring a crop to maturity, except in a very early
feafon. The practice has never been general here: very
little land has been hurt by it: and it feems now to be
wholly given up.

Sect. III.—*Manures.*

Dunghills are here made and ufed in the fame manner
as in Roxburghfhire. Great attention is paid, of late, to
collect and preferve dung; and in different places to form
composts. Marl is mixed with mofs; and lime with earth,
weeds, and the fluff dug out of ruins, or gathered from
roads.

Lime is chiefly ufed in the north-eaft part of the county,
and brought from Middleton in Mid-Lothian, which is fixteen miles from the neareft, and not lefs than thirty from
fome places whither that manure is carried. From fix to
eight

* By fome plan of the fame nature, rats and other vermin might be fup-
preffed, or rendered lefs numerous and ruinous to grain. It might alfo be
extended to diminifh the havoc made by pigeons, crows, fparrows, and
other birds, among corns, when newly fown, and while advancing flowly
to maturity.

eight carts of three bolls* each is the common allowance
for an acre. Some do not lay on fo much. There is reafon to believe that the ufe of lime to any confiderable extent
as a manure was firft introduced by the Reverend Mr Alex-
ander Glen †, now at Dirleton, while he was minifter at Galafhiels from the 1757 to 1769.

During that period, the late Lord Alemoor drained a
morafs, on the confines of Roxburghfhire ‡, and brought
confiderable quantities of marl to different fields, which
ftill retain the benefit of it. This example, however, was
not followed by thofe who had marl in their eftates or
farms; and it could not be followed by others, till marl
was expofed to fale about the 1772 at Whitmoorhall § in
Roxburghfhire, within three miles of lands belonging to
the burgh of Selkirk and its burgeffes. From the pits
there it was carried to different farms at the diftance of
feven or eight miles. About the fame time, marl was dug
on the eftate of Sintoun, and foon afterwards on other e-
ftates in that neighbourhood, but the ufe of it was either
confined to the tenants, or the fale was not extenfive. It
is only within thefe very few years, that moraffes were
drained, and marl taken out of them, except on the very
extremities of the county; and in none of thefe more cen-
tral places is it open for fale. When Mr Currie left the
farm

* The boll is four Linlithgow firlots, and cofts 1 s. at the kiln. See
p. 139.

† He was likewife the firft, or amongft the firft, who drained and fallowed land, ftraightened ridges, and made other improvements in hufbandry.

‡ Clofe by the *Hairmrfs* toll-bar, on the road from Selkirk to Hawick.
The marl was brought to Haining three or four miles diftant from the pit,
Before his time fmall fpots had been marked at Brownmuir and around Sel-
kirk.

§ See page 135.

farm of Carterhaugh, and purchased the lands of Green-
head (in Roxburghshire) about a mile east from Selkirk, he
had the spirit to buy and to drain, at the vast expence of
L. 1000 Sterling, a small lake full of marl, lying between
his estate and that burgh; which has furnished him with
abundance of that useful manure for all his own fields, and
a vast surplus to supply his neighbours in this county. His
marl and that at Whitmoorhall are of the richest quality,
and sell this year (1797) at 1 s. for the single-horse cart,
which is supposed to contain two bolls or sixteen cubic-feet,
but the proprietors do not strictly confine purchasers to that
measure. The same quantity is laid upon an acre as upon
the light lands in Roxburghshire. Farmers have found,
from experience, that less than forty bolls is of little avail,
and they seldom give more than sixty. Instances occurred
sometime ago, of their greatly exceeding that quantity, but
there is not much danger now of their putting themselves
to such unnecessary expence and trouble *.

Lime

* I transcribe the following note, with the alteration of a few immaterial words, and the omission of others, from the margin of one of the
original reports, as containing matter worthy of public attention.

" SHELL-MARL, a fossil substance used as a manure, is found in great
" quantities, in almost all the mosses (which have formerly been lakes) in
" the south parts of this county and in the neighbouring county of Rox-
" burgh. This substance has evidently been produced from the accumu-
" lated remains of immense quantities of fresh-water snails; and must
" therefore consist, partly of animal matter from the bodies, and partly of
" a pure calcarious earth from the shells of their animals.

" It is perhaps one of the richest manures that has yet been discovered.
" People, at first, were very little acquainted with its powers as a ma-
" nure, and generally applied much greater quantities than were necessary
" or proper to be laid upon the land at one time. It has not been un-
" common to lay on from 100 to 200 bolls and upwards upon an acre of
" land at once; and the consequence has uniformly been, that the crops,
" from their excessive luxuriance, did not yield a quantity of grain any
" way proportionate to what might have been expected, from their appear-
" ance

Lime and marl, remain in heaps till they are reduced to a state of pulverization, when they are carried out in carts, and

" ance upon the field or even in the barn-yard, and that the grain itself
" was of an inferior quality. Besides, where particular care has not been
" taken to prevent the tenants from over-cropping the land, after such ex-
" cessive applications of marl, the fertility of the soil has been almost en-
" tirely destroyed ; and it is actually of much less value at this time than
" it was before the marl was laid upon it. And, even where some care
" has been taken to prevent the tenants from reducing the land by over-
" cropping it, it will be found that they have deprived themselves of the
" advantage they might have derived from a repetition of this manure :
" for it is a well-known fact, that when a large quantity of marl is laid
" upon land at one time, it cannot be again repeated, with any confide-
" rable degree of advantage, for many years thereafter. It seems there-
" fore to be a duty, which proprietors owe to themselves and the public,
" to prevent their tenants from abusing a blessing bestowed by Providence
" for the improvement of the country, and restrict them in the use of it
" to such moderate quantities as may render it perpetually useful.

" It is believed, that it has never yet been ascertained, by actual expe-
" riments, what is the most proper quantity of marl to be applied as ma-
" nure upon an acre of land. For an English acre, it is supposed that
" from twenty to forty or forty-five bolls may be sufficient. This is, how-
" ever a subject that well merits the attention of gentlemen, who have
" marl in their estates, or have land in the neighbourhood of it ; and it
" would be a consequential service done to the country in general, if any
" gentleman of correct observation would take the trouble of making the
" experiment, by laying on different quantities of marl upon equal quanti-
" ties of land (never marled before) of the same nature and quality, at the
" rate of from twenty to sixty bolls per acre, and weigh accurately the
" grain produced on each of these pieces of land, upon which the different
" quantities of marl have been laid. It must, however, be observed, that
" it is not perhaps the quantity of marl, which is found to produce the
" greatest weight of grain in the first instance, that ought to be applied
" in common use. For example, supposing it should be found, from
" these experiments, that the land, which had been manured at the rate of
" forty bolls to the acre, produced the greatest weight of grain, it would
" perhaps be more advisable to restrict the common use of it to thirty-five
" or even to thirty bolls per acre ; because, it is supposed, that either of
" these quantities could be more frequently repeated than forty bolls to ad-
" vantage."

Some

and spread on the fields by shovels *. On land that has been newly broken, fallowed, or in potatoes, this operation

Some of these observations must not be permitted to pass unnoticed. The first paragraph contains the commonly-received opinion concerning the nature and formation of marl. The assertion in the second, of the immense quantity of it laid upon an acre, applies not, as far as I can learn, to a single field in this county. On some cold and deep soil in Roxburgh-shire, about an hundred carts have been given to an acre ;—but I know only of one instance ; the farmer is both judicious and enterprising, has not overcropped the land, and is well repaid for his expence. Marled land may certainly be materially injured by overcropping ; but I am warranted to assert, that no part of this county has been so severely scourged by a succession of white crops after being marled, as the whole outfield-land in it has been and some of it still continues to be thus scourged, without receiving a particle of marl ; and that, at this moment, there are very few marled fields which have suffered from being overcropped. The proposed restriction on tenants, with respect to the quantity of marl to be laid upon an acre, I should apprehend to be entirely unnecessary ; because none of them will put himself to the expence and trouble of carrying a single boll more than his own experience or that of his neighbours teaches him to be sufficient ; and though he should, the land would not suffer, provided he was prevented from overcropping it. Restrictions to that effect are certainly very proper. The experiment recommended could not be of general utility, as the soil of contiguous fields, and sometimes of the same field, may require very different doses of marl. For all the sharp soil in this county and Roxburghshire, from twenty to twenty-five carts, or from forty to fifty bolls of marl, are found to be the most eligible quantity. As to repeating the manure, the oftener that is done, and the more of it that is given at a time to land subjected to severe cropping, the sooner is the land brought to poverty ; but when land, after being once marled, is judiciously and gently managed, the experience of this county has not yet had time to ascertain how long it may remain in good condition without marl, and how soon it may be marled a second time to advantage. The idea, however, of applying little of it at a time, and having recourse to it again after a short interval, certainly deserves a fair trial ; though few tenants may be disposed to make this trial on the longest leases usually given.

* Marl is often laid upon the land in small heaps from the cart, and afterwards spread.

tion takes place in the beginning of winter, that the foil
may receive greater affiftance from the manure in producing a white crop. With a crop of peas or turnips, thefe
manures are thought to have a better effect, when applied
about the time that the feeds are fown : And the quickeft
lime is always preferred, as operating foonest in warming
the ground, promoting a rapid vegetation, and preventing
the fly from attacking the turnips. In other cafes, it is
not reckoned any difadvantage to land, that the lime fhall
lie a confiderable time in the heap before it is fpread and
tilled down, provided it is not too much exhaufted, by being expofed to an alternate fucceffion of froft and rain,

SECT. IV.—*Weeding.*

Too little attention is paid to the fuppreffion of weeds,
both in thofe lands which are kept in conftant tillage, and
in thofe which are fown up with graffes for pafture. Where
the turnip-hufbandry prevails, farmers are, indeed, at pains
to make their fields clean, and put them in good order for
barley and clover. But along with the feeds of the clover
a ' different graffes, are very often mixed the feeds of
docks and other pernicious weeds, which never fail to fpring
up, and few are at the trouble of eradicating thefe or cutting them over. Some are fo flovenly as even to neglect
their turnip-fields, and to leave their peas and white crops
to ftruggle with a multitude of weeds. Others, at the fame
time, are fo careful as to dig up docks with a fpade, to cut
thiftles and fimilar upright weeds with a hook made for
the purpofe, and even to employ people to pull up with
their hands fuch as are branchy and crawling.

SECT.

Sect. V.—*Watering:*

Mr Curror of Brownmuir, a proprietor in Selkirk-shire, obferving, in the Agricultural Reports of fome coun-ties in England, the vaft advantage of watering land, and perceiving that it muft be of equal importance to fheep-far-mers here, made an attempt, in the beginning of the 1796, to introduce this improvement on five or fix acres of coarfe heathy ground, lying in a corner of an extenfive farm, which he has in this county, immediately adjoining to his dwell-ing-houfe which ftands in Tweeddale. He was at great pains, without receiving any advice or directions except what he derived from thefe reports, to catch rivulets and fprings, to make levels, and to conduct water over every part of a very irregular furface; and he was perfectly con-fcious, during that feafon, of making a vifible progrefs in leffening the heath, and of increafing the quantity and the quality of the natural graffes which grew on the field. But he had the mortification to find all his ingenious la-bours, in a great meafure, overturned or altered, by the Meffrs Stephens, father and fon, who had been completely inftructed in that art in England, and who were generouf-ly fent by the Duke of Buccleuch, on hearing of the rited undertaking, to direct and carry it forward. The fpot felected for their operations, not lying within this county, it belongs not to my province to defcribe what has been done. Yet I cannot forbear to make mention of a practice, altogether new in this part of Scotland, which is called *rafter-levelling*, and which confifts in cutting rows of fods, in a ftraight line on the furface, and diagonally below it, in taking away and leaving a row alternately, and in preffing together, with the foot, a fpade, or a mallet, the rows that are left, fo as to preferve a large portion of the

P p   fward

fward unbroken, and bring that on the different rows nearly into contact. After they become united and compact,
the operation can be repeated if neceffary. The fods are
cut more or lefs obliquely, and made deeper or fhallower,
according to the quantity of earth requifite to be removed,
and are laid, with their graffy furface uppermoft, on low
parts of the field to raife them to the proper level. It is
obvious that this method can only be practifed, where the
inequality to be levelled is fmall, and where there are no
obftructions in the foil.

Two advantages are expected from watering land: early
grafs at a time when it is fcarce and of the greateft fervice
to ewes while pregnant or nourifhing their lambs; and a
heavier crop of hay fooner in the feafon and of a better
quality. The experience of a few years will determine how
far thefe advantages fhall be gained by the perfevering efforts of Mr Currer.

CHAP.

CHAP. XIII.

LIVE STOCK.

SECT. I.—*Black Cattle.*

ALTHOUGH there is not a greater number of black cattle, in proportion to their relative extents, in this county than in Roxburghshire, yet here the rearing of them is more an object of attention and profit. Few cows are requisite to supply a thin population with milk and butter. The small quantity of arable land can be employed to better purpose, than in keeping them for the sake of making these articles and cheese for sale. And all the turnips, hitherto raised, are scarcely sufficient to preserve the necessary stock kept on farms during winter in a proper condition. From all which, it would appear that the number of black cattle, kept for real use, or fattened for the market, must be very inconsiderable. But in most farms there is

more

more or less, and in many there is a great deal of land, producing luxuriant crops of coarse grasses, of which sheep are not fond, but which are much relished by cattle both when green and made into hay; and, on such land, it is the evident interest of farmers to rear young cattle, which they can sell to advantage from two and a half to four or five years old, according to circumstances. The number of cattle in the whole county must exceed 2200, of which about one-sixth will be sold annually, exclusive of calves and what may be fatted for the butcher.

No partiality is entertained for any particular breed; and hitherto little attention has been shewn to improve the stock upon the different farms by purchasing or rearing handsome bulls, though several farmers are excellent judges, and always buy such cows, and keep such calves, as are most likely to give plenty of rich milk, and to be good breeders. In this selection, more regard is shewn to shape than to kind. Small and long horns, a thin shoulder and neck, a round body, neat, tight, and broad bones, and large milk veins, are preferred to the boasted progeny of the most celebrated breed. If they were equally careful to provide proper bulls*, their cattle would give more and better milk, and fetch higher prices.

All the butter made in the county is little more than sufficient for the consumpt of the inhabitants, and for salving the sheep. The quantity carried out of it is nearly balanced by what is brought into it for these purposes.

Very

* A bull of the noted Tees-water breed, and remarkably handsome, was lately brought down a few years ago to Riddell, by Sir J. B. Riddell, Baronet. The descendants of this bull are rising to so great esteem among tenants, in the lower parts of this county, that some are purchasing heifers, and others sending cows to bulls, begotten by him. It is to be hoped that this spirit will spread.

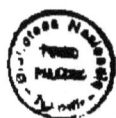

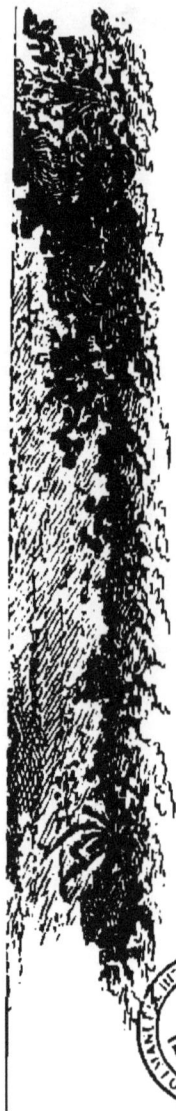

BLACK-FACED or SCOTS RAM

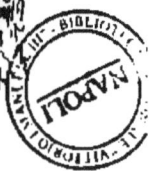

Very few cheeses are made of pure cow-milk : but a good many of cow and ewe milk mixed.

Sect. II.—*Sheep.*

It has already been observed that this county is wholly flocked with white-faced sheep, except a tract towards the sources of Ettrick and Yarrow-waters, of which Hindhope is the lowest point on the one, and Ladhope on the other. Few of these, however, are of the genuine Cheviot breed. The change, from the black-faced kind, was effected in most places by using Cheviot tups, for a succession of years, till all traces of the coarse wool, short bodies, black faces and legs, disappeared. This plan was extremely plausible in theory. There was every reason to expect that some of the good qualities of the mother might be retained, and her chief defects corrected ; that her hardiness, her height in the forequarter, and her round body, might descend to her progeny, with finer wool and greater weight of carcase. But the event is a striking proof that the most species theoretical reasoning may be delusive. The present white-faced flocks in Selkirkshire do indeed possess the hardiness of the race from whence they sprung in the female line, and their wool is considerably improven. But still even in wool, and much more in shape and size, they are greatly inferior to true Cheviot sheep.

Some tenants ventured to purchase lambs or ewe-hogs from approved flocks of the Cheviot kind, and, after seasoning them to the soil and climate of their new pasture, procured rams for them of the same breed. Considering the danger, which always attends the removal of young sheep to a distant pasture, this experiment has been abun-

dantly

dantly fuccefsful, although the permanent effect of it is loft,
by allowing the progeny to mix with the reft of the flock,
and giving the whole promifcuoufly the fame rams. One
or two had the boldnefs to bring flocks of old Cheviot
fheep, and fome young wethers, upon ftrange and very expofed ground, in very unfavourable circumftances, and have
hitherto had no caufe to repent. In finenefs of fleeces, and
weight of carcafe, thefe fheep excel all that have been hitherto mentioned. Nor are they lefs hardy, or more fubject to difeafes and mortality, than their predeceffors were
upon the fame farms.

In falving, more tar is ufed than in Roxburghfhire, which
affects not a little the weight of fleeces. There, only two
gallons of it are mixed with a ftone or twenty-four pounds
Englifh of butter for fixty fheep [a]. Whereas, here, the
common allowance for that number is no lefs than five gallons
of tar and thirty-fix or perhaps thirty-eight pounds of butter.
This quantity is laid upon fifty young, and upon feventy
old fheep: the latter being more numerous, it muft, at an
average, falve rather more than fixty; but this is the cafe
equally in both counties. For that number fome farmers
here give lefs butter, but the quantity of tar is never di-
minifhed; and feveral of them, who are very intelligent,
after trying various proportions of thefe ingredients, have
fixed upon twenty-five pounds of butter and ten pints of tar,
(both Scotch, and equal to $37\frac{1}{2}$ pounds and five gallons
Englifh) as the moft proper mixture both for the fheep and
wool of this county. An addition of $2\frac{1}{2}$ ounces Englifh is
thus made to each fleece by the tar alone, exclufive of the
duft, fand, &c. which infeparably adhere to it; and confequently, about $6\frac{1}{2}$ fleeces, at an average, will weigh a
ftone, inftead of $7\frac{1}{4}$ [b] as in Roxburghfhire, though the animal

fnal itſelf is leſs than a true Cheviot ſheep, and its fleece would be lighter if both were freed from ſalve.

Few wethers are reared, except for the farmer's own uſe; and, when fattened on his common paſture, they will weigh about twelve or thirteen pounds per quarter; in a rich incloſure they may reach fifteen pounds [*]. Ewes on the hill are about nine or ten pounds [*], often not ſo much, and ſometimes more. Wool, though nearly as fine in the pile as that of Roxburghſhire, ſells, on account of the great quantity of tar in it, at one-fifth [†] leſs price. Its average in 1795 was about 16 s., and in 1796 might be 20 s. or a guinea, excluſive of the wool of the true Cheviot ſheep, which was 20 s. in 1795, and 26 s. in 1796.

The male lambs are all cut, except the few kept to become rams, and, after being weaned, are ſold to farmers in the lower parts of Roxburghſhire, Berwickſhire, and Northumberland. The ſurplus or *draught* ewe-lambs, after the beſt are picked out for ſupplying vacancies in the flock, go to the ſame market, or ſometimes find purchaſers in butchers, when tolerably fat.

Caſt or draught-ewes are an important article of ſale. Such of them as do not bring forth a lamb, or ſoon loſe it, grow quickly fat on the top of the graſs, and fetch a good price as early mutton, or to be fattened on better paſtures. The reſt, as ſoon as they get into decent condition after ſuckling their lambs, are diſpoſed of to graziers.

Black-faced ſheep are managed in a manner ſomewhat different. Inhabiting a higher and more expoſed country, they require more tar in ſalve; a large proportion of their male lambs are not cut; and moſt of the lambs, not neceſſary

---

[*] All Dutch weight, the pound equal to ſeventeen and a half oz. Engliſh.

[†] See p. 153, 155. the ſtone is twenty-four pounds Engliſh.

ceffary for the flock, and of their caft or draught-ewes, are
made fat for the fhambles.

The quantity of tar and butter, moft commonly mixed,
applies not fo accurately, without fractions, to fixty as to
forty-five fheep. For that number, only twenty-four pounds *
of butter are ufed with five gallons * of tar, which is nearly 6¼ gallons * for the three fcore. Few or none give lefs
tar; and feveral allow fix gallons * of it to twenty-four
pounds * butter for forty-five, which is precifely equal to
eight gallons * and thirty-two pounds * for fixty fheep.
One or two retain the old practice of making the quantities of tar and butter equal, a gallon of tar being fuppofed
to weigh nearly the fame with two Scotch or three Englifh
pounds of butter, and to meafure no more than the butter
when melted. Even the leaft of thefe quantities appears
enormous on a fuperficial view; but though the practice
may not be altogether defenfible, it is far from deferving
the condemnation and ridicule to which it has been expofed. For it is allowed that the coarfe wool of thefe fheep
is extremely open and thin at the bottom, and readily admits rain or melted fnow. Now this wetnefs, lodging in
the fleece, would hurt the wool, incommode the fheep by
its weight, and occafion a conftant and unhealthy dampnefs on the fkin, if the animals were not defended by a
thick and warm covering, which moifture and cold cannot
eafily penetrate. At the fame time it muft be granted, that
this covering may be made, by unfkilful hands, as cumbrous and intolerable as the evils which it is intended to
prevent. And it cannot be denied, that the wool, from
this treatment and from its natural coarfenefs, reaches only
about two-fifths of the price of the other. It commonly
                                                    fells

* All Englifh weight and meafure; but the Englifh pound is fuppofed
to contain fixteen Englifh ounces.

fells at about 6 s. or 6 s. 6 d. when the wool of white-faced
sheep is 15 s. or 16 s.; and fix or fix and a half fleeces of it
will at an average weigh a stone.

The lambs, coming into the world with more wool, are
less apt to suffer from severity of weather when newly
dropped, than those of the white-faced kind. The males,
from not being cut, grow larger and stouter; and, from
sucking longer, and sometimes too getting sweet and tender grass, are sold fat at 1 s. 6 d. a-piece above the current
price of other lambs. The females, also, are thereby put
into excellent order, either for being kept on the farm,
or for accompanying their brothers to the markets of Edinburgh or Dalkeith. In this case little or no cheese can be
made, as the mothers, brought low by giving milk so long,
require rest and nutritive food to recover their flesh and
strength, for standing the winter, or for being sold to advantage. Such lambs, as are cut and early weaned with
a view of making butter for salve or cheese for sale from
their mother's milk, as well as the cast ewe-lambs, are dif-
posed of in the same way with the white-faced lambs.
Both are sometimes kept over winter and sold about Whitsunday under the name of *hogs*.

Being kindly feeders, ewes, uncumbered with lambs,
grow soon fat, and even many, after being reduced by
nursing, pick up so quickly as to become excellent mutton towards the end of the season. Their average weight
then will be from nine and a half* to ten and a half pounds
per quarter. On turnips, and even on grass in fertile and
sheltered fields, they will reach two pounds more. The
rich juice and admirable flavour of their mutton secure to
them a ready market and a good price.

Q q   In

* Dutch weight.

In several farms, flocked some with white and others with black-faced sheep, great ewes are sold. Instead of being sent to market towards the close of the season, they are kept till spring, and fetch when big with young 3 s. or 4 s. of additional price. To accommodate them with food during winter, fewer other sheep either old or young must be kept on the farm. For this mode of management, two reasons are assigned; the profit of wintering a part of the draught-ewes, and the advantage of lightening the pasture in spring and leaving more food for the remaining ewes and lambs. But these reasons can only apply to a few farms, where there is little grass early in the season when lambs make their appearance, and when the heath, on which ewes feed through winter, becomes unfit for their use. For on most sheep-walks there is as much more grass in summer than in winter, as will sufficiently maintain all the lambs brought forth by the breeding flock, and, as it gradually fails, the mouths upon it are lessened by the sale, first of lambs, and afterwards of cast-ewes. Not to dispose of these cast-ewes at such a price as they will bring must be attended with one of two disadvantages: it must either diminish the number of breeding ones or of young ones to supply their places, or it must overstock the farm. To sell them before the commencement of winter is certainly the most simple and natural method, and it is becoming daily more prevalent [a].

Ewes of both white-faced and black-faced flocks are milked from three to eight weeks, according to circumstances.

---

[a] I understand the practice of selling great ewes was introduced at a time, when both wool and lambs were of little value: And farmers were willing to forego the trifling profit arising from them, for the sake of selling their ewes at a higher price, and of avoiding all risk of diseases and mortality among both sheep and lambs.

ftances. Some butter is made of their cream, chiefly for
falving; and a good many cheefes are made of their milk,
mixed in different proportions with that of cows, of the
fame fize and weight, and much in the fame manner, as in
Roxburghfhire.

Though the fame difeafes alfo prevail, and may be ar-
ranged in the fame order with refpect to prevalence and
fatality, yet it deferves to be mentioned, that, in particular local fituations, this arrangement admits of fome variety; of which the following inftances are the moft common and ftriking. In one farm, the difeafes are thus clafs-
ed, *ficknefs, rot, braxy, fturdy, louping-ill.* In a neighbouring farm, *louping-ill, ficknefs, rot, fturdy, braxy.* In
one at the diftance of four miles from the laft mentioned,
ficknefs, rot, fturdy, little braxy, or louping-ill. Thefe three
inftances are all taken from farms on the north of Ettrick
water. In feveral places on Yarrow water, the *louping-
ill* takes place of the *ficknefs.* But it is remarkable, that,
where this laft difeafe is not the moft prevalent, it always
holds the fecond place, except in a fingle inftance, in which
the fturdy * comes before it; a fact which clearly efta-
blifhes

* Concerning the fturdy, I have been favoured with the following curious information, of which I gave a hint, page 163. A medical gentleman, of acknowledged ability and anatomical knowledge, writes to this
purpofe: "In my young and inquifitive days, I examined feveral difeafed
"heads of fheep, none of whom, however, was allowed to die of the
"difeafe, and found one having thirteen cifts with water in different parts
"of the brain, one larger than the reft behind the horns, where moft
"commonly that cift is feated between the lobs of the brain, which, when
"full of water, by its preffure thins the fkull. The brain feems not to
"fuffer otherwife than from being compreffed by the watery cift. If
"there is only one large cift of water between the lobs of the brain, and
"if it could either be burft by fomething thruft up in the noftril, or taken
"out by trepanning the fkull, a cure may be effected; but if there are
"more

blishes its claim to a decided precedence among all the ma-
ladies incident to sheep.

From the preceding pages it may be collected, that,
through the whole of this county, five acres will nearly
maintain four sheep. Reckoning the average rent of an
acre at 2 s. 9 d. and the grass eat annually by every sheep
at 3 s. 6 d., the former multiplied by five amounts to 13 s.
9 d. and the latter multiplied by four to 14 s. According
to this calculation, there are 118,400 sheep on the 148,000
acres in pasture. We shall arrive pretty much at the same
conclusion, by supposing, with several judicious farmers,
that, throwing all the poor land together, there may be
fully one-third of the pasture-district, of which a sheep will
eat the produce almost of two acres, and that 50,000 acres
will scarcely maintain 30,000 sheep, that there is about
another third, of which four sheep will confume five acres,
and that, on the remaining third, an acre will afford sufficient food for a sheep, and some favourite spots may even
do more. There will thus be

50,000,

" more than one, I fee no prospect of a cure." The same gentleman
told me in conversation, that he is assured by several shepherds, who are in
use to trepan skulls, and to examine the heads of sheep either cut off by
this disease or killed upon its being found incurable, that they frequently
have seen more than one cist or bag of water in a head.

To ascertain how far this disorder is hereditary, it would be a patriotic
attempt, if any farmer would pick out a few ewes and a ram who have
been cured of it, keep these by themselves, and watch their offspring; or
make the same experiment with a ram and ewes, one of whom had recovered from it and the other had never been affected by it. The state of
their progeny, compared with that of other sheep in the flock of the same
age, would probably solve this question. It is of equal importance to determine whether other diseases are transmitted directly from one genera-
tion to another. To know the cause is always one essential step towards
preventing or at least mitigating a mischievous effect.

		Sheep.
50,000 acres for — — —		30,000
49,000 acres at five acres to four sheep,		39,200
49,000 acres at one sheep to each		49,000
148,000 acres, maintaining		118,200 sheep.

It is admitted, that there is not one-third of the whole
sheep in the county black-faced. Estimating them at
36,000, and allowing thirteen fleeces to weigh two stones,
they will yield annually about 5538 stone of wool, which,
at the average price of 6 s. 6 d. is nearly L. 1800 Sterling.
Taking 200 less than the lowest of the two preceding calculations, and supposing the whole sheep in the county to
be only 118,000, there will remain, after deducting 36,000
black-faced ones, precisely 82,000 of the white-faced, whose
fleeces at 7 to a stone, will weigh upwards of 11,700 stone,
and the wool, at the average of 15 s. *per* stone, brings a
little more than L. 8770 Sterling.

For other particulars relative to sheep, the reader is referred to what is mentioned on this subject in the Account
of Roxburghshire. Perhaps it should be noticed, that the people here are not reckoned so nice in mixing the ingredients,
laying on the salve, and shearing the sheep, as they are
there. But this remark already admits of some exceptions,
and, it is hoped, will, in a few years hence, cease to be
applicable to a single individual *.

SECT.

* A singular instance of longevity in a sheep occurred lately in this
county. As far as I can judge, she must have been of (what Mr Culley
calls) the *Herdwick* breed, though rather larger, perhaps from getting better pasture, or having a *heath* or black-faced ram for her father. The
mother was presented, by the late Archibald Douglas Esq; of Cavers,
some years before his death which happened in the beginning of 1774, to
John

Sect. III.—*Horses.*

The few horses, requiſite for cultivating the arable diſtrict, are partly of the Lanarkſhire, and partly of the Northumberland breed. The former were in higher eſtimation ſome years ago than they are now. They are naturally too weighty to ſtand the fatigue of long journies, and of late this inability has increaſed by the great length and conſequent ſlackneſs of back, which they have acquired from the inattention or injudicious management of the breeders. Their ſtallions ſtill frequent this county, and are employed in the higher parts of it, where young horſes are chiefly reared. But in the lower parts, horſes from the north of England are preferred, becauſe, having all more or leſs blood, they can be ridden as well as wrought, they are admirable travellers with loaded carts in a hilly country, they have ſufficient ſtrength to draw a plough through light ſoil, and their foals partake of their mettle and ſpeed. Some Iriſh horſes are alſo uſed for draught. Farmers do not ſo much regard the kind or breed, when purchaſing horſes, as their ſhape, their tractability, their ſuitableneſs for a particular purpoſe, and, if mares, their being likely to bring good foals. Several of them, as well as the reſident proprietors, keep ſaddle-horſes with a conſiderable portion of blood, and ponies as drudges. But

horſes

John Elliot Eſq; late of Borthwickbrae, when with lamb of this ewe, which lived till March 1796. The preciſe year of her birth cannot be certainly aſcertained. The ſhepherd alleges, that ſhe was on the eve of twenty-ſeven years when ſhe died, and ſhe muſt have been at leaſt twenty-four. Moſt people, who had acceſs to know her age, agree that ſhe was twenty five if not older. But even twenty four, which is undiſputed, is an extraordinary period for a ſheep to live.

horses of full blood, though sometimes used for the chace and for the road, are not numerous.

More horses are reared in the county, than are purchased from other places; but the number of both fluctuate so much annually, that it cannot be easily ascertained. There were, in 1796, 574 saddle, carriage, and draught horses, in the whole county, charged with duty to Government, and only 22 exempted from it, not including foals.

Sect. IV.—*Hogs.*

Swine are reared only by a few gentlemen and farmers for their tables, and by millers for the market. In some seasons, one or two of them are fattened by other farmers, cottagers, and artificers, on the offals of their stack-yards, gardens, and tables, during the winter months, either for the use of their families or for sale. Their number varies so much from year to year, that no average can be formed of it; but though it is never great, yet a small quantity of bacon or pickled pork is sent annually from Selkirk to Berwick. The large breed are chiefly kept about mills; a middling kind, weighing when fat from twelve to fixteen stone, are in greatest esteem through the county in general, and a few of the Chinese are likewise used.

Sect. V.—*Rabbits.*

Sect. VI.—*Poultry.*

Sect. VII.—*Pigeons.*

The reader must be referred to what is said concerning these particulars in the Account of Roxburghshire. Rabbits burrow in several places. A few of them are kept

tame;

tame; but they are not any where an object of much attention. As corn is essential to the maintenance of poultry and pigeons, there must be few of both, except in the arable district and its immediate vicinity. The reverse is the case with bees. They thrive and yield plenty of excellent honey in the wildest as well as in the most cultivated places. In a favourable season, their produce must be a considerable source of profit to the lower class of people, by many of whom they are managed with much skill. There can be no doubt that many more of them might be kept with equal advantage. Every shepherd, cottager, and mechanic, especially in remote situations, would find pleasure in paying attention to them, and generally may make an addition to his yearly income. There is no place from whence heath or white clover is far distant: Bees are remarkably fond of both; and both give a rich flavour to honey. The culture of bees is attended with little expence or trouble: They are not subjected to many accidents; and their honey is sure of bringing a good price either in combs or in a fluid state.

CHAP.

CHAP. XIV.

RURAL ECONOMY.

Sect. I.—*Labour, Servants, Labourers, Hours of Labour.*

THE only works done by the piece, are drains, ditches, and buildings.

In some soft spots, drains have been made of two feet, both in width and depth, so low as at 4 d. When carried through light soil on a bottom of till approaching towards gravel, they cost 6 d. and when the till is very hard, or when huge stones are to be removed or cut through, they cost 8 d. and sometimes 10 d. That price has been paid for digging and filling up drains, both wider and deeper, where such obstructions did not come in the way: the undertakers, however, seldom fill the drains: that is commonly done by their employers. Branches, to convey

small

small springs into the main drains, are from sixteen to twenty-four inches, and cost less in proportion to their narrowness, their shallowness, and the facility of making them. Open drains, in sheep-walks, from fourteen to twenty inches broad, and from seven to fourteen inches deep, seldom exceed 1 d. and are often not so much.

The rate paid for ditches varies according to their width, and the nature of the ground. When not above three feet or even three and a half feet wide, and from twenty to twenty-four inches deep, 5 d. or 6 d. is about the average price of making them and planting thorns. They are seldom broader and deeper, because the good soil is in general shallow and the substratum hard.

Stone-walls, without mortar, are built four and a half feet high for 1 s. 8 d., when the stones are brought to the spot; to cope them with sods, costs 2 d. more, and to add eighteen inches of a Galloway top to their height, advances the price to 2 s. All the above prices relate to the rood of six yards. The rate of building with lime and of slating by the piece is the same as in Roxburghshire.

To the account already given of that county, a reference may be made for information concerning the other particulars in this section. But I think it necessary to correct a small mistake which I made with respect to the supper of reapers. Bread and milk is rarely given them since the introduction of potatoes. Their common supper, in both counties, is, either porridge and milk, or mashed potatoes and milk ; or else a penny each evening, or a certain quantity of oatmeal or grain through the whole harvest, to provide one for themselves. It may not be improper to add, that ewe-milking being reckoned the severest and most unpleasant of all female labours, the women, who are employed in it, receive from 50 s. to L. 3 of wages for the

summer

summer half year; while during the winter half year they get only from a guinea to 30 s.

The wages of shepherds, also, deserve to be particularly mentioned, as they are nearly the same in both counties. They are commonly eight *soums* of grass, or what the parties reckon equivalent in value to these. A *soum* is the grass eaten by one cow or ten sheep. Supposing a shepherd to receive his whole wages in the grass of eighty sheep, their amount, according to the preceding calculations, would be as follows :

His 80 sheep will bring 54 lambs, of which, after keeping
  a proportion for his flock, he will sell 36 at
  5 s.   -   -   -   -   -   L. 9   0   0
He will sell 12 or perhaps 13 old or cast-ewes,
  at 11 s. say only 12,   -   -   -   6 12   0
Besides 75 fleeces, which, of white-faced sheep,
  will produce, at 2 s. each,   -   -   7 10   0
The skins and carcases of his dead sheep, his
  cheese and butter, and his udder-locks, will
  be   -   -   -   -   -   -   2   0   0

                                 L. 25   2   0

In this calculation, there is a sufficient allowance for casualties; but from the sum total must be deducted the interest of the original price paid for his flock, which, at 13 s. each sheep, will be L. 52, and will reduce his wage to L. 22, 10 s.

The more common wages of shepherds, however, are 40 or 45 sheep; a cow kept through the whole year; a house and garden; his master's horses to bring home his fuel; and a stone of oatmeal every week. According to
                                        the

the above statement, his profit on the 40 sheep

will be	–	–	–	–	–	L. 11	5 0
His cow is commonly valued at			–	–	3	0 0
His stone of meal, at the average of 2 s. is		–	5	4 0
His house, garden, and use of horses,		–	2	2 0

L. 21 11 0

But his cow will yield him double the sum that is here af-
signed, besides maintaining his family. He is careful to
provide a good one; she fares well both in summer and
winter, and brings into his pocket of clear gain generally
L. 6, and sometimes L. 10. In some places he is allowed
forty-five sheep, for the summer's grass of a steer or heifer;
but in these places the pasture generally is coarse, the chance
of mortality is great, or the fleece is of inferior value. The
number of sheep is always reckoned at the time of calving.

It deserves the special notice of sheep-farmers, that this
last is the most profitable plan both for themselves and
their shepherds. Masters pay, as rent, 3 s. 6 d. for every
sheep kept by their shepherds. At this rate, it may be
thought, that, in the former case, they are only L. 14 out
of pocket to the shepherd for his eighty sheep. But it is
evident that they likewise lose all the profit which he makes,
after every reasonable allowance for risk and the interest
of stock. In the latter case, he has a sufficient number of
sheep to interest him in the welfare of the flock, he has
more conveniency for his family, and by frugal management his annual income may be larger. Farmers, at the
same time, have the profit arising from forty more sheep,
are not put to so great expence by what they give to the
shepherd in lieu of these, and have a sure pledge that proper care shall be taken of their flocks. It should be a max-
im with them to give a shepherd maintenance for no more
sheep

sheep than will enfure his attention, and to make up his wages from other fources lefs connected with the grand object of emolument to themfelves.

SECT. II.—*Provifions.*

MEAL and flower, which conflitute the chief food of the inhabitants, are rather dearer here than in the arable diftrict of Roxburghfhire, but not fo dear as in Peebles or Dalkeith.　On account of the fmall quantity of grain raifed, no *fiars* * *are ftruck,* as in the neighbouring counties The monthly returns fent to Government of the prices of grain are as follows, by the county boll :

---

* To *ftrike the fiars,* is the common phrafe in Scotland for fixing the average price of grain.　See note, p. 194.

TABLE

T A B L E.

	Wheat.			Peas.			Barley.			Oats.			Oatmeal.		
	L.	s.	d.	L.	s.	d.	L.	s.	d.	L.	s.	d.	L.	s.	d.
1791, last 4 months, –	1	6	1	0	19	5	0	19	5	0	15	4	1	8	0
1792, first 6 months, –	1	6	1	0	16	9¼	1	0	1¼	0	15	0¾	1	6	0
—— last 6 months, –	1	8	2	0	19	1½	1	0	9¼	0	16	1¾	1	7	0
1793, first 6 months, –	1	8	9	1	3	3	1	5	2¼	0	19	1	1	11	10
—— last 6 months, –	1	11	7	1	10	0	1	1	8	0	19	5	1	13	4
1794, first 6 months, –	1	9	8¼	1	1	3	1	1	5¼	0	19	9½	1	12	2
—— last 6 months, –	1	12	1	1	2	7½	1	6	6½	1	1	3½	1	11	10
1795, first 6 months, –	1	15	7	1	2	0½	1	5	5¼	0	18	10½	1	11	2
—— last 6 months, –	2	15	2½	1	9	6	1	8	8	1	9	0	1	15	8
1796, first 6 months, –	2	14	7½	1	7	9	1	13	8½	1	6	7¼	2	1	4
—— last 6 months, –	2	2	4½	1	7	4½	1	8	1	0	19	11¼	1	14	2

There

There are butcher markets both at Selkirk and Galashiels, where beef, mutton, veal, lamb, and pork are all sold
in their different seasons, nearly at the same prices as at the
neighbouring markets in Roxburghshire. None of these
articles is to be got regularly through the whole season.
From the beginning of August until March, the mutton in
excellence will yield to none in the kingdom. Lamb is
plentiful and very good from the middle of June until the
end of September. Beef, fed on grass, abounds from September till Martinmas, and is soon succeeded by similar
beef fattened on turnips, which continues till May. From
that time till August every kind of butcher-meat is rather
scarce except lamb. Little pork or veal is killed for sale;
though both are favourite dishes at the tables of some gentlemen and farmers, who are at the trouble, either of feeding them, or of providing them from other markets. The
southern part of this county is supplied with every kind
of provisions from Hawick. And such farmers as are far
from markets, as well as most of the gentlemen, use their
own mutton and lamb. A number of very good salmon
are caught in that part of Tweed which intersects this
county, and sold at 6 d. *per* pound (Dutch) till they begin to fall away, when they are sometimes so low as 1¼ d.
and are purchased by the poorer class to be salted and eat during winter with potatoes. Herrings, however, are a cheaper,
a more common and a more agreeable seasoning to that popular and nutritive root. Salt herrings seldom cost more
and generally less than 9 d. *per* dozen. And those, who
do not raise enough of potatoes for themselves, can always
be supplied with plenty at the average price of 10 d. or
1 s. the Linlithgow firlot. Onions being annually exposed
to sale at a reasonable rate, milk being every where abundant and cheap, and butter and cheese being easily within
their

their reach, the poor, while meal does not rife to an exorbitant price, live comfortably on thefe wholefome and fa-
voury difhes. There is a great differe ce between the
price of poultry in the northern and fouth. rn parts both of
this county and Roxburghfhire, owing to the one being
nearer to the capital, nd having eafy communication with
it by excellent roads. In 1791, the prices were as under :

	NORTHERN.	SOUTHERN.
A good hen, -	1 s. o d.	— o s. 7 d. or 8 d.
A chicken, from 3 d. to	o s. 5 d.	— o s. 1½ d. to 3 d.
A duck, from 1 s. to	1 s. 2 d.	— o s. 8 d. or 9 d.
A duckling, 8 d. or	o s. 9 d.	— o s. 5 d. feld fold.
A goofe, - -	2 s. 6 d.	— 1 s. 8 d.
Pigeons, *per* dozen, -	2 s. o d.	— 1 s. 6 d.
Eggs, *per* doz. from 3 d. to o s. 8 d.		— o s. 3 d. to 6 d.

In both diftricts, thefe prices are on the increafe, and
the difference now is not fo ftriking, though it is ftill very confiderable.

Sect. III.—*Fuel.*

The northern part of this county is fupplied with coals
from Middleton, and the fouth-eaft corner of it from Canoby in Dumfries-fhire. Their weight, meafure, and prime
coft, at both places, have been already mentioned *. And
to it, an addition may be made of 2 d. *per* cwt. for every
five miles that they are carried. It is chiefly in thefe parts,
too, and efpecially towards the north, that the thinnings
of wood are ufed for fuel. In all the higher diftrict,

                                        peats

* See p. 196.

peats are burnt; and to make and prepare them, confti-
tutes the principal work of the inhabitants during fummer. They would gladly bring coals, notwithftanding the
diftance, if the roads were fitter for wheel-carriages. I
am forry to add, that turfs, thofe inveterate foes, to the
foil, are not entirely laid afide.

CHAP.

CHAP. XV.

POLITICAL ECONOMY, AS CONNECTED WITH OR AFFECT-
ING AGRICULTURE.

SECT. I.—Roads.

IN consequence of an act of Parliament, obtained in 1764, a road of twelve miles was made from Crofslee toll-bar on the confines of Mid-Lothian, through Selkirk, to Haremofs toll-bar towards Hawick, with a branch of three miles to the village of Galashiels. Part of the road from Kelfo to Peebles, to the extent of six or seven miles, runs also through this county from Galashiels bridge, to Gait-hope-burn beyond Hollilee toll-bar. The expence of these roads, and of a substantial bridge over Tweed at Fairnilee, was L. 6560. And the produce of the tolls has hitherto been barely sufficient to defray the annual charge of keeping the roads, bridges, and toll-houses, in proper order.

Substantial

Subſtantial and laſting roads could eaſily be made on the gravelly and ſtony bottom of this county, eſpecially near its running waters. Yet few of the crofs or county roads have ever been put in proper order. An excellent road was indeed made, about thirty years ago, from Selkirk along the banks of Yarrow for five miles, when it aſcends Minchmoor, and proceeds towards Peebles. Attempts have ſince been made to amend and alter the direction of the roads on the ſides of Ettrick and Yarrow waters, both of which might be carried forward to Moffat, and open up the neareſt line of communication from the northern parts of Roxburghſhire, the ſouthern extremity of Mid-Lothian, and a large tract of Berwickſhire, to (Dumfries and the circum-jacent country. A little attention to improve another crofs-road, from Aſhkirk in Roxburghſhire to Roberton church, and from thence through a corner of this county in a line towards Mofspaul, would ſave about five miles to a conſiderable diſtrict of both counties, which is furniſhed with coals, lime, and other articles from the neighbourhood of Langholm. Much remains to be done to all theſe crofs-roads, and to one between Galaſhiels and the county town. If theſe were put into a reſpectable condition for allowing an eaſy paſſage to wheel-carriages, a very little expence, beſtowed on the bad ſteps of the others, would render them much ſafer and eaſier to travellers on horſeback, for whom alone they ſeem to be deſigned.

A trial has lately been made of a ſmall piece of road on an inclined plane. Roads, made on this plan, may be very durable, and anſwer the purpoſe extremely well in mild weather; but during the ſeverity of winter, froſt may render travelling upon them highly dangerous, eſpecially in thoſe places of this hilly and cold country which then feel not the influence of the ſun.

SECT.

Sect. II.—*Canals.*

In a hilly county, whose lowest point is 300 feet above the sea, and upwards of thirty miles distant from it, and whose extent, population, and produce are small, the practicability of making a canal may reasonably be doubted, and the advantages attending one would be trifling.

Sect. III.—*Fairs.*

At Selkirk there are two considerable fairs; one upon the 5th of April for hiring servants especially ewe-milkers, paying rents, feu-duties, taxes, and other debts, and selling great ewes, and different grains for seed; the other on the 21st August for cattle, paying rents, and receiving the price of sheep, and seed-corn sold at the former one. At both there is a good deal of linen and woollen cloth. Four lesser fairs are likewise held there, and three at Galashiels for various purposes, according to the season of the year, the chief of which are seed-corn, great ewes, wool, cheese, sickles, hiring reapers, and settling accounts. It may be proper to mention, that all grain for seed is sold by sample, great ewes, wool, and cheese, by their known state and the character of the farm where they are raised or made, and that cattle alone are brought personally to the fairs. It will readily occur to every reader, that the farmers here regularly attend the neighbouring fairs at Earlstoun, Melrose, St Boswell's, and Hawick. Some of them also

also go to other fairs, particularly to Langholm on the 26th July, where wool and lambs are fold, to Peebles on the first Tuesday of March, reckoned the largest fair in the neighbourhood for great ewes, besides two or three other fairs there, and to fairs in Mid-Lothian, Lanark, and Dumfries-shires for horses and black-cattle. One or two of the most enterprising among them frequent fairs in England, and have been for some years successively as far as Boroughbridge.

Sect. IV.—*Weekly-Markets.*

The only weekly market in the whole county is at Selkirk on Wednesday. It has generally a tolerable supply of butcher-meat, and is pretty well attended by the neighbouring farmers; but most of them towards the south prefer the market at Hawick on Thursday; and a few towards the west and north-west go to the market at Peebles on Tuesday.

Sect. V.—*Commerce.*

This county, neither raising wheat nor fattening cattle sufficient for its consumption, is obliged to import these, besides the necessaries and luxuries imported into Roxburgh-shire. But, at the same time, being more thinly peopled in proportion to its extent, less is to be deducted from its exports for maintaining the inhabitants, and something may be added to them on account of its manufactures. The following statement is the most correct that the slender materials,

terials, with which I am furnished, enables me to give of the principal articles of its produce and expenditure:

Oats, 4800 acres, at 3½ bolls *per* acre, and at 15 s. *per* boll, or L. 2 : 12 : 6 *per* acre, 16800 bolls, — — — — L. 12600 0 0

Barley, 1000 acres, at 4½ bolls *per* acre, and L. 1 *per* boll, or L. 4, 10 s. *per* acre, 4500 bolls, — — — — — 4500 0 0

Peas, 600 acres, at 4 bolls *per* acre, and at L. 1, 10 s. *per* boll, or L. 6 *per* acre, 2400 bolls, — — — — — 3600 0 0

Black-cattle, 360, (being nearly one-sixth of 2200), lean and fat, young and old, at L. 7 each, — — — — 2520 0 0

Horses, 50, young and old, at L. 12 each, 600 0 0

Ewes, 19600, at 11 s. each, — — 9800 0 0

Lambs, 56200, at 5 s. each, — — 14050 0 0

Wool, 82000 fleeces, at 2 s. — — 8200 0 0

Cheese, 36000 fleeces, at 11 d. about — 800 0 0

Cloth manufactured, 79000 yards, at 2 s. 6 d. — — — — 9875 0 0

Clear profit on other manufactures, as tanned-leather, inkle, &c. supposed about 800 0 0
———————
Total produce of the county, — L. 68995 0 0

From this sum, are to be deducted,

The rent of the county, L. 28000 0 0
———————
Carried forward, — L. 28000 0 0 L. 68995 0 0

Brought forward, L. 28000 0 0 L. 68995 0 0

Grain for the inhabitants, at
the rate of one-half ftone of
meal to each *per* week, at
2 s. *per* ftone, 4646 people, — — L. 2323 0 0

Oats for 574 horfes, at the
rate of thirteen bolls to
each, and of 15 s. *per* boll, 5596 0 0

Butcher-meat, and wheaten-
bread, for 4446 people, at
the rate of 8 d. *per* week
for each, — — 8052 0 0

Prime coft of 412 pack, or
34608 fleeces, at the average of feven to a ftone,
and at the average price
of 2 s. *per* fleece, — 3460 0 0
                                    —————— 47432 0 0

Which leaves a clear gain to the county, ————→
of — — — — — L. 21563 0 0

after paying rents, and maintaining the inhabitants and their
cattle. The reader will obferve that it is greater, in proportion to the real rent, than that of Roxburghfhire, which
is to be afcribed chiefly to the flourifhing manufactures at
Galafhiels. For while all the cloth and tanned leather
made in the one county, with the furplus of profit arifing
from tawed-leather and carpets, will be barely fufficient
for clothing the inhabitants, it may be fafely affirmed, that,
in the other county, the number of yards mentioned in the
text are annually fold of woolen-cloth, befides what the
people wear, and that there is at leaft the amount there ftated

ted of clear profit on other articles actually manufactured,
after a fair allowance for what are used in the county, and
for the prime cost of materials. It is, however, to be remembered, that the wages of manufacturers are high, and
that they consume fully more butcher-meat and wheaten-
bread, than the quantity specified. Neither beef nor wheat
being produced in the county in any respect adequate to its
consumpt, instead of deducting, as in Roxburghshire, a fifth
part of the live-stock annually sold, I hope to come nearer
to the truth, by allotting a small portion of each weekly to
every soul in the population, and by supposing that the
gentlemen and their servants, the farmers, the manufacturers, and the wealthier inhabitants of Selkirk and Galashiels, eat as much more than the assigned quota, as infants
will fall short of it, and those labourers and peasants who
seldom regale themselves with such sumptuous fare. It
may be thought, as most of the black-cattle are sold at or
below four years old, that more than one-sixth of them
ought to be charged to the produce of the county. But
most of the inhabitants of Selkirk and Galashiels, and many tradesmen and cottagers, who keep cows for their families, rear no calves, except a few fatted ones, and seldom part with their cows except in exchange for younger
ones, so that one-sixth of the whole cattle will be fully equal
to one-fourth of those which are actually reared. The same
rule cannot be applied to horses, because those, employed
for draught and the saddle, require so great an annual supply as to leave no more than a surplus of fifty, if so many,
to increase the general account. The quantity of cheese
made here is rather greater in proportion to the number of
sheep than in Roxburghshire *, and the consumpt by the
thin

* Even there more cheese is made than consumed; but it is not stated, because of the higher value put upon both sheep and lambs.

thin population being much lefs, another fmall addition arifes from this article. I hope the prices fpecified will be
found a tolerably juft medium between the higheft and
loweft which have been given for fome years paft, and fuch
as may be reafonably expected, at a fair average, for a fe-
ries of future years.

SECT. VI.—*Manufactures.*

THE chief manufactures are woollen-cloth, flockings, tanned-leather, inkle, and different implements of hufbandry,
or wood *blocked* out for making them.

Woollen cloth is moftly made in Galafhiels; and its fub-
urbs in Roxburghfhire which were all built during the laft
twenty years. It is of different degrees of finenefs, from
600 to 1300 threads in breadth, and from 1 s. 4 d. to 7 s.
of price *per* yard to wholefale dealers. The average will
run from 2 s. 4 d. to 2 s. 9 d. The wool, in general, is
rather coarfe, and will not, at an average of eight or ten
years, exceed 14 s. or 15 s. *per* ftone, though fmall parcels
of it have been ufed as fine as 45 s. and feveral are annually manufactured from 21 s. to 30 s. The gradual increafe and improvement of this manufacture may be feen
from the following facts. In 1775 *, there were only 722
ftones of wool manufactured, every kind of machinery for
preparing and fpinning it was unknown except the common cards and wheels, and there was little or no cloth
made above 3 s. *per* yard. In 1790 *, the number of ftones
manufactured was 2916, there were two *jennies* for fpinning yarn, and cloth was frequently made at 5 s. *per*

T t   yard,

* Stat. Acct. Vol. II. p. 708, 9, 10, 11.

yard, fome of it even higher. In 1797, the quantity of
wool purchafed is 4944 ftone, the number of fpinning-jennies has increafed to 18 *, four different houfes have been
built with water-machinery for teafing, fcribbling and card-
ing the wool, broad looms have been procured for making
blankets eleven-quarters wide when finifhed, machines have
been erected, for raifing the pile upon them, and alfo on
cloth that it may be more equally fhorn, and for brufh-
ing cloth free from all coarfe piles and all rough fubftances
which may adhere to it, both before it is fubjected for the
laft time to the fhears, and after it comes from the prefs.
There are, likewife, improved preffes, larger and ftronger
than the common ones, with plates heated in an oven,
which, being placed among the cloth at the fame diftances,
diffufe the heat more equally than a fire below, and fave
the neceffity and trouble of fhifting the pofition of the different pieces and bringing them alternately near to the
heat. A cylinder, too, has been juft purchafed for glazing
worfted ftuffs. Thefe and other acquifitions, all made in
the courfe of feven years, have coft about L. 3000 Sterling, befides the aid afforded by the Honourable Board of
Truftees for Manufactures, &c. in Scotland,—a trifling fum,
indeed, in comparifon of what has been laid out in other
places, but a great deal for poor people, who began bufinefs
without any capital, to earn in a fhort time by their own
induftry and enterprife, and to fink in buildings and pe-
rifhable machinery. They are now enabled to make a
much greater quantity of cloth, on a fhorter notice, and of
a better quality. Pieces are fometimes expofed to fale as
high as 8 s. per yard, from 7-8ths to very nearly a full
yard wide, and thofe at 5 s. and even at 4 s. 6 d. are rather
better and fomewhat broader than what fome time ago
brought

---

* There will probably be twenty-four before the end of the year.

brought thefe prices. An attempt has been made to efta-
blifh a Hall for felling cloth, and a commodious houfe has
been built for that purpofe, which, in a few years hence, it
is hoped, will meet with the encouragement it deferves.
Here, too, as well as at Selkirk, a good deal of *country-
work* is done. The wool and yarn of private families
are made into cloth, flannels, blankets, and worfled-ftuffs
for womens gowns, to an extent fully equal to the demand
of the county itfelf. There are eight fulling-mills pretty
conftantly employed, feventeen clothiers who manufacture
cloth on their own account for fale, and about fixty-four
hands in all daily working at fome branch of this bufinefs,
befides thofe who fpin wool at their own houfes and weavers, whofe joint number will exceed 300. In 1790, the
clothiers in Galafhiels employed 241 women to fpin yarn
for them. Their number is rather leffened fince the introduction of fpinning-jennies, but thefe and the other machines afford work to feveral hands, and many fpin in different parts of the county for themfelves, for the families
where they are fervants, or for thofe who furnifh them with
wool properly prepared and pay them at the rate of 6 d.
for every *flip* or *bank* of twelve cuts. That quantity of
yarn fpun by the machines, cofts only 4¼ d. There were
then forty-three looms in that village, and there are fifty-
four at prefent, befides a few at Selkirk and other places in the county; and though fome of them conftantly,
and others occafionally, are employed in weaving cotton
and linen-cloth, yet by far the greateft part of them are
entirely, or at leaft moftly, filled with woollen-webs, which
fometimes, though very rarely, belong to the weaver himfelf, and are in general the property either of manufacturers or private families in the neighbourhood. Thefe circumftances

* See p. 212.　　† Stat. Acct. Vol. II. p. 309.

cumstances prove that the number of people affigned to the woollen-manufactory is not exaggerated.

The quantity of stockings made annually, after supplying the county, is extremely trifling. But an inkle manufacture, carried on with spirit, employs fifty hands*, and must bring a very handsome return. There are, also, two tanworks which paid L. 124 : 1 : 11¼ of excife-duty in 1795. The tawers in Galashiels have all removed to its suburbs in Roxburghshire, and an account of the duty paid by them has already been given †. There are none now in the county. Two candlemakers pay annually about L. 53 to Government; but do not furnish nearly enough for the inhabitants, several of whom make candles for themselves, or are supplied from other places. Implements of husbandry, especially ploughs, carts, hay-rakes, and of late thrashing-machines made here, are carried to the neighbouring counties. A good deal of timber, also, was some time ago *blocked* or shaped coarsely for different purposes, particularly for carts, and sold in that state to be dressed and put together elsewhere; but the cartwrights find now more constant and profitable employment. The clear profit gained on the articles mentioned in this paragraph are estimated at L. 800 in the preceding section.

Sect. VII.—*Poor.*

EVERY thing of importance relative to this subject has already been anticipated. The number of the poor, the way and the amount of their maintenance, and their ability in general to earn something for themselves, have been mentioned in Chap. IV. Sect. 4. p. 254 : And the remarks made

* Stat. Acct. of Selkirk, Vol. II. p. 349.   † p. 117.

made on vagrants, in the Account of Roxburghshire, p. 218,
hold equally true with respect to this county. Beggars of
that description become always the greater nuisance, in proportion as places are lonely and remote from aid. Their
tales impose upon the simple, or their numbers and their
appearance overawe the timid. It would appear, that a
spirit of extravagance and dissipation has infected the lower
ranks in the parish of Selkirk *, and that they expend most
of their wages on finery and pleasures, in a dependence on
receiving support from the parish in poverty and old age.
Though a few instances may occur of a similar spirit in
other places, yet this is not the general character of the poor
through the county. They consist mostly of such as are
infirm, from constitution, fixed diseases, or hard labour;
or of the old, whose frugal savings have been all expended
on the education or perhaps distresses of a numerous family, or on their own sustenance after having been set aside
from work. It cannot, however, be doubted, from the
experience of a neighbouring kingdom, that poors-laws
have a tendency to relax diligence and economy among the
lower orders of society, though this baneful effect has hitherto been only slightly felt in this corner. Other evils,
also, arising from them, have sometimes appeared here.
Children, brought up by the parish, when in circumstances
to spare a little of their earnings, have refused to assist an
aged mother, under pretence that she has no occasion to
be ashamed of applying for subsistence to herself, as she
discovered no shame in asking it for them. The idea is
daily taking a deeper root, that maintenance from the parochial funds is not charity but the legal right of the poor,
as much as the possession and rents of their estates, are the
rights of the rich: and it is manifest that this idea, when
cherished by the poor, must naturally overcome all delicacy

in

* Stat. Acct. Vol. II. p. 444, 5.

in demanding what is accounted their own. Many of the middling classes, who pay little or no poors-rates, are forward both to encourage the claims of the poor, and to urge an enlargement of their allowance, from a defire of touching the purfes of rich proprietors who do not attend the church, and of their tenants, who in general are able to bear thefe burdens. But the influence of thefe various confiderations is only beginning to operate in this county, and its fmall progrefs is evinced by the little decreafe that has as yet taken place in the weekly collections in the Eftablifhed Church, which continue to bear a very fair proportion to the number and circumftances of the audience. It is an object of national importance to preferve thefe voluntary contributions as large as poffible, and it is particularly the intereft of thofe in the higher ranks of life, who cannot or at leaft do not attend public worfhip, to fhew a pattern of liberality in this refpect. They may be affured that the poor, till their minds are perverted, have an honeft pride, which makes them fhy of accepting charity, but forward to claim a right.

Sect. VIII.—*Population.*

There is no fmall difficulty in afcertaining the precife ftate of the population, both in 1755, when Dr Webfter made his inquiries, and at prefent. No regard was paid to the limits of different counties, either in the returns made to him, or in the Statiftical Accounts lately poblifhed. In conftructing the fubjoined table, I have therefore been reduced to the neceffity of having recourfe to conjecture and calculations, equally applicable to both periods, the foundations of which it is my duty to explain. By the valued rents of the parifhes of Afhkirk and Roberton, only about two-fevenths of them belong to this county, and that proportion

portion of their population in the two periods is affigned to
it. The inhabitants of thofe parts of Selkirk and Galafhiels parifhes, which lie in Roxburghfhire, having been
lately enumerated, are fubtracted from the population in
1790,-1, and a proportionate deduction is made from the
population in 1755. A computation is made of the probable number prefently refiding in Stow and Innerleithen
parifhes within this county, and the fame number is allowed to that diftrict of thefe parifhes in the 1755. The whole
of Ettrick and Yarrow parifhes being in this county, their
population is given as in the Statiftical Account.

PARISHES.	POPULATION		VALUED RENT.		
	in 1755.	1790, 3.			
			Scots.		
			L.	s.	d.
Selkirk, – –	1650	1650	14644	13	4
Galafhiels, – –	850	780	5891	6	8
Yarrow, – – –	1180	1230	31377	9	8
Ettrick, – – –	397	470	15958	3	6
Roberton, ⅗, – –	186	180	3475	13	4
Afhkirk, ⅘, – –	179	156	1866	13	4
Stow, – – – –	150	150	4910	2	4
Innerleithen, – –	30	30	1841	0	0
Peebles, – – –	none.	none.	343	13	4
	4622	4646	80307	15	6

Increafe fince 1755,——24.

I: muft give fincere pleafure to every friend of his country to find, that, amidft the ruinous confequences afcribed
to large farms, and all the common fubjects of murmuring
and complaint among the difcontented, her population is
increafing,

increafing, not only in diftricts where manufactures and commerce flourifh, but in an inland county where there is little of either, and in thofe parts of that county which are almoft entirely paftoral. For it is not a little remarkable, that, in the parifhes of Ettrick and Yarrow, where a very fmall quantity of corn is raifed, and where every kind of manufacture is altogether unknown, there are more inhabitants than there were forty years ago, while there are fewer in Galafhiels, where there is a thriving manufacture. This is one of many curious facts, which deferves to be brought forward to public notice, as the beft anfwer to fpeculative declaimers on our national decline. It is the general opinion, that, by the union and extenfion of farms, the country is depopulated and ruined, while the inhabitants, driven into great towns, and employed in manufactures, lofe their health and their morals. The latter part of this opinion may be well founded; but the former part of it is not confirmed by the increafing population of thofe diftricts, both of this county and of Roxburghfhire, where the accumulation of farms is moft prevalent. I mean not either to juftify the practice, or to deny that it is frequently the caufe of depopulation. I mean only to affert that this is not always the cafe, and, by holding out a ftrong exception in this corner to an opinion which feems to have obtained currency without examination and proof, to affift others who have better opportunities in their inquiries into its truth. Perhaps it will be found, that large farms, and in fome cafes two farms in the hands of one man, are rather an advantage than an injury to fuch counties as thofe of Roxburgh and Selkirk, but that the practice, when carried too far, degenerates into an abufe, and becomes truly hurtful to population, the fundamental fupport of fociety. There is always a happy medium between oppofite and dangerous extremes.

AGRI-

AGRICULTURAL SURVEY

OF

ROXBURGH AND SELKIRK SHIRES.

CHAP. XVI.

OBSTACLES TO IMPROVEMENT.

THE principal obstacle to improvement is distance from fuel, manure, and markets. Farmers are obliged to occupy their horses so much, in carrying the grain and wool which they export, from twenty to forty-five miles according to local situation and particular circumstances, and in bringing most of the necessary articles for the use of their families and the melioration of their fields from afar, that they are unable to enrich and keep in tillage as many acres, and pay as high a rent as might otherwise be expected. The number of work-horses in Roxburghshire is stated at 3684. But from the Surveyor's remarks it appears that most of the carriage and saddle-horses and some horses under size are frequently employed in husbandry, which, by a moderate computation, will swell the number of actual work-horses to 4496, and still leave 500 for the sole purposes of riding and going in chaises. The number of acres

supposed

supposed to be annually in tillage being 98,422. (Chap. VII Sect. 4.) the average is scarcely forty-four acres for each pair of horses, without any deduction for what may be ploughed by 20 or perhaps 25 pair of oxen: whereas, if freed from long carriages, every farmer knows that a pair could manage at least sixty acres of easy-wrought soil like that which mostly prevails in these counties. In Selkirkshire, the number of draught-horses is 474, and the acres annually in tillage are about 7809; there are consequently not quite thirty-three acres to each pair of horses. And were the horses of carriers, cadgers, and jobbers, taken out of the account in both counties, the averages would not be much affected, because most if not all of these people have more or less land, and besides their horses are often employed in bringing coals and manure and in other kinds of labour, all of which would otherwise devolve on the horses of farmers. This evil has been in part remedied by the excellent roads made in many different directions; but it never can be entirely removed till fuel and manure are obtained at a reasonable rate and with little labour, in the centre, and in different parts of the counties.

It is obvious that this inconvenience must be more severely felt in particular local situations than in others. The roads to several places are almost impassable during a great part of winter, and the inhabitants are obliged to devote the whole time and labour of their horses and servants, through summer, to lay in their annual provision of fuel. Hence weeding corn, hoeing drilled crops, fallowing and manuring land, and every improvement in husbandry, for which summer is the proper season, become only secondary operations. Farms, in these circumstances, cannot yield as high a rent as they would do if this necessary article was brought within their reach at every period of the year: and it is, therefore, the interest of proprietors to bestow

the

the fame laudable attention upon the crofs-roads, which they have already paid to the great and direct ones. Farmers in other places labour under the difadvantage, of being denied accefs to marl in their immediate neighbourhood, becaufe it belongs to another proprietor, and of being reduced to the neceffity of wanting that ufeful manure altogether, or of bringing it from a great diftance at a prodigious expence. They muft confequently manure a lefs extent of ground annually, give a lefs allowance of marl to the acre, and pay lefs rent, than their more fortunate neighbours. And, in fuch cafes, when landlords cannot purchafe the privilege of getting marl from the contiguous pits, they will increafe their rents, by paying the prime coft of all the marl laid upon their land during the firft three or four years of a leafe, and by keeping the road in good order by which it is carried. Some local hardfhips cannot be overcome without much difficulty and expence. The river Tweed is a formidable bar to the improvement of that large track, which lies along its fouthern banks from the village of Laffuden towards the neighbourhood of Kelfo. Moft of it is fufceptible of being fubftantially benefited by marl, and a copious fund of that valuable fubftance is now opened for fale at Whittrig, on the oppofite fide of the river, fcarcely three miles from fome and not more than fix miles from any part of the track to which I allude. Yet carts, from thofe parts of Roxburghfhire which lie north of Tweed, can go one journey each day to the pit more than carts from places at the fame diftance on the fouth of it, and confequently muft fave from one-half to one-fourth of the labour, according to the number of journies made in a day. The different proprietors of this track will act a wife part by uniting their endeavours to throw a bridge over Tweed at fome fafe and convenient fpot, in which they cannot fail to be vigoroufly fupported by the proprietor of the marl,

who

who thereby muſt gain L. 400 or more annually for many years, and in which they will receive countenance and aſſiſtance from all the neighbourhood as a meaſure of public utility.

Theſe obſtacles by no means prevent improvement: they only circumſcribe its limits, and retard its progreſs; and other obſtacles, more eaſily ſurmounted, lend their aid to clog its wheels. Scarcity of labourers has frequently prevented many fields from being incloſed, cleared, and drained ſo quickly, the fences and drains kept in ſuch good order, the drilled crops ſo regularly and completely hoed, and the grain ſo ſoon thraſhed, as the tenant wiſhed. There have alſo been inſtances of labour ſtopping, till a carpenter or ſmith came from a diſtance to mend ſome implement, or till the implement was carried to their workſhops and brought back. To remove theſe inconveniencies, gentlemen ſhould encourage labourers and artificers to ſettle on their eſtates, by accommodating them with decent dwelling-houſes and workſhops; and tenants ſhould aſſiſt them in bringing home their fuel and neceſſary proviſions. This indeed would increaſe the labour of their horſes: but the leſſer evil muſt be borne to avoid the greater.

The practice of ſelling ſtaple commodities of the counties, by contract at the ſame ſtipulated price for a number of years, deſerves reprehenſion, as hurtful both to improvement and to the intereſt of farmers. They ceaſe to beſtow pains upon meliorating the quality of the hay, grain, or wool thus ſold, and are only anxious to deliver a large quantity to the purchaſer in ſuch a ſtate, however coarſe, as he cannot legally challenge. Wool eſpecially is liable to ſuffer materially from the load of tar uſed to increaſe its weight. When ſuch bargains are diſadvantageous to farmers, they are always rigorouſly exacted by the contractor, or by his creditors ſhould he fail; and when favourable to

farmers,

farmers, they are fulfilled by the other party with a grudge; some abatement is expected, many shifts are tried to elude or break them, and in case of his bankruptcy, they are at end. They are less pernicious when the price is left to be regulated annually by the common rate of the market. But the true spirit of agriculture, as well as of commerce, condemns every kind of shackles upon buyers and sellers, till the goods are ready to be produced; and it is then the mutual interest of the one to give and of the other to take the current prices of the day.

The progress of improvement is also retarded by the shortness of leases on arable farms, and by absurd restrictions on them. This subject being of national importance, I hope the public will receive with indulgence the following general observations upon it:

One great object with gentlemen, when letting their farms, should be the character of tenants for good sense, agricultural skill, and successful management. They should also have regard to the education, which young farmers have received in other arts as well as husbandry, and to the indications which they give of application and relish for the employment. It is not probable, that such men will suffer themselves to be outbid by the ignorant and unskilful, where there is a reasonable prospect of sufficient profit. In all competitions, they may be supposed to offer as much as the land, by every exertion of ingenuity and judgment, can be expected to afford. And landlords will find it more for their interest, on the whole, to prefer them, on somewhat of a less rent, to others, who may either hurt their farms by injudicious cropping, or bring them into disrepute by becoming bankrupts.

With tenants of this description, restrictions are not only unnecessary, but cumbrous fetters on industry and genius. When

teroft on the farms thus laid out, and with one-half of the expence of upholding the fences. With the same view, I would suggest the propriety of a progressive instead of a fixed rent, in every case, where it is requisite to lay out a good deal of money on the improvement of a farm, and where some time must elapse before an adequate return can be obtained. On a lease, for example, of twenty-one years at L. 300 a-year, the proprietor will receive during its currency precisely L. 6300 Sterling. What an advantage would it be to the tenant, were he to pay only L. 200 annually for the first five years when he is much out of pocket meliorating his farm, L. 300 for the next six years when it begins to repay his expence and labour, and L. 350 for the last ten years when he reaps the full benefit of it? The sums and the terms may be varied, according to circumstances. It is the principle for which I contend. For the use of a little money, when a tenant is at great expence improving land, is the most essential service which he can receive from his landlord. He will be much abler to pay a large rent towards the close of his lease, than a small one at the commencement of it.

Much has been said concerning the duration of leases; but nothing should depend more on the nature and condition of different farms. In sheep-pastures, which admit of little improvement except open drains, the length of leases is of less consequence; though even for these, farmers will give more rent, and will bestow more attention on their houses; their gardens, and the fields around, when secured against all risk of soon changing their residence. Nor is a long lease of much importance in an arable farm already brought into high cultivation, especially if there be a command of dung either in the farm itself or in the neighbourhood. Three full rotations, whether of four or five years, may amply recompense the tenant, and afford the landlord an

opportunity

opportunity of going again to the market for an advance of rent. But such short leases, besides rendering tenants indifferent about the decoration of places which they may soon be compelled to quit, really shut the door against all useful experiments, and in a manner forbid all deviations from the beaten path. As the best lands are susceptible of the speediest and highest improvement, they are fittest for trying the success, both of foreign grains and plants brought from a warm climate or rich soil, and of new modes of rearing common crops to greater perfection. But who would run the risk, without a sufficient length of lease, to indemnify him in case of failure, and to reward him in case the undertaking should prosper?

The leases, then, of all arable farms should be of considerable length, but the precise period of their continuance must be determined by the state and extent of the ground, the expence, and the time requisite for its melioration. An extensive farm, whether in a state of nature, or impoverished by bad management, cannot be put into good order in a few years, or at a trifling expence. At an average through the whole of these two counties, from L. 6 to L. 15 Sterling must be allowed for manuring and labouring every acre of this description; and a pair of horses could not fetch the medium allowance of lime or marl to more than fixteen acres in a year, give these the necessary ploughings, remove the stones, and straighten the ridges. Supposing a farmer to keep ten extra horses for the sole purpose of carrying manure, they could only lime or marl properly from 130 to 160 acres, and fix horses more would find it hard work to ridge and dress these as they ought to be, for a year or two till they are reduced to a manageable form and mould. Now when fixteen horses can only thus break and put in order at most 160 acres annually, it is easy to compute the time when farms of different extents, according-

ing

ing to the ſtrength of horſes in each, can be completely brought under a regular and profitable ſyſtem of huſbandry, and the vaſt expence which tenants muſt lay out for many years before they can be reimburſed. Hence ariſes an argument for proportioning the length of leaſes to the time and coſt of enriching all the land with manure, giving it the neceſſary tillage, freeing it from weeds and ſtones, draining and incloſing it. After a reaſonable allowance of crops to refund the expence of theſe ſpirited and beneficial operations, the tenant ſhould enjoy at leaſt three if not four complete rotations of every acre he has improven. And in general, the farther that ſuch farms are from the means of improvement, the greater that the difficulties are which muſt be ſurmounted, ſo much the longer ſhould be the leaſe, or elſe ſo much the lower will be the rent.

Here it may not be improper to obſerve, that want of attention to theſe conſiderations, on the part both of maſters and tenants, has driven many of the latter to the pernicious expedient of obtaining money, by diſcounting bills payable at a ſhort date. Setting aſide the difficulty under which they often laboured to procure real ſignatures, and the neceſſity to which at other times they were reduced of affixing fictitious names to theſe bills, it was certainly, in its moſt favourable ſhape, an unwiſe meaſure to borrow money, at the extravagant rate of paying 5 *per cent.* of intereſt ſix or ſeven times in the year, inſtead of once, and of having it deducted out of the ſum they received, inſtead of enjoying the uſe of both principal and intereſt till the ſtipulated term of payment ſhould arrive, beſides being ſubjected to the expence of all the ſtamped paper required, and of frequent journies to the neareſt market-town to tranſact the buſineſs. A caſh-account with ſome Bank or Banking Company, to which many of them have recourſe, is a more reputable and leſs expenſive mode of attaining the

ſame

fame end, but is only within the reach of those who find fufficient fureties. In both thefe ways, a very great deal of money has been raifed to be laid out on the melioration of land; and tenants, while thereby they improved the face of the country, have been amply compenfated for their rifk, except in a few inftances, where their refources failed before their farms had time to yield profitable returns. In fuch cafes, though the fupport of friends and the indulgence of creditors have faved from impending ruin a few worthy characters, whofe perfevering induftry has now placed them in eafy circumftances; yet the evils, which fome have brought on themfelves by getting too eafy credit, and others by dabbling in the ruinous traffic of accommodation-bills, ftrongly fuggeft the propriety of granting lenient terms to tenants at the beginning of their leafes, that they may not be fo much expofed to thefe dangers. The more money that is then allowed to remain in their pockets, the lefs occafion will they have to borrow it on difadvantageous conditions.

Leafes for one or more lives are common in England, but have feldom excited a fpirit of improvement either there, or in fome parts of Scotland where the fame practice was adopted. A few proprietors, however, and farmers here are of opinion, that fuch leafes may be added to thofe for a fixed period, at an advanced rent and upon a plan of farming beneficial to the land, much to the advantage both of mafters and tenants. The former, it is alleged, get their lands put and preferved in fuch excellent order, and all the buildings fitted up in fuch a commodious and fubftantial manner, as to enfure them of a great increafe of rent upon the tenant's death, or of a handfome price in cafe of a fale. While the latter fit down with the comfortable thoughts of not being driven away, in old age, from the fields which by their exertions had become beautiful

tiful and fertile, from the habitations which they had been at pains to render convenient and agreeable, and which to them have additional charms from having been the scene of conjugal felicity and domestic endearments. After having passed the meridian of life, and entered into the vale of years, how hard is it to be under the necessity of seeking a new home, and of beginning the laborious and persevering improvements of agriculture upon a strange soil! How much pleasanter to be secure of remaining, during the whole of their lives, even at a stretched rent and under severe restrictions, in the place where they spent the prime and strength of their days, and where every surrounding object recalls to remembrance the joys that are past * !

To the force of these considerations I am not insensible, though they certainly are addressed more to the feelings than to the reason of men, and are better calculated to move than to convince. They represent a lease for his life as a desirable object to a tenant. But in deciding the general question concerning the propriety of such leases, the

---

* This language is held by Mr Dawson, so often mentioned, who himself took a lease for a certain number of years with the addition of his lifetime at a higher rent, and under a strict system of management highly favourable to his farm, and who, from his perfect knowledge of the subject, could recommend the plan more clearly and forcibly, than from the recollection of his arguments I have done in the text. It is with regret that I differ from him on this point as well as on many others. But I cannot take my leave of him, without expressing, in this public manner, my thanks for his liberal information and corrections, which difference of opinion did not provoke him to withhold. Every lover of agriculture must be pleased to hear, that this acknowledged Father of it, in these parts of the united kingdoms, lives in ease and affluence, the just reward of his patriotic exertions for the good of his native country. What nobler encomium can be bestowed on our excellent constitution, than the protection and security, which every man of merit enjoys, in thus reaping the happy fruits of his talents, his knowledge, and his labours !

the interest of both parties must be equally and fairly regarded : And that they are advantageous to a landlord is by no means clear : the contrary may rather be inferred from the tenor of the argument in their favour. A great increase of rent is held out to him upon the tenant's decease ; and yet the tenants are supposed to pay rents that are amply sufficient for their farms, and even somewhat exorbitant, for the privilege of having the remainder of their lives added to the fixed length of their leases ! Is there not a manifest contradiction here ? Must not the tenants for life sit on very easy terms, when their successors can afford to give much higher ones ? Or if the former tenants actually paid the full value of the lands, who would be so foolish as to give more ? If farms, at the expiration of such leases, fetch a considerable advance of rent, is it not evident that the preceding tenants have had lucrative and the proprietors losing bargains ? It is only, therefore, where the rent is stationary or the advance is trifling, that the latter can be gainers by giving leases during the lives of the former. Nor can the increase of rent be justly attributed to the gentle treatment of farms prescribed to such lessees. For the mode of management, which during any considerable length of time is most favourable to land, is also most beneficial to the occupiers of it. And, in this respect, the possessors of farms, formerly held on lifetime leases, generally exceed their predecessors. Besides, on every sound principle, all covenants should be explicit and express, and subjected to limitations both as to their extent and duration. The quantity of goods and length of time are always distinctly and precisely specified by sensible and sure dealers. In no contract is it more essential to adhere to this rule than in a lease; and while every other condition in it is accurately and positively expressed, why is its continuance, of all its clauses the most important, left inde-

finite

finite and dependent on accidental circumſtances? A leaſe
of this nature, at a low rent, is perhaps the moſt delicate
compliment, which can be paid to a truſty ſervant or an
unfortunate friend, becauſe it is an independent eſtabliſh-
ment during the remainder of their lives. But ſuch a leaſe
to a ſtranger, who, however deſerving, has no particular
claim to favour, though he may offer more for it than appears at the time to be a full equivalent, is objectionable
on the ſcore of its uncertain termination. The proprietor
or his heir knows not when he ſhall be at liberty, to build
a dwelling-houſe for himſelf on ſome eligible ſpot in this
farm, to include a part of it in his pleaſure-ground, to alter its boundaries ſo as to render it and other farms on his
eſtate more compact and commodious, or to proſecute ſome
favourite ſcheme to the completion of which it is neceſſary. If he ſhould expoſe it to ſale, who would give an
adequate price for a place, however charming, when the
period of entering into poſſeſſion of it is altogether inde-
terminate? Had the length of the leaſe been fixed, both
ſeller and purchaſer could know how long they had to wait.
Or the proprietor might calculate its value, and try to buy
it at a reaſonable rate to carry forward any of his projects.
But what price can tempt a leſſee to give up a place for
which he has a ſtronger attachment than what ariſes from
its intrinſic worth, and whoſe chief inducements for retaining it are, the pleaſure of rejoicing in the works of his former days, and the deſire of deſcending into the grave a-
midſt objects, which have become the companions and ſo-
lace of his declining years? Theſe conſiderations render it
at leaſt doubtful how far leaſes ought to be granted during
the lives of tenants. The intereſt of the proprietor muſt
be laid in the balance againſt that of his tenant, and the
hardſhip, to which the one is ſubjected by being ſecluded

from

from poffeffing his own, muft be contrafted with the hardfhip of turning the other adrift in his old age.

If in thefe obfervations I rather appear to lean towards
the fide of the landlords, in another article, which they
commonly infift upon in leafes, I am decidedly againft
them. Why fhould a tenant, after expending a good deal
of money, and beftowing much pains upon the improvement of a farm, be fecluded from difpofing of his leafe either for a ftipulated fum or at an advanced rent? In point
of juftice, he fhould be allowed to turn his capital, his induftry, and his time to the beft account. In point of found
policy, he fhould be encouraged in his laudible exertions
to extend the practice of good hufbandry, by enjoying the
full rewards which it yields in whatever manner he may
prefer, that is not unfair or injurious to others. And, in
point of humanity, he himfelf if in bad health, or, in cafe
of his death, his widow and young children, or his heirs
whoever they are, fhould not be compelled to retain in
their own hands a leafe, which may be unprofitable, from
his inability to fuperintend the farm, or from their ignorance and unfkilful management, but which could be fold
to great advantage. To thefe powerful motives, nothing
of any folidity is oppofed, but the chance of the purchafer,
or *fubtenant* as he is here called, proving a difagreeable
neighbour to the proprietor or the farmers around. But
this objection will lofe much of its weight, when we call
to mind, that people are very likely to become bad neighbours, when conftrained to remain in a place againft their
inclinations and contrary to their pecuniary interefts; that
the prefumption can fcarcely be fo ftrong againft any purchafer or fubtenants, becaufe farmers of good character, efpecially for ingenuity and diligence, are generally the higheft offerers, that there is at leaft equal if not greater probability of their being good neighbours than bad ones, and
that

that even fuppofing the worſt, the hardſhip is leſs upon a
landlord to have a troubleſome fellow faſtened upon him
for a few years, than upon a tenant to be debarred from
accepting an advantageous propoſal, by which he would be
enabled to puſh forward ſimilar operations in agriculture
elſewhere with greater ſucceſs, or upon his ſurvivors to have
the fruits of his expenſive labours ſnatched out of their
hands. In every view, therefore, of juſtice, policy, and
humanity, tenants ſhould be allowed to make the moſt of
their leaſes, under the reſtrictions previouſly mentioned,
and with the reſervation of giving the firſt offer to the landlord of ſuch as are expoſed to ſale, at the expected ſum or
advanced rent.

On the bad policy of giving no leaſes, I have ſaid enough
in Chap. IV. Sect. 5. p. 255, 6. of the Survey of Selkirk-
ſhire : And the pernicious practice, of taking a ſum of money from a tenant at his entrance to a farm, and giving a
proportionable deduction of the rent, is ſo diametrically oppoſite to thoſe liberal principles which I have attempted to
eſtabliſh as to require no further notice. I have only to
add, that, in the preceding reflections on leaſes, I have paid
no further regard to the intereſt either of landholders or
farmers, than appeared to me, on a general view of the
ſubject, to be for the real good of the country. No prejudices on either part, no temporary accommodation of individuals ſhould obſtruct the advancement of agriculture, that
primary ſource of national nouriſhment and proſperity.

CHAP.

CHAP. XIV.

MISCELLANEOUS OBSERVATIONS.

Sect. I.—*Agricultural Societies.*

SEVERAL Agricultural Societies were formed in different parts of these counties, but they were all of short duration. While they lasted, they were pleasant meetings, and of confiderable ufe in diffufing information and exciting a fpirit of emulation. Though a variety of accidental circumftances in different places contributed to put an end to them, yet all of them every where fell into one common error which accelerated their downfal. They were held on the market-day, with a view of accommodating the farmers who had occafion to be in the place that day on other bufinefs; the confequence of which was, that from the beginning to the end of the meeting, the fervants were continually calling out one member after another, who naturally preferred the fettlement of a heavy account, the making of an advantageous bargain, and above all the receipt

of

of money, to the most interesting debate or conversation, from which they could only eventually derive profit at a future period. This inconveniency was not removed by the Society dining together: for the calls were generally as frequent after dinner; and the company sometimes sat so late that it was archly said they did more service to the inn than to agriculture. To this sarcasm it may be replied, that they who are fond of a glass will seldom want a specious pretence for taking one, and that, of all pretences, the acquirement of useful knowledge in the line of their occupation is undoubtedly the most tenable.

An association of a different nature, though intimately connected with agriculture, was lately formed in Roxburgh-shire, and there is a prospect of its being extended to the other county. The object of it is to detect and prosecute felons, and the following is the substance of its principal regulations:

1. " That it shall be binding for seven years.

2. " That a fund shall be raised, by annual subscrip-
" tion, for defraying the expence of apprehending, and
" prosecuting to conviction, any person or persons, suspect-
" ed of murders, robberies, or any other kind of felonies,
" or petty thefts, committed on the persons or property of
" any of the subscribers of this association.

3. " That the sums subscribed shall be regulated by the
" rent of the respective possessions of subscribers; and to
" be, for the ensuing year, at the rate of 2 s. 6 d. for each
" L. 100 Sterling: Subscribers possessing less than L. 100
" also to pay 2 s. 6 d.; and subscribers possessing more than
" L. 50 above any even L. 100, to pay for an additional
" L. 100. The first year's subscription to be paid at the time of
" subscribing; and the subscriptions for the following years
" to be paid to the treasurer for the time, within three

" months

" months after the general annual meeting on the fecond
" Tuefday in the month of April.

4. " That any perfon of the defcription before-mention-
" ed, (*i. e.* heritors and farmers) may, upon obtaining the
" confent of the committee and fubfcribing, be admitted
" members of this affociation. And if any fubfcriber, du-
" ring the faid period of feven years, fhall remove with
" his property out of the coun:y, in that cafe the affocia-
" tion fhall have no further claim upon him, nor fhall he
" have any benefit from the faid fund or inflitution.

5. " That A. B. &c. &c. or any five of them, be a
" committee for the enfuing year, to carry into execution
" the refolutions herein contained, and to tranfact every
" other neceffary bufinefs of this affociation, to meet at
" Jedburgh upon the fecond Tuefday in the months of Ju-
" ly, October, and January next; the committee to be
" chofen annually at the general meeting of fubfcribers.
" And if the affociation fhall become general through the
" county, it is propofed that one member of the committee
" fhall be chofen from each parifh.

6. " That in cafe any murder, robbery, or theft fhall at
" any time during the continuance of this affociation be
" committed on the perfons or property of any of the hinds,
" herds, or other fervants or cottagers belonging to fubfcri-
" bers, the committee fhall carry on profecutions at the ex-
" pence of the affociation.

7. " That for more effectually preventing any of the
" faid crimes, if any member of this affociation fhall, at
" any time during the faid term, lodge, harbour, or con-
" ceal any perfon or perfons fufpected of being guilty of
" any of the crimes above mentioned, or any ftrolling va-
" grants, or other loofe, idle, or diforderly perfons, fuch
" fubfcriber fhall, in that cafe, forfeit all right to the
                                        " funds

" funds of the affociation, and fhall no longer be confider-
" ed as a member thereof.

8. " That the committee fhall have power to call a ge-
" neral meeting of fubfcribers, at any time they may find
" neceffary, to alter thefe or add new regulations as may
" be thought proper; and any three members may call an
" extra meeting of the committee for the time.

9. " That when any member of this affociation fhall
" have any of his property ftolen, he fhall be allowed 3 s.
" per day for each fervant and horfe employed in fearching
" for the fame, if they are not a night from home; and if
" they fhall be one or more nights from home on that bu-
" finefs, they fhall be allowed 5 s. per day. Thefe allow-
" ances to include every expence.

10. " That any member, having property ftolen, may
" offer a reward of L. 5 Sterling, in the name of the affo-
" ciation, to the perfon or perfons who will difcover the
" offender or offenders; and if the property ftolen be fheep
" or horfes, he may offer a reward of L. 20 Sterling.

11. " It is recommended to fubfcribers to be particular-
" ly attentive to the marks of their horfes and other pro-
" perty, fo as to be able to defcribe them with precifion;
" and upon any of them being ftolen, to fend immediately
" as many of their own fervants as they can fpare in the
" purfuit and fearch, carrying with them defcriptions of
" the property ftolen, to be left at the turnpike-gates and
" other places they may think proper; the fervant or
" fervants to be entitled to the reward offered, upon appre-
" hending and convicting the offender or offenders.

12. " That thefe refolutions fhall be printed, and diftri-
" buted in the different parifhes of the county, in hopes of
" preventing any of the above crimes being committed,
" by fhowing offenders the great improbability of efcaping
" the

" the punifhment due to them, the affociation having unani-
" moufly agreed to enforce their refolutions to the utmoft
" of their power."

The defign of this affociation is undoubtedly laudable,
and the regulations are well adapted to promote it. The
rent, indeed, in fome inftances, is difproportionate to the
ftock or property on the farm which is liable to depredations; yet, in general, it is the beft rule which can be
adopted for afcertaining the annual rates to be paid. It
might be an improvement on the plan, if *heritors* (proprietors of land) were to pay, not only as farmers for what
property in cattle or corn they may have upon the land in
their own poffeffion, but alfo fome trifle more or lefs according to the rents they receive, as this would both intereft them more in protecting their tenants, and be a greater
check upon offenders. There is perhaps fomething narrow
and exclufive in confining the privilege and benefits of the
affociation to a fingle county, efpecially to one irregular like
Roxburghfhire, where feveral places in other counties are
much nearer to the county-town than a large portion of itfelf is. Yet it is extremely difficult to fix on any other limits fo diftinct and proper. And on the whole, though
there may be fome room for amendment, there is certainly
much more for commendation.

Sect. II.—*Weights and Meafures.*

A Table of thefe in both counties is given in the introduction. It may not be improper to mention, that, with
refpect to all articles fold by the heavy Scotch or troue
weight, purchafers have feldom caufe to complain of in-
juftice.

juftice. In buying large quantities of hay, wool, or cheefe, the fcale is always largely turned in their favours, befides what is fpontaneoufly thrown into the bargain. But they receive very little or no allowance of this nature when any other kind of weight is ufed.

The abfurd practice of giving an addition *gratis*, generally of the one and twentieth part of the quantity fold by meafure, weight, or numbers, and fometimes more or lefs, which once univerfally prevailed in all this neighbourhood, is not wholly given up. Twenty-one bolls of grain were regularly delivered, though the price of twenty was only received, probably to anfwer the multure which either feller or buyer were bound to pay at a particular mill; and fuch families, as are thus adftricted, continue at this day to fend as much grain of every kind, as will fatisfy the demands of the miller, above the quantity to be ground for their own ufe; though now a boll is feldom added to the fcore when grain is fold. It is ftill ufual in feveral places to give a pound of *incaft*, as it is here called, to every ftone of wool, and a fleece to every pack fold, a fheep or lamb to every fcore, and an additional one to every hundred. Part only of this incaft is allowed by many fheep-farmers, and moft of them have very judicioufly abolifhed it altogether. It is reprehenfible, as being a fallacious way of felling their moft valuable commodities, thereby deceiving ftrangers with regard to their real price, and likewife as being impolitic, by leading landlords to form too high ideas of their profits and to expect too great an increafe of rent. By felling five fcore of fheep at L. 20 *per* fcore and delivering 106, they get only 18 s. 10$\frac{44}{105}$ d. for each fheep inftead of 20 s. the nominal price. In like manner, by giving 17 pounds for every ftone of wool they lofe a feventeenth part of its weight, and every fleece added to a pack is a further deduction more or lefs from the price,

which

which they appear to receive in the eyes of every perfon
unacquainted with the manner of managing the tranfaction.
Whereas, by abolifhing this injudicious practice, and by
felling a greater number of fheep at a lower rate, they
would not be reputed fo great gainers, and yet put more
money into their pockets.

The propofal of felling all grain by weight inftead of
by meafure, if carried into effect, would be productive of
many advantages. It would prevent much of the confu-
fion which is occafioned by the prefent diverfity of meafures; it would afcertain the quality of grain by its weight
in a common tub or veffel; and it would check abftraction
and fraud by letting every body know to a trifle what return he had a right to expect from the mill. To extend it to
vegetables alfo would render it a ftill greater fervice to
the public.

CONCLUSION.

MEANS OF IMPROVEMENT AND THE MEASURES CALCULA-
TED FOR THAT PURPOSE.

To remove the obftacles to improvement is certainly the
firft ftep to promote it: To what has already been obferved on this fubject, little remains to be added.

Entails are commonly reckoned the bane of agriculture,
and the abolition of them has been frequently fuggefted and
warmly recommended. But how can this be effected, when
fo many great families poffefs entailed eftates and ftand in

the

the entail of others? If every inch of property in the
kingdom was subjected to a strict entail, and rendered incapable of coming in any shape to sale, perhaps the general
inconveniency, thus created, might reconcile all parties to
the repeal of the acts authorising entails and to the total
extinction of the practice. In an agricultural view, entails
may be more or less hurtful according to the restrictive
clauses they contain. And a late act of Parliament, made
with a view of improving entailed estates for the benefit
both of the present proprietor and his heirs of tailzie, im-
poses so many and such hard terms on tenants, that no farmer of sense and spirit would take a lease under it. That
a law might be made to mitigate the mischievous effects of
entails on good husbandry, without altering their nature or
their spirit, I cannot take upon me to affirm or deny. But
a law putting an end, to such entails as forbid leases of a
moderate length to be granted without absurd restrictions,
and to the disgraceful practice of selling a long lease at a low
rent for a large sum, to enrich the present proprietor and to
impoverish his successors, might undoubtedly contribute, in
various respects, towards the improvement of the country.
Tenants, on such estates, would be on a footing with their
neighbours, would obtain leases on the same equal and encouraging terms, and would not be tempted to give away
their substance and live meanly themselves, for the sake of
purchasing and leaving a long lease of a fine farm at less
than half its value to heirs, who, by having little rent to
pay, would be deprived of one great motive to industrious
exertions, and might sink into inactivity, sloth, and dissipation. All proprietors should be perfectly free to let their
lands on such equitable and meliorating conditions, and
during such a competent period, as would make their tenants easy and comfortable, and secure a gradual and reasonable

fonable increafe of rent to themfelves, and thofe who are to come in their place.

Intercourfe by good roads, to places where the produce of the counties might be difpofed of to advantage, is an important encouragement to improvement. And befides thofe already made the following ones would be of great utility. There is already a pretty good road from Canoby (about fix miles fouth of Langholm on the road between that place and Carlifle) to the lower parts of Liddefdale, and it is propofed to apply immediately for a turnpike act, to make a road from thence to Jedburgh by Hermitage bridge and Note of the Gate, which is already nearly completed, and alfo a line from faid bridge over Hermitage, by the Lime-kilns to Hawick, by which a confiderable diftrict of country will be fupplied with coal and lime with lefs trouble and expence than at prefent; and the above line from Jedburgh will fave travellers in going to Carlifle a diftance of 12 miles. A road from Jedburgh, in the neareft line to Wool-er, would open up a communication to Morpeth and the moft fertile and beft cultivated parts of Northumberland, and faci-litate the exportation of fat cattle, fheep, and wool, and the importation of feveral neceffary articles. A bridge thrown over Tweed, as already fuggefted, befides affording ready accefs to the marl at Whitrig and a fhorter cut to Edin-burgh from feveral places, lies very much in the line be-tween Jedburgh and Greenlaw, and might eventually lead to the formation of a direct road between them. If the road, lately made from Kelfo to St Bofwel's Green, was continued to Selkirk and from thence to Moffat, a good deal of grain would find a new and profitable market in the higher parts of Dumfries-fhire. With the exception of Liddefdale, no part of thefe counties ftands more in need of good roads, than Lilliefleaf and thofe places on both fides

of

of Ale-water which lie between it and Ancrum. This want might be in a great measure supplied by a road from Selkirk to Jedburgh, crossing Ale-water near Clarilaw, and keeping its south bank to Ancrum, from which there is a good road to Jedburgh. There should also be a good road made from Lilliesleaf by the west end of Bowden to the bridge over Tweed near Melrose. Coals and lime might then be brought, both from Mid-Lothian and the N. E. parts of Northumberland, and corn carried to the markets of Dalkeith, Peebles, Kelso, and Berwick, with great ease at any season, whereas at present the access to and from that district is often difficult and precarious during winter.

There seems to be a serious resolution of striking out a road from Kelso to join the road to Edinburgh by Cornhill about five miles W. from Greenlaw, which will be more level and nearer than the present one by Smaillholm and Lauder. A road has also been talked of from Edinburgh to Langholm, in a new and direct line, leaving the one by Selkirk and Hawick at Middleton, and proceeding through the lower parts of Tweeddale and the higher parts of Selkirkshire, either to Moss Paul, or along the Esk by Esk-dalemuir to Langholm. But such a road, through a hilly country thinly peopled, little of which is susceptible of cultivation, though it would certainly be a saving of 12 or perhaps of 15 miles, and might be of much service to the inhabitants near the sources of Yarrow and Ettrick waters, cannot be attended with advantages in any degree commensurate to the vast expence of throwing bridges over several considerable waters and numerous brooks, all of them rapid, and most of them apt to swell at times to a prodigious size, of cutting banks to lessen steep ascents, and make the road of sufficient breadth for carriages, and of fetching materials to the bridges, and in some places to the roads, from a considerable distance.

Z z

Though

Though the fafe and fpeedy conveyance of letters is of greater confequence in a mercantile and commercial than in an agricultural view, yet it certainly ought to be extended to every corner of the kingdom, where the correfpondence of any clafs of fubjects, efpecially of farmers, can produce the fmalleft gain to the ftate, after defraying the neceffary charges of eftablifhing a regular poft. Yet fuch appointments, in this diftrict, have hitherto taken place in a very flow and capricious manner: and there can be no doubt, that a laudable though miftaken zeal, to increafe the revenue by a pitiful retrenchment of expenditure, more than a regard for the accommodation of the public, dictated the prefent circuitous and unproductive route. The only poft, allowed to thefe counties either to the S. or the N. is by Berwick. Intelligence from London, or any part on the E. coaft of England, thereby reaches them more fpeedily than by any other practicable mode. But, though they certainly carry on a good deal of bufinefs with different places in that quarter, yet nine-tenths of their poftages arife from their correfpondence with the capital of Scotland, and its neighbourhood. Edinburgh, being the feat of juftice, of education, and of amufements, having populous environs, and requiring a large fupply of the ftaple commodities produced in the fhires of Roxburgh and Selkirk, every farmer, and indeed almoft every inhabitant in them of any confideration, has a regular correfpondent there, and very many of them are conftant readers of one or other of its newfpapers. Yet are they precluded, by a prepofterous regulation, from all intercourfe with it, except by Berwick, which is farther from Edinburgh than any place in either county where there is a poft-office; although it is demonftrable, that, by an alteration in the arrangement at a fmall additional expence, letters would come fo much more conveniently and expeditioufly as to enfure a valuable increafe

of

of revenue. There can be no doubt, that the more directly and quickly they are conveyed, there is the greater encouragement to use and pay for that conveyance. On this
undeniable principle, I would propose that all letters and
newspapers from Edinburgh, to every part of these, counties, should be sent by the post who comes regularly to
Lauder, and to dispatch two runners from thence, one to
Kelso, and the other by Melrose and Selkirk to Hawick,
with a byebag from Melrose to Galashiels. This would
occasion no additional charge, except for the runner from
Lauder to Kelso, 17 miles, and from Lauder to Melrose,
11 miles; all the rest of the proposed route being travelled
at present: and I submit to all concerned, if there be not
a strong presumption of this additional charge being amply
compensated by the greater number of letters and newspapers carried by a shorter road, through a more extensive
range of inhabited country. This matter will be placed in
a just and strong light, by the following table, exhibiting,
at one view, in different columns, the real distance of every
post-office from Edinburgh,—by the common turnpike-
road,—by the present route of the post,—and by the one I
propose: other two columns are added, shewing the usual
time of the post's arrival at the several offices, and the difference in point of earliness that might be expected from
the suggested arrangement.

Places.	Distance from Edinburgh,			Time of his arrival now.	His arrival would be ear-lier.
	By the com-mon turn-pike-road.	As the post now travels.	As by the proposed al-teration.		
Kelso,	42 miles.	76 miles.	42 miles.	4 or 5 m.	by 6 hours.
Jedburgh,	45	85	51	6 to 8 m.	
Hawick,	47	97	54	9 or 10 m.	10 ditto.
Selkirk,	36	108	43	12 noon.	14 ditto.
Melrose,	34	115	36	1 or 2 ev.	16 ditto.
Galashiels,	30	119	40	3 or 4 ev.	16 ditto.

Jedburgh

Jedburgh is the only place which would derive little or
no benefit from this plan : for as the post, calculating from
the present time of his departure from Edinburgh, would
arrive there at midnight, it might be found more eligible,
to detain him at Kelso for six or seven hours, to forward
his bag along with the English mails, which makes no alteration with respect to Jedburgh, and to send himself back
to Lauder with all letters and newspapers from the S. for
that burgh, and for several gentlemen and farmers near the
high road, whose servants now go for them to Kelso.   The
English mails, proceeding as they do at present to Hawick,
would there be delivered to the runner from Selkirk, &c.
whose horse and himself, after resting ten or eleven hours,
would be sufficiently refreshed to return at a brisk pace, so
as to reach the remaining stages rather before the usual
hour, and would carry with him answers, from Hawick,
and from the several offices in his way, to the letters received the preceding day, to be forwarded from Lauder to
Edinburgh that very evening.   It would be a further advantage to these counties, if a post was established from
Hawick by Langholm to Carlisle.   But I have not the
same sure grounds to assert, that such an establishment
would be lucrative to the revenue.   The runner from Lauder to Kelso may be discontinued, if experience shall prove
that part of the plan to be unproductive : And other alterations may be adopted, or other measures devised, more
simple, and of more extensive public utility.   But no sound
judgment can be formed, concerning the real effect of any
particular arrangement, either with respect to general convenience or profit to the State, without a trial for such a
competent time, as will enable the country to understand
its nature, and to feel its complete operation.

The improvement of the country, and the interests of
agriculture, are more deeply involved in this subject, than

superficial

superficial inquirers may imagine. For, setting aside the useful hints and valuable information on rural affairs, often contained in periodical publications and private letters, in the conveyance of which, the delay of a day or two may be of little consequence, are there not many particulars concerning which early intelligence is of vast importance to farmers? Intimation of any sudden change in the prices of grain, cattle, or sheep, in the leading markets, of any kind of grain for seed, or of animals for rearing, of peculiar excellency, of the acceptance or rejection of an offered bargain, of the failure or suspected solvency of a debtor, and of various other matters, which it would be tedious as well as difficult to specify, cannot surely be too speedily conveyed. There is, besides, an indefinite number of local and incidental circumstances of more or less moment continually arising among his neighbours, for a distinct account of which, any farmer would rather pay the postage of a letter, than send a servant and a horse ten or a dozen of miles. And there are numerous pecuniary transactions, which exact and honest dealers could easily manage by a cross post, and thus save to one of the parties the expence of a journey or an express. In short, the loss of time and of labour, in a critical season, the injury done to horses, and the travelling charges of servants, all of which are grievous impediments to agriculture, could in many instances be lessened, and in some almost wholly done away, by a judicious arrangement of direct and cross posts.

I forbear to say any thing concerning the abolition of *thirlage*, or adstriction to a particular mill, where tenants are bound to grind the corns upon their farms at a higher rate than what is commonly given at other places, because it is generally allowed, by all the proprietors and tenants with whom I have conversed on the subject, to be a grievance, which, in the progress of improvement, will be gradually

dually leffened, and at laft ceafe to be felt *. To this general conviction, which is daily becoming ftronger, all motives of felf-intereft muft foon give way. The time, we
ardently hope, is not far diftant, when, freed from all the
incumbrances which the pride or miftaken policy of our
anceftors impofed upon agricultural improvements, our
land, under the aufpices of a juft and mild government,
fhall attain a high ftate of cultivation, and fhall abundantly
reward the fkill and labour of the farmers, and the liberal
maxims adopted by their landlords.

* It is believed, that an act for the abolition of thirlage, is fpeedily
to be brought in, under the aufpices of the Highland Society, and with
the concurrence of Government.

A D.

ADDENDA.

THE following particulars have either occurred since the preceding pages went to press, or information concerning them was not communicated to me in time to be taken notice of in the proper place. To each article is prefixed the page, where it ought to have been introduced either into the text or a note.

I.

P. 58.—ON the fuppofition made in this page of a machine with two horfes thrafhing fifteen bolls each day for 26 days or 390 bolls, a friend has favoured me with the following full and accurate ftatement of the expence and faving arifing from it ; and, at the fame time, has fubjoined other calculations and obfervations worthy of public attention.

It requires fix hands, viz.—a boy to drive the horfes,—two women to unloofe and hand the fheaves to the feeder, —a man to feed, that is, to fpread out the loofened fheaves fo as to be caught equally by the whole length of the rollers,—a woman to riddle the grain when thrafhed,—and a

man

man or woman to take away the ſtraw. The expence will be as under:

A man and a pair of horſes, for 26 days,
   at   —   —   —   5 s. 4 d. L. 6 18 8

A man, for 26 days, at   —   1 s. 2 d.   1 10 4

Three women, 26 days, at 10 d. each or 2 s. 6 d.   3 5 0

A boy, 26 days, at   —   0 s. 8 d.   0 17 4

A man, three women and a boy, cleaning the
   grain, by a common fan, after being winnowed from the chaff by the machine, meaſuring and putting it up in ſacks, eleven
   days, at the above wages,   —   2 7 8

Intereſt at 10 per cent. of L. 50, the prime
   coſt of the machine and fans,   —   5 0 0

Annual expence of greaſe, &c.   —   1 0 0
                          L. 20 19 0

A thraſher's wages and maintenance, ſuppoſing him to be
   a houſe-ſervant, is eſtimated at   —   L. 18 0 0

One man and three women aſſiſting to win-
   now, clean, meaſure, and put up the corn,
   one-half day every week, or 26 days through
   the year, at the above wages,   —   4 15 4
                          L. 22 15 4

Hence there is, after every deduction, a clear
   ſaving by the machine of   1 16 4

Again, ſuppoſing the thraſher to work by the piece, and to receive 1 s. per boll for thraſhing and bundling the ſtraw, the ſaving will be greater.

Thraſhing

Thrashing 390 bolls at 1 s. - L. 19 10 0
Expence of winnowing, &c. as before, 4 15 4

L. 24 5 4
The same quantity done by the machine, 20 19 0

Saving by the machine, - - L. 3 6 4

The reader will be pleased to observe, that the machine is calculated to go only 8 hours in the day, and that all the hands, receiving a full day's wage, have two hours each day to bundle up the straw. It must be obvious that this saving will always be greater, in proportion both to the number of days during which the machine is employed more than the 26 reckoned upon, and to the quantity of grain thrashed more than 15 bolls in a day. From some experiments lately made, by adding a horse to the pair usually yoked, one machine thrashed a little more than 4 bolls in an hour, and another thrashed $3\frac{1}{12}$ of a boll in the same time. In the latter case the straw was very rank and somewhat damp. A third machine, drawn only by two horses, went with so much smoothness, ease, and velocity, as to be able, in the opinion of very experienced judges, to thrash at least 5 if not 6 bolls in an hour, without any extraordinary fatigue to the horses. It was made by a mill-wright in the suburbs of Galashiels, who increased the velocity, by enlarging the circumference of the wheels and giving them more teeth or cogs, and, at the same time, diminished the friction, by placing the switchers or beaters a little diagonally upon the drum or cylinder, instead of horizontally or in a straight line. The precise degree of obliquity, or departure from the straight line, that ought to be preferred, must be determined by experience. But the difference of six inches, which he has brought forward one end of his beaters, has a visible effect in giving the machine a soft and easy motion, while it completely separates the grain from the

A a straw.

straw. By such a machine, thrashing only four bolls in an hour, going eight hours in the day, and one day every week from the 12th. of October to the 1st of June, being nearly 33 weeks, the quantity thrashed, the expence, and the saving, will all be as follows:

The quantity thrashed at four bolls an hour for eight hours, will be 32 bolls each day for 33 days, or 1056 bolls. A man and a pair of horses for 33 days,

at	—	—	5 s. 4 d.	L. 8 16	0
A man, for 33 days, at	—		1 s. 2 d.	1 18	6
Three women, at 8 d. each, for 33 days,					
at	—	—	2 s. 0 d.	3 6	0
A boy, for 33 days, at	—		0 s. 8 d.	1 2	0
Interest, and expence of grease *,	—	—		6 10	0
A man, three women, and a boy, cleaning the grain, measuring, and putting it up in sacks, 33 days, at the above wages,			—	6 6	6
				L. 27 19	0

Thrashing 1056 bolls by the flail, and shaking the straw, at 11 d. per boll,   L. 48 8 0
Winnowing, cleaning, measuring, and putting it up, calculated from the expence stated above, of winnowin., &c. the 390 bolls,   —   * 12 18 0

	61 6	0
Sum as above,	27 19	0
Hence the saving by the machine is L. 33 7	0

Instances

* Lest the reader should think these calculations are founded on different and unfair principles, it may not be improper to explain some of the particulars

Inſtances may occur, when, from a ſmall want of exactneſs in ſome of its parts, or from ſome of them going out of order; the machine may not be eaſily drawn by two horſes. In ſuch caſes, an additional horſe might be added
at

ticulars which ſeem to countenance this ſuſpicion. The firſt calculation, relative to the 26 days, was accommodated to the ſuppoſed work of a thraſher with the flail through the year, both as a houſe-ſervant, and as a worker by the piece, or *by lot* as it is here called. In both caſes he is ſuppoſed to bundle the ſtraw, and therefore only 1¼ of a boll is expected from him each day; and he is allowed 2 s. *per* boll when working by the piece. In the contract with his thraſhing, the machine is ſuppoſed to go eight hours each day, to thraſh fifteen bolls, and to require ſix hands, whoſe wages are reckoned for ten hours work; two of theſe hours being allotted for bundling the ſtraw. This calculation was merely intended to ſhew the ſuperiority of the machine, even upon the moſt moderate computation of its efficient powers. The ſecond calculation proceeds upon the quantity of grain which ſeveral machines have actually been found to thraſh in a day, and upon the number of days during which one of them muſt be employed, during a great part of the year, to furniſh fodder for the cattle upon a farm which has above 250 acres annually in tillage. In it the bundling of the ſtraw is omitted: the women are only charged at the rate of 2 d. *per* hour for the time they attend upon the machine; and the thraſher is allowed only 11 d. *per* boll; which conſiderably leſſens the ſaving by the machine, becauſe an additional 1 d. on 1056 bolls is L. 4. 6 s. whereas an additional 2 d. to three women for 35 days, amounts only to 16 s. 8 d. To have made the contraſt perfectly fair, a deduction of two hours from ten, or of one-fifth, ſhould alſo have been made from the wages of the two men and the boy employed at the machine, which would have increaſed the ſaving by it about 10 s. The charge for greaſe or oil for the machine is made ¼ more on account of the additional days it is worked, and the greater velocity with which it moves. In both calculations, the expence of cleaning the corn by the flail is ſtated fully at double what it is repreſented to coſt by the machine, becauſe one-half of that work is done by a fan attached to the machine and by the woman who riddles. And beſides, the large quantity thraſhed at once, and winnowed by the machine, muſt be dreſſed for the market in a ſhorter time, than the ſame amount made up of ſmall quantities thraſhed by the flail, and cleaned regularly as it is thraſhed. The very time, conſumed in aſſembling the neceſſary hands and putting the barn in order as often as a few bolls are thraſhed, is precious to a judicious farmer.

at 2 s. *per* day, or two pairs might be kept, to be yoked four hours alternately, and the pair, not employed in the machine, set to any easy work about the farm. But, as the average of stacks contains only from 16 to 20 bolls, and as very seldom more than one are thrashed in a day, one pair of horses, with the allowance of an hour to rest and to eat a little corn, will in general manage one of them without much difficulty, besides doing some lighter and necessary jobs during the rest of the day.

It is but justice to add, that there are very few, if any, instances of grain being so completely beat from the straw, by the flail, as by the machine. This seems to be generally allowed by every person, who has made frequent and careful comparisons of the straw thrashed by both.

II.

P. 82.—Owing to the unfavourable season at the end of 1796, wheat was not dibbled to such an extent as was proposed. Mr Church at Mosstower gave one furrow of 9 inches to a field which had lain two years in clover. The soil was a sandy loam, and the subsoil was hard gravel, with an intermixture of barren earth. His son, who had lately returned from Norfolk, got dibbles made, taught some people how to use them, and had the operation performed exactly according to the practice of that county. The dibbles are about 3¼ feet long, and are used without stooping; their stalk is of iron, with a handle or top like that of a spade; their lower end conical, very sharp and steeled at the point. The dibblers moved backward, making two rows of holes at once with one of these instruments in each hand, by thrusting both into the ground at the same instant, and pulling them out with a quick circular motion inward or outward,

ward, to fmooth the fides of the holes, and prevent loofe
earth from tumbling in, without which precaution the work
would have been imperfectly done. The furrows, being
all exactly equal, and nicely flattened with a roller, ferved
the dibblers for a rule or line to keep the rows pretty
ftraight. An acre had two rows on every furrow, and they
were confequently 4¼ inches diftant from each other: Upon
¼ of an acre only one row was made in the furrow. The
holes in the rows in both cafes were about 3 inches afunder,
and from 1½ to 2¼ inches deep. Four boys or girls followed each dibbler, dropping from 2 to 4 grains into each
hole, as nearly as could be guefled; for their young fingers
were fo benumbed with cold, that they could not always
be quite certain of the number they let fall; though the
¼ of an acre was rather more accurately done than the
other. The feed was covered by a common harrow bufhed
with thorns. The quantity ufed was 3 pecks 1½ gallons
Englifh meafure, or about 3 pecks to the acre. This operation was performed in November; and the weather not
permitting more to be dibbled, the reft of the field was
fown broadcaft, about the fame time, with the fame wheat,
pickled in the fame manner. The broadcaft was talleft,
and ripened a few days earlier. The dibbled, from the
land being very clean, required neither hoeing nor weeding; it tillered more than the other; its ftraw was thicker,
flouter, and fooner ready for inning after being cut; the
grain was large, well publifhed and heavy; and the produce of the acre was 36 bufhels, that of the ¼ of an acre
was at the rate of 42 bufhels. The boll beft known in Roxburgbfhire is rather more than 6 bufhels.

III.

III.

P. 97.—Potatoes were planted with the plough before the 1760, by the late Mr Scott of Wool, and he was among the first to adopt the improved method of preparing ridges for them, or of dropping them into every third furrow. He likewise brought feed from Langholm of the common white kind, before Dr Macknight came to the county ; but they were fo little known in the neighbourhood, that a few, with which Dr Macknight favoured me in 1772, were looked upon as a novelty by moft people who faw them. I am happy in an opportunity of doing juftice to the memory of a very ingenious and worthy gentleman ; and I moft fincerely regret that I had it not in my power to trace every fpecies of improvement in thefe counties to its true origin.

IV.

P. 120.—Since this page was printed, I have been favoured with the following meafurement of 3 trees, fuppofed to be the largeft of their refpective kinds in the county.

An oak, on the eftate of Fernieherft near Jeburgh, called from its majeftic appearance the *King of the Wood*, is 78¼ feet high, and has a ftraight trunk of 42 feet, which meafures, at the bottom 11 feet 5 inches, at the height of 6¼ feet 10 feet 3 inches, and nearly as much at the height of 10 feet, when it fends out its firft branches. This part of the trunk contains about 65 feet of wood, and, as the remaining part of 32 feet will admit of an average circumference of 3¼ feet, it will probably contain about 55 feet, befides much valuable wood in feveral large branches.

An

An elm, at Friars, between Roxburgh Castle and Kelso, known by the name of the *Tryfting-tree*, is 79 feet high, and has a trunk of 10 feet in height, which measures at the bottom 18¼ feet, and at the top 22½ feet. But, as this greater compass at the top is owing to an excrescence of spongy or fungous matter, and as the trunk rather tapers a little from the bottom to the place where this excrescence begins, the average circumference cannot be reckoned above 17 feet, which makes its solid contents a little more than 180 feet. The quantity of wood in its branches I am unable to estimate.

Both these trees are greatly inferior to an ash at Cesford, called the *Crow-tree*. The height of its trunk is 18 feet; its circumference at the bottom 26¼ feet, at 9 feet above the ground 15 feet, and immediately below the clefts 18 feet 2 inches. Calculated in the common way, by two lengths of 9 feet each according to Hoppus, this trunk contains nearly 397 solid feet. At the height of 18 feet three huge limbs branch out from it, each of them equal to a large tree: These are calculated to contain at least 676 feet, making the whole tree 1073 feet, besides several smaller branches not measurable. I was not favoured with the height of this tree.

The larix at Haining, mentioned p. 286, as measuring 11 feet 5 inches, was planted in 1746, and measured in 1769, at 2 feet above the ground, 5 feet 2 inches; and, in 1791, at the same height, 7 feet 2 inches. A fine silver fir was lately cut down there, which, at the same height, measured, in 1769, 6 feet; and in 1791, 7 feet 5 inches.

V.

V.

MISCELLANEOUS PARTICULARS.

A farmer in Roxburghſhire has, for ſome years, made a few cheeſes from the butter-milk of cows, and finds them to be remarkably well flavoured, and much richer than any cheeſe made from cow-milk after the cream is taken from it. The milk is coagulated, and the cheeſes are made in the common way.

It may not be improper to mention, that ſince the account of Roxburghſhire went to preſs, ſome alteration has taken place in the ſtate of property there, by which a larger ſhare of it now belongs to Peers.

Much damage was done to part of the crops in ſeveral places, by a prodigious fall of ſleet and rain on the 20th and 21ſt October 1797. The potatoes eſpecially ſuffered ſeverely. The waters of Gala and Leeder were ſwelled to an unuſual ſize; many damheads were ſwept away; ſome bridges were ſhattered; ſeveral houſes were rendered uninhabitable; and a good deal of fine arable land was deſtroyed. After receiving them, the Tweed roſe ſo high, as to carry off the bridge at Kelſo. It was fortunate that Tweed itſelf, and the waters which run into it on the ſouth, were not ſwelled in the ſame proportion, otherwiſe the moſt alarming miſchiefs might have been apprehended.

EX.

i

The Sides are 2 feet 2.3. or 4 in. apart at the handle of the Mouldboard, 11 in. wide at top, 9 in. at bottom, measuring from the land side of the plough.

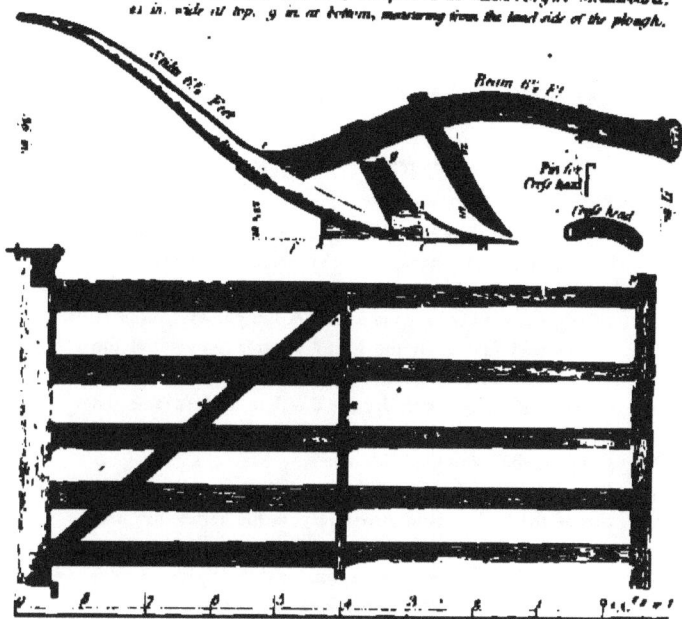

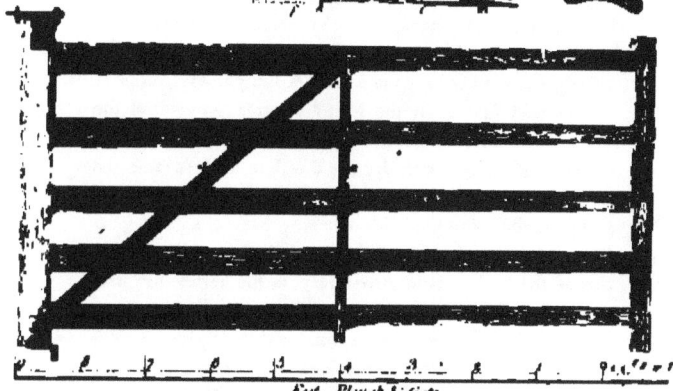

Side 6½ Feet

Beam 6½ Ft

Pin for Cross head

Cross head

Feet. Plough & Gate

Form of the joint where the cross bars meet the top rail of the gate

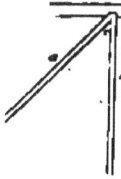

Sling for connecting stretchers &c.

Tip for the middle and ends of stretchers.

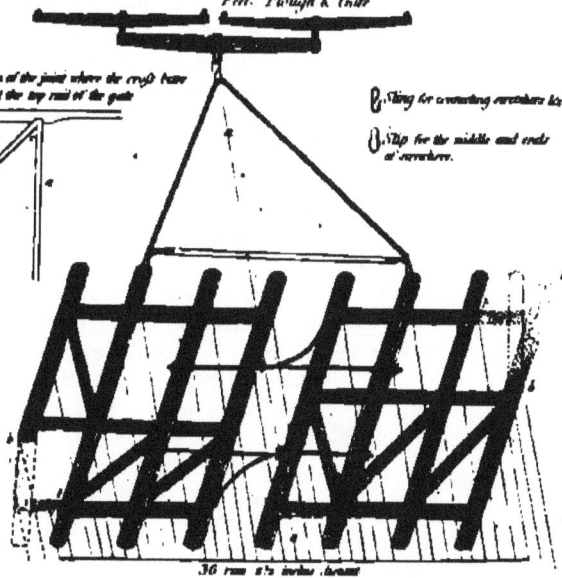

36 runs 2½ inches asunder

EXPLANATION OF THE PLATE.

1. The plough is reprefented without the ftilt or handle, held by the right hand, and the mould or mould-board which leans or refts upon the lower part of that ftilt. The principal dimenfions are marked. A ftraight edge, applied to the land fide from the heel *l* towards the point of the beam muft clear that point an inch : this is done by cutting the mortoife in the beam for the fheath a little nearer the land fide before than behind, and is intended to keep the plough inclining to the land, where it meets the greateft refiftance. When forming ridges for drilled crops, an alteration of the bridle becomes neceffary, as the horfes then cannot go in a line with the plough. In many cafes, more or lefs breadth of furrow may be wanted than is given by this inclination of the heel to the land fide, for which purpofe the bridle may be turned more or lefs to the land or furrow fide as circumftances require, and is always kept fteady by the hooked pin put into one or other of the holes in the horizontal crofs head. The coulter is regulated by wedges to the length of the iron fock *m* which covers the head or peak, and its lower point is placed about 1¼ inch above, and a very little behind that of the fock, fo as to clear the land fide of it about 1¼ inch. When land is clayey, or free from ftones, thefe diftances muft be leffened, and in very ftony land muft be increafed.

2. The bind-poft of the gate is made broad and heavy, not only as a counterpoife to the bars and fore-poft, but that the bars, by having long tenons in it, may be kept more

fteady.

steady. The whole weight of that post is behind the hinge. The fore-post *b* is as light and slender as the dimensions of the rest of the gate will allow. The mid-post *a* is not above 1¼ inch broad, but so thick as to admit of mortoises for he bars. The diagonal bar, likewise marked *a*, is 2½ inches broad, and as thick below as the hind-post is, and above as the top bar is. Its lower end rests upon the hind-post, and is cut at right angles, to prevent it from sliding by the pressure of the weight of the gate. The joint of that bar, at the top, rests upon the upright bar its whole breadth ; and the upright bar is let up its whole breadth about ¼ inch into the top-rail, so that till the wood fail, it is impossible for the gate to move out of its proper position.

3. In the harrows, the line *a a* is extended beyond the tooth, of which it represents the rut, through the two hinges to the junction of the chain with the two horse-tree, merely to shew the line of draught. If two crooked bars, here called *bulls*, be used for the outside of the harrow, as represented by dotted lines *b b b* at each extremity, four more ruts at equal distances may be obtained, and the harrows will be much stronger, than when the outside bulls are kept short according to the part of the plate that is deeply shaded. The dotted parts, both straight and crooked, are added in the plate, to shew one of them the strength which the harrow would gain, and the other both the strength and the advantage of four additional ruts.

N. B. A pair of harrows, with crooked bulls, and four additional teeth, have been used at Langlee, (p. 67, 68), and found to answer even in rugged and stony fields, and still more in smoother ones, fully better, than a pair made under Mr Dawson's direction.